FOOD ALLERGY
Methods of Detection and Clinical Studies

FOOD ALLERGY
Methods of Detection and Clinical Studies

Editor

Anas M. Abdel Rahman

Department of Genetics, Research Center
King Faisal Specialist Hospital and Research Center (KFSHRC)
and College of Medicine
Al-Faisal University
Riyadh
Saudi Arabia

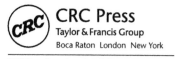

CRC Press
Taylor & Francis Group
Boca Raton London New York

CRC Press is an imprint of the
Taylor & Francis Group, an **informa** business
A SCIENCE PUBLISHERS BOOK

CRC Press
Taylor & Francis Group
6000 Broken Sound Parkway NW, Suite 300
Boca Raton, FL 33487-2742

First issued in paperback 2020

© 2017 by Taylor & Francis Group, LLC
CRC Press is an imprint of Taylor & Francis Group, an Informa business

No claim to original U.S. Government works

ISBN-13: 978-1-4987-4357-0 (hbk)
ISBN-13: 978-0-367-78203-0 (pbk)

Library of Congress Cataloging-in-Publication Data

Names: Abdel Rahman, Anas M., editor.
Title: Food allergy : methods of detection and clinical studies / editor,
Anas M. Abdel Rahman, Department of Genetics, Research Center, King Faisal
Specialist Hospital and Research Center (KFSHRC), and College of Medicine,
Al-Faisal University, Riyadh, Saudi Arabia.
Description: Boca Raton, FL : CRC Press, 2017. | "A science publisher's book."
| Includes bibliographical references and index.
Identifiers: LCCN 2017000361| ISBN 9781498743570 (hardback : alk. paper) |
ISBN 9781498743587 (e-book : alk. paper)
Subjects: LCSH: Food allergy.
Classification: LCC RC596 .F6585 2017 | DDC 616.97/5--dc23
LC record available at https://lccn.loc.gov/2017000361

Visit the Taylor & Francis Web site at
http://www.taylorandfrancis.com

and the CRC Press Web site at
http://www.crcpress.com

Preface

Bridging the gap between the clinicians and basic science researchers in food allergy was the idea of writing this book. A few dozen of authors from around the world were invited to share their bedside and bench top research experience in the field of food allergy. We tried to cover all the clinical updates in the first seven chapters starting from nomenclature to immunotherapy. The other half of the book includes state of the art technology role in enhancing the molecular knowledge in food allergy research and the updated experience of the authors' laboratories. The authors of these chapters introduced their expertise in the novel technologies such as mass spectrometry and biosensors, bioinformatics and databases, and the food labeling regulations. This book will be a useful reading material for the young and expert scientists in food allergy with the theme of introductory to the basic knowledge and literature updates, respectively.

Contents

CHAPTER 1

Food Allergy Nomenclature

Sten Dreborg

Introduction

Nomenclature is the basis for appropriate communication between scientists and clinicians. Studies should be performed using defined methods, grouping populations of patients with given characteristics, using words which describe patients clearly enough to be understood by others. Results can be applied to similar patients using the same methodology and patient characteristics using established nomenclature. This makes nomenclature crucial to both investigators as well as to clinicians to convey the message from research to the clinic. Allergists as well as other scientists interested in allergy, and not least lay persons and lay organizations must have a common language when communicating.

The nomenclature of allergy and allergic diseases has varied from time to time. However, within some areas confusing terms have been used such as "non-atopic atopic dermatitis", i.e., a dermatitis, clinically resembling that of so called "atopic dermatitis" (with allergen specific IgE antibodies also called eczema (Johansson *et al.*, 2004)), but without allergen specific IgE antibodies. That was, and still is, confusing. Accordingly, Gunnar O. Johansson formed a task force within the European Academy of Allergy and Clinical Immunology, EAACI, to write a position paper expressing the meaning of the Academy of allergy nomenclature (Johansson *et al.*, 2001). To make the message general he later formed a group within the World Allergy Organization, WAO to discuss the EAACI position paper (Johansson *et al.*, 2001), adding views from other continents and to agree on a common nomenclature for the worldwide allergy community (Johansson *et al.*, 2004). One of the main achievements was to start using "eczema" instead of "atopic dermatitis". However, as often happens,

Professor emeritus, Child and Adolescent Allergology, Women's and Children's Health Uppsala University, Academic Hospital, SE-751 85 UPPSALA, Sweden.
Email: sten.dreborg@kbh.uu.se

conservatives maintained atopic dermatitis as a parallel option to eczema, why "non-atopic atopic dermatitis" could not be eradicated. Since then, many people have tried to implement the new nomenclature. However, allergy and thereby allergy nomenclature, concerns not only allergists, but even specialists within adult and pediatric gastroenterology, dermatology, Ear, Nose and Throat (ENT), and respiratory medicine, who therefore have an interest in allergy nomenclature. All these related specialists and even lay persons and lay organizations must be involved to implement the allergy nomenclature to achieve global mutual understanding.

Recently, a Nomenclature Review Committee was set up by the WAO Board of Directors (Rosenwasser *et al.*, in prep.) for the purpose of updating the present nomenclature (Johansson *et al.*, 2004).

This chapter presents the existent nomenclature (Johansson *et al.*, 2004) discussing possible changes of the Food Allergy Nomenclature (Johansson *et al.*, 2001; Johansson *et al.*, 2004).

General considerations

Hypersensitivity is the global term describing not tolerating an environmental factor tolerated by the majority. Hypersensitivity can be mediated either by an immunological mechanism, i.e., allergy, or by non-immunological mechanisms. It does not include infection, autoimmunity or toxic reactions (Johansson *et al.*, 2004).

The WAO nomenclature 2004

The WAO nomenclature describes hypersensitivity as "objectively reproducible symptoms or signs initiated by exposure to a defined stimulus at a dose tolerated by normal persons".

Hypersensitivity is either mediated by an immunological mechanism or not, dividing hypersensitivity into immunologically mediated hypersensitivity or allergy and non-immunologically mediated hypersensitivity, Fig. 1.1.

Immunologically mediated food hypersensitivity or allergy

Originally, allergy was defined by Clemens von Pirquet in 1906 as "changed reactivity", based on the old Greek words "allos" (different or changed) and "ergos" (work or effect) (von Pirquet, 1906). The WAO nomenclature defines allergy as "an immunologically mediated specific hypersensitivity" and this definition is still accepted by the allergy community (Fig. 1.1) (Johansson *et al.*, 2004).

Immunologically mediated symptoms and diseases are named allergic. The WAO definition is: "Allergy is a hypersensitivity reaction initiated by specific immunologic mechanisms" (Johansson *et al.*, 2004). Allergy includes many mechanisms caused by environmental influences. "Allergy can be

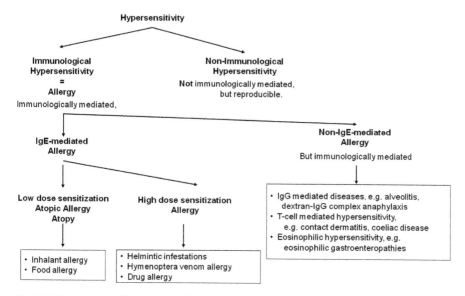

Fig. 1.1: Principles of Allergy nomenclature. Modified after (Johansson *et al.*, 2001; Johansson *et al.*, 2004).

antibody-mediated or cell-mediated. In most patients with allergic symptoms from mucosal membranes in the airways and gastrointestinal tract, the antibody belongs to the IgE isotype, and these patients may be said to have an IgE-mediated allergy or atopic allergy" (Johansson *et al.*, 2004). Even diseases/symptoms with obvious inflammatory components but without known mechanism should be classified as allergic.

The WAO position paper classifies allergies mediated by IgE antibodies as IgE-mediated allergy (previous paragraph). Atopic allergy is caused by low dose of allergen exposure to mucosal membranes in genetically predisposed individuals causing long standing sensitization. IgE-mediated allergy consists of atopic allergy and high dose dependent IgE-mediated allergies. Doses are discussed later.

Atopic allergy

Atopic allergy is due to an immunological response induced by very low doses of seemingly harmless proteins (mainly) in the environment, stimulating the immune system to respond with a humoral response of Th2 type with production by B-cells of allergen specific IgE antibodies.

High antigen dose IgE-mediated allergy

To this category belong, e.g., IgE mediated reactions to Hymenoptera venoms and IgE reactions against helminths (Fig. 1.1).

Comments

According to the WAO nomenclature (Johansson *et al.*, 2001; Johansson *et al.*, 2004), there are two types of IgE-mediated allergy, low dose sensitization (atopic) and reactivity and high dose sensitization and reactivity.

Low doses of allergen sensitizing via the mucous membranes is typical for atopic sensitization. **Atopy** was introduced by Cooke and Coca in 1923 (Coca and Cooke, 1923). Individuals with a predisposition to develop diseases like asthma, rhino-conjunctivitis, eczema and urticaria, combined with a hereditary predisposition to be sensitized to proteins that they were exposed to, were classified as atopic. In 1975, Pepys defined atopy as a tendency to develop IgE antibodies when exposed to low concentrations of environmental, normally harmless, proteins called allergens (Pepys, 1975). The diseases caused by sensitization were called atopic diseases. The WAO position paper (Johansson *et al.*, 2004) states: "The term atopy should be reserved to describe the genetic predisposition to become IgE-sensitized to allergens commonly occurring in the environment and to which everyone is exposed but to which the majority do not produce a prolonged IgE antibody response. Thus, atopy is a clinical definition of an IgE-antibody high-responder. The term atopy cannot be used until an IgE sensitization has been documented by IgE antibodies in serum or by a positive skin prick test". And, "Allergic symptoms in a person of the atopic constitution may be referred to as atopic, as in atopic rhinitis. A positive skin test or the presence of IgE antibody to a less common allergen, especially if the exposure is not low dose or does not occur via mucosal membranes, is not a diagnostic criterion for atopy. Typical examples are Hymenoptera sting allergy and most drug allergies. Such patients should be referred to as skin test positive and IgE-sensitized, respectively" (Johansson *et al.*, 2004). This is confusing, since not all cases of atopic diseases are caused by IgE sensitization and reactions involving allergens, allergen specific IgE and mast cells. In fact, patients with long standing atopic eczema (atopic dermatitis) or asthma show a neutrophil inflammation (Johansson *et al.*, 2004). The use of the "atopic diseases" concept has led to the term "atopic dermatitis" for infantile eczema, even present in adults. However, since many patients with that disease do not show any IgE-sensitization, i.e., are not atopic, the term "non-atopic atopic dermatitis" was coined that is causing confusion. As mentioned, this was one of the reasons for starting the nomenclature discussions that led to development of the present WAO nomenclature (Johansson *et al.*, 2001; Johansson *et al.*, 2004).

Comments on doses

Inhalant allergies belong to the low allergen exposure group, reactions to parasites to the high exposure group of IgE-mediated diseases. Insect venom allergy and penicillin allergy and the like were considered to be high dose allergy (Johansson *et al.*, 2001). However, the oral dose of penicillin is at the milligram to gram level, a little higher than that of ordinary food allergens (Eller *et al.*, 2012). The injected dose of Hymenoptera venom is 100 mg of venom, corresponding to 6–10 mg of major allergen.

This should be compared to the doses of food allergen that food allergic patients are exposed to and are reacting to in double blind placebo controlled food challenges, i.e., for hen's egg, hazelnut and peanut with a 95% confidence interval between 42 and 190 mg of fresh, solid food, for cow's milk 1.5–5.4 ml corresponding to 30–200 mg protein. It can also be compared with the amount of inhalant allergen eliciting a reaction in the skin, conjunctiva or bronchi that ranges from 0.001 to 1 mg of major allergen (Dreborg *et al.*, 1987; Dreborg and Einarsson, 1992).

The concentrations of inhalation allergens causing sensitization are difficult to establish. However there are some data from the MAS study (Wahn *et al.*, 1997). During the first 3 years of life, children sensitized to mite or cat were exposed to significantly higher house dust mite (median, 868 ng/gm vs. 210 ng/mg; $p = 0.001$) and cat (median, 150 ng/gm vs. 64 ng/gm; $p = 0.011$) allergen concentrations in domestic carpet dust compared with the group without sensitization. Thus, lower concentrations in the environment of children can be expected to sensitize than those causing asthma attacks, i.e., between 2 and 8 µg/g of carpet dust. However, the doses of airborne inhalant allergens causing increase in bronchial hyperreactivity are much lower, less than 1 ng/day (Dreborg and Einarsson, 1992; Ihre and Zetterstrom, 1993).

In conclusion, there is a floating dose level causing sensitization and reactivity, between allergens and administration forms. The concentrations causing sensitization are more difficult to define.

Non-IgE-mediated allergic diseases

Non-IgE-mediated allergic diseases are caused by other mechanisms than allergen-IgE-mast cell interaction. Most non-IgE-mediated allergic diseases are due to induction of allergen specific T-cells. Another mechanism is by IgG-antibodies complement binding to dextran (Richter and Hedin, 1982), etc., Fig. 1.1.

Comment

Since 2004 (Johansson *et al.*, 2004), several diagnostic entities have been recognized, Figs. 1.2 and 1.3.

Non-immunologically mediated mechanisms

The non-immunologically mediated diseases and symptoms were not given any short name, are easy to understand and use.

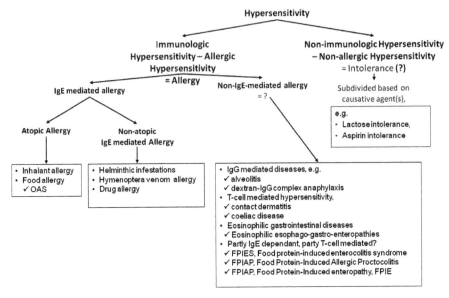

Fig. 1.2: The WAO nomenclature modified including recently defined diagnostic entities.

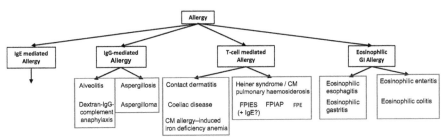

Fig. 1.3: Proposed preliminary grouping of non-IgE-mediated allergies. The T-cell mediated diseases can be partly further differentiated according to T-cell mechanism.

Comments

Recently, it has been proposed to use the word "Intolerance" to describe non-immunological/non-allergic hypersensitivity conditions (Dreborg, 2015). Intolerance has been used to describe the two most important groups of diseases under this heading, i.e., not tolerating di-saccharides (lactose, sucrose, fructose) (Durand, 1960; Holzel *et al.*, 1962) due to enzyme deficiency in the intestine and sometimes intolerance is used describing not tolerating aspirin, e.g., aspirin induced asthma (Samter and Beers, 1967).

Auto-immune diseases

Auto-immune diseases are not included within allergy, since the causative agents are not environmental but internal/of human origin. However, the limit between autoimmunity and allergy is floating, since, e.g., with time, asthma and atopic eczema shift from an eosinophilic inflammation to an inflammation dominated by neutrophils with not fully understood mechanisms.

Food allergy nomenclature modification

The general principles applied to food allergy are those of the general allergy nomenclature, Fig. 1.1.

IgE-mediated food allergy

The contact with food allergens is mainly after oral intake, sometimes via the skin.

Comments

After oral intake, symptoms can be induced in every organ system, mostly gastrointestinal and skin symptoms, but even respiratory symptoms.

IgE-mediated food allergic symptoms appear within 2 hours of intake but can appear immediately after intake of minute amounts of allergenic food. Mostly, symptoms do not appear after intake of pg., ng or µg of allergenic protein as is the case for inhaled allergens, even inhaled food proteins, but rather after intake of mg to grams of whole food material (Eller *et al.*, 2012). Whether the difference in amount inducing a reaction is due to difference in route of administration including digestion, difference in timing or difference in mechanism, is not clear. See also above doses of food, injected, ingested or inhaled allergen needed for induction of reactions.

Very seldom, allergic symptoms appear after inhalation of food protein. It has been described in very sensitive food allergic patients and when handling crops (Mason *et al.*, 2015).

Contact via the skin of cold-buffet managers has caused a form of IgE-mediated contact dermatitis, "IgE-associated allergic protein contact dermatitis" (Cronin, 1987) that is a serious occupational allergy in cold-buffet managers in restaurants.

A special form of food allergy is the local reaction in the oral mucosa, sometimes spreading to the nose, eyes and larynx after ingestion of foods containing allergens mostly cross-reacting with allergens in pollens (Juhlin-Dannfelt, 1948), "para-allergies", nowadays named Oral Allergy Syndrome, OAS (Ortolani *et al.*, 1988), Fig. 1.2. With the exception of laryngeal involvement (Pastorello *et al.*, 1999), these reactions are not life-threatening. The laryngeal mucosa is as much part of the local oro-facial mucosa as the conjunctiva, lips and the salpinges. If OAS symptoms escalate within minutes, involving organs at distance, there is a high risk of severe anaphylaxis (Cox *et al.*, 2010; Dreborg, 2013).

Non-IgE-mediated or non-atopic food allergy

Non-IgE-mediated food allergy is not discussed in detail in the WAO nomenclature document (Johansson *et al.*, 2004), stating: "If IgE is involved in the reaction, the term IgE-mediated food allergy is appropriate. All other reactions should be referred to as non-allergic food hypersensitivity", thus not mentioning, e.g., the non-IgE-mediated mechanisms involved in some, probably T-cell mediated food induced gastrointestinal diseases. On this point, the newly instituted "WAO Nomenclature Review Committee" will update the present nomenclature.

Opposite to IgE-mediated allergic reactions, most reactions caused by non-IgE-mediated mechanisms do not start until 2 hours after ingestion of the food.

Comments

Since non-IgE-mediated diseases were not clearly pointed at in the WAO document (Johansson *et al.*, 2004) this must be updated.

In addition to the diseases mentioned in the WAO and EAACI nomenclature documents (Johansson *et al.*, 2001; Johansson *et al.*, 2004) a number of diseases have been identified that are immunologically mediated without obvious IgE involvement, although the mechanisms involved are not fully understood (Nowak-Wegrzyn *et al.*, 2015), Fig. 1.3. Furthermore, eosinophilic oesophagitis (Furuta and Katzka, 2015), enterocolitis (Nowak-Wegrzyn *et al.*, 2015) and proctocolitis (Lake, 2000) can be IgE-mediated but even other mechanisms have been proposed.

To this group also belongs Heiner syndrome, also known as pulmonary haemosiderosis (Heiner *et al.*, 1962).

Although not IgE-mediated, the mechanism causing gluten allergy (formerly gluten intolerance or coeliac disease) is immunological. Therefore, it should be considered allergic, i.e., belonging to the non-IgE-mediated, mostly T-cell mediated, allergic diseases. It should not be confused with IgE mediated wheat and gluten allergy. Furthermore, contact dermatitis belongs to this group.

Non-immunologically mediated food hypersensitivity

The main alimentary disease among diseases/symptoms that are not caused by an immunological hypersensitivity/allergy is lactose intolerance, i.e., primary or secondary enteric lactase deficiency (Durand, 1960; Sicherer and Sampson, 2014), leading to bacterial fermentation of lactose in the gut. Lactose in dairy products not digested in the intestine are fermented in the gut leading to acid loose stools. Similarly, inherited lack of enzyme for digestion of sucrose (Weijers *et al.*, 1961) and fructose (Cox, 1990) leads to similar symptoms. The other major cause of non-allergic food hypersensitivity is aspirin intolerance (Samter and Beers, 1967).

Comments

It is proposed to use the term intolerance to describe the non-immunologically mediated hypersensitivities.

Non-acceptable entities and terms

Among laypersons, gastrointestinal symptoms of different kinds are named allergy or intolerance.

The basis for classification should be according to mechanism, i.e., according to the WAO nomenclature. As mentioned non-atopic atopic dermatitis is still used by some dermatologists, but should, in my opinion, be avoided.

Some gastroenterologists are using terms that cannot be accepted from an allergological point of view such as cow's milk protein allergy/intolerance, CMPA/I and "cow's milk related symptoms".

Comments

For some years, Yves Vandenplas and colleagues used the term cow's milk protein allergy/intolerance, CMPA/I (Vandenplas *et al.*, 2011; Vandenplas *et al.*, 2013). The same group of mainly pediatric gastoenterologists (Vandenplas *et al.*, 2015; Vandenplas *et al.*, 2016a) launched a series of non-proven stepwise hypotheses, supporting the use of the non-defined diagnosis "cow's milk related symptoms". The 10 steps are:

1. Double Blind Placebo Controlled Food Challenges, DBPCFC, are the gold standard for diagnosis of food allergy. However, this is expensive and not possible to perform in primary care. Therefore, elimination and reintroduction should be the standard diagnostic procedure when diagnosing CMPA in primary care.

2. The next step is claiming simple gastrointestinal symptoms like infantile colic, regurgitation and constipation may be due to CMPA (Vandenplas, 2015; Vandenplas *et al.*, 2011; Vandenplas *et al.*, 2016a), based on the fact infantile colic, regurgitation and constipation sometimes are present in infants with CMPA.

3. Since these symptoms sometimes are seen in children with CMPA, children with such symptoms may have CMPA.

4. Thus, CMPA should be diagnosed in these children. Primarily they proposed an elimination diet, followed by reintroduction at home in those improving after some months.

5. To "easily" diagnose CMPA in infants, they worked out a non-validated scoring system mainly based on the common symptoms, infantile colic, regurgitation and obstipation (Vandenplas *et al.*, 2015).

6. Those improving on an elimination diet and not relapsing when normal formula is re-introduced are said to have "cow's milk related symptoms" (Vandenplas *et al.*, 2016a).

7. The treatment recommended is an elimination diet, in this age group a hypoallergenic formula.

8. Since, in infants, the common symptoms mentioned are self-limited, the therapeutic success will be marked.

9. The parents will be stigmatized and the "diagnosis" of "CMPA/I" (or CMPA) will follow the child.

10. Furthermore, parents without economic resources will suffer from economic loss to the benefit of formula companies.

The terms CMPA/I and "cow's milk related symptoms" may not be used, especially since the concept is not evidence based and has been developed in cooperation with formula industry (Vandenplas *et al.*, 2014). It should be regarded a marketing concept.

The GI Committee of the European Society on Paediatric Gastroenterology, Hepatology and Nutrition, ESPGHAN, does not mention CMPA/I or "cow's milk related symptoms" in their practical guidelines on the management of CMPA in infants and children (Koletzko *et al.*, 2012). Recently, a committee within ESPGHAN has banned the widespread use of partially hydrolyzed formulas among non-diseased children (Vandenplas *et al.*, 2016b).

Future Perspectives

I reviewed (Dreborg, 2016) the paper by the group of gastroenterologists led by Yves Vandenplas (Vandenplas *et al.*, 2015). At the same time, I wrote the con paper on "Intolerance does not exist" (Dreborg, 2016) for the WAO Journal. Simultaneously Vandenplas wrote the "pro intolerance" paper (Vandenplas, 2016) in a series of pro-con debates in the WAO J. I found the reasoning of the gastroenterologists to be threatening the present nomenclature. Therefore, I asked the World Allergy Organization, WAO Board of Directors to initiate an update of the old nomenclature document (Johansson *et al.*, 2004) that resulted in the formation of a "WAO Nomenclature Review Committee" that has started its work. It can be foreseen that the new version of the allergy nomenclature will mainly follow the design of the old nomenclature document and this summary, but if possible be more detailed (Rosenwasser *et al.*).

Furthermore, reactivity is not limited to the organ that gets sensitized. Patients react to the sensitizing allergen in other organs than that causing most symptoms, e.g., a majority of patients with asthma also report rhinitis (conjunctivitis) (Passalacqua *et al.*, 2006). Furthermore, in asthmatics, the skin, conjunctiva and bronchi (Dreborg *et al.*, 1986) react, in rhinitis patients the nose or conjunctiva and skin (Dreborg *et al.*, 2016; Østerballe, 1982) and in food allergic patients the skin, gut and conjunctiva (Kvenshagen *et al.*, 2010).

These references were chosen since they exemplify documentation of the fact allergic inflammation is universal, i.e., is not limited to the organ showing most symptoms.

Like IgE-mediated diseases non-IgE-mediated allergic diseases should be split up according to their partly understood mechanisms as illustrated in Fig. 1.3.

To assure well defined diseases are continuously evaluated, a permanent committee on allergy nomenclature should be set up. The group should govern allergen nomenclature with the responsibility to evaluate and register new syndromes-diseases when their mechanisms have been elucidated.

Summary

The allergy nomenclature is based on mechanisms. Most important is to differ between allergy, i.e., immunological hypersensitivity and hypersensitivity due to other mechanisms. Furthermore, it will be of importance to reveal immunological mechanism involved in different types of allergic diseases, phenotypes and genotypes. To assure new terms are in accordance with the new WAO system it is proposed to register of accepted disease entities with proposed mechanisms within the area of allergy.

Keywords: Hyperreactivity, Allergy, IgE, non-IgE, Immunological hypersensitivity, Non-immunological hypersensitivity, non-IgE-mediated allergy, Intolerance

References

Coca, A. F., and Cooke, R. A. (1923). On the classification of the phenomenon of hypersensitiveness. Journal of Immunology 8: 163–182.

Cox, L., Larenas-Linnemann, D., Lockey, R., Passalacqua, G., Bernstein, D., and Valovirta, E. (2010). Speaking the same language: the World Allergy organization subcutaneous immunotherapy systemic reaction grading system. The Journal of Allergy and Clinical Immunology 125: 569–574.

Cox, T. M. (1990). Hereditary fructose intolerance. Baillieres Clin Gastroenterol 4(1): 61–78.

Cronin, E. (1987). Dermatitis of the hands in caterers. Contact Dermatitis 17(5): 265–269.

Dreborg, S., Agrell, B., Foucard, T., Kjellman, N. I., Koivikko, A., and Nilsson, S. (1986). A double-blind, multicenter immunotherapy trial in children, using a purified and standardized Cladosporium herbarum preparation. I. Clinical results. Allergy 41(2): 131–140.

Dreborg, S., Basomba, A., Belin, L., Durham, S., Einarsson, R., Eriksson, N. *et al.* (1987). Biological equilibration of allergen preparations: methodological aspects and reproducibility. Clinical of Allergy 17(6): 537–550.

Dreborg, S., and Einarsson, R. (1992). The major allergen content of allergenic preparations reflect their biological activity. Allergy 47(4 Pt 2): 418–423.

Dreborg, S. (2013). When should adrenaline be given and by whom? Pediatric of Allergy Immunology 24(1): 97–98.

Dreborg, S. (2015). Debates in allergy medicine: food intolerance does not exist. World Allergy Organization Journal 8: 37. doi: DOI: 10.1186/s40413-015-0088-6.

Dreborg, S. (2016). Cow's milk protein allergy and common gastrointestinal symptoms in infants. Acta Paediatr 105(3): 253–254. doi:10.1111/apa.13311.

Dreborg, S., Basomba, A., Löfkvist, T., Holgersson, M., and Möller, C. (2016). Evaluation of Skin Reactivity during (Immuno-) Therapy. Validation of Methods for Estimation of Changes in Skin Reactivity and Correlation to Shock Organ Sensitivity. Immunotherapy. Open access 2: 109. doi:10.4172/imt.1000109.

Durand, P. (1960). Intolerance to lactose. Insufficient intestinal hydrolysis of lactose. Pediatrie 15: 407–409.

Eller, E., Hansen, T. K., and Bindslev-Jensen, C. (2012). Clinical thresholds to egg, hazelnut, milk and peanut: results from a single-center study using standardized challenges. Annals of Allergy, Asthma and Immunology 108(5): 332–336.

Furuta, G. T., and Katzka, D. A. (2015). Eosinophilic esophagitis. The New England Journal of Medicine 373(17): 1640–1648. doi: 10.1056/NEJMra1502863.

Heiner, D. C., Sears, J. W., and Kniker, W. T. (1962). Multiple precipitins to cow's milk in chronic respiratory disease. A syndrome including poor growth, gastrointestinal symptoms, evidence of allergy, iron deficiency anemia, and pulmonary hemosiderosis. Am J Dis Child 103: 634–654.

Holzel, A., Mereu, T., and Thomson, M. L. (1962). Severe lactose intolerance in infancy. Lancet 2(7270): 1346–1348.

Ihre, E., and Zetterstrom, O. (1993). Increase in non-specific bronchial responsiveness after repeated inhalation of low doses of allergen. Clinical and Experimental Allergy 23(4): 298–305.

Johansson, S. G. O., Hourihane, J. O., Bousquet, J., Bruijnzeel-Koomen, C., Dreborg, S., Haahtela, T., and Wuthrich, B. (2001). A revised nomenclature for allergy. An EAACI position statement from the EAACI nomenclature task force. Allergy 56(9): 813–824.

Johansson, S. G. O., Bieber, T., Dahl, R., Friedmann, P. S., Lanier, B. Q., Lockey, R. F., and Williams, H. C. (2004). Revised nomenclature for allergy for global use: Report of the nomenclature review committee of the World Allergy Organization, October 2003. The Journal of Allergy and Clinical Immunology 113(5): 832–836.

Juhlin-Dannfelt, C. (1948). About the occurrence of various forms of pollen allergy in Sweden. Acta Med Scand 131(Suppl 206): 563–577.

Koletzko, S., Niggemann, B., Arato, A., Dias, J. A., Heuschkel, R., and Husby, S. (2012). Nutrition. Diagnostic approach and management of cow's-milk protein allergy in infants and children: ESPGHAN GI Committee practical guidelines. Journal of Pediatric Gastroenterology and Nutrition 55(2): 221–229.

Krane Kvenshagen, B., Jacobsen, M., and Halvorsen, R. (2010). Can conjunctival provocation test facilitate the diagnosis of food allergy in children? Allergol Immunopathol (Madr) 38(6): 321–326.

Lake, A. M. (2000). Food-induced eosinophilic proctocolitis. Journal of Pediatric Gastroenterology and Nutrition 30 Suppl: S58–60.

Mason, H., Gomez-Olles, S., Cruz, M. J., Smith, I., Evans, G., Simpson, A., and Smith, G. (2015). Levels of soya aeroallergens during dockside unloading as measured by personal and static sampling. Arh Hig Rada Toksikol 66(1): 23–29.

Nowak-Wegrzyn, A., Katz, Y., Mehr, S. S., and Koletzko, S. (2015). Non-IgE-mediated gastrointestinal food allergy. The Journal of Allergy and Clinical Immunology 135(5): 1114–1124.

Østerballe, O. (1982). Nasal and skin sensitivity during immunotherapy with two major allergens 19, 25 and partially purified extract of timothy grass pollen. Allergy 37(3): 169–177.

Ortolani, C., Ispano, M., Pastorello, E., Bigi, A., and Ansaloni, R. (1988). The oral allergy syndrome. Annals of Allergy 61(6 Pt 2): 47–52.

Passalacqua, G., Bousquet, P. J., Carlsen, K. H., Kemp, J., Lockey, R. F., Niggemann, B., and Bousquet, J. (2006). ARIA update: I—Systematic review of complementary and alternative medicine for rhinitis and asthma. The Journal of Allergy and Clinical Immunology 117(5): 1054–1062.

Pastorello, E. A., Pravettoni, V., Farioli, L., Ispano, M., Fortunato, D., Monza, M., and Ortolani, C. (1999). Clinical role of a lipid transfer protein that acts as a new apple-specific allergen. The Journal of Allergy and Clinical Immunology 104(5): 1099–1106.

Pepys, J. (1975). Atopy. pp. 877–902. In: P.G.H. Gill, R.R.A. Coombs and P.J. Lachmann (eds.). Clinical Aspects of Immunology, 3rd ed. Oxford: Blackwell Scientific.

Richter, A. W., and Hedin, H. I. (1982). Dextran hypersensitivity. Immunology Today 3(5): 132–138.

Samter, M., and Beers, R. F., Jr. (1967). Concerning the nature of intolerance to aspirin. Journal of Allergy 40(5): 281–293.

Sicherer, S. H., and Sampson, H. A. (2014). Food allergy: Epidemiology, pathogenesis, diagnosis, and treatment. The Journal of Allergy and Clinical Immunology 133(2): 291–307.

Vandenplas, Y., Veereman-Wauters, G., De Greef, E., Devreker, T., Hauser, B., Benninga, M., and Heymans, H. S. (2011). Gastrointestinal manifestation of cow's milk protein allergy or intolerance and gastrointestinal motility. Journal of Pediatric Gastroenterology and Nutrition 53 Suppl 2: S15–17.

Vandenplas, Y., Gutierrez-Castrellon, P., Velasco-Benitez, C., Palacios, J., Jaen, D., Ribeiro, H., and Alarcon, P. (2013). Practical algorithms for managing common gastrointestinal symptoms in infants. Nutrition 29(1): 184–194.

Vandenplas, Y., Group, A. S., Steenhout, P., and Grathwohl, D. (2014). A pilot study on the application of a symptom-based score for the diagnosis of cow's milk protein allergy. SAGE Open Medicine 2.

Vandenplas, Y., Benninga, M., Broekaert, I., Falconer, J., Gottrand, F., Guarino, A., and Wilschanski, M. (2016a). Functional gastro-intestinal disorder algorithms focus on early recognition, parental reassurance and nutritional strategies. Acta Paediatr 105(3): 244–252. doi:10.1111/apa.13270.

Vandenplas, Y., Dupont, C., Eigenmann, P., Host, A., Kuitunen, M., Ribes-Koninckx, C., and Von Berg, A. (2015). A workshop report on the development of the Cow's Milk-related Symptom Score awareness tool for young children. Acta Paediatrica 104(4): 334–339.

Vandenplas, Y. (2016). Debates in allergy medicine: food intolerance does exist. World Allergy Organization Journal 8; 36.

Vandenplas, Y., Alarcon, P., Fleischer, D., Hernell, O., Kolacek, S., Laignelet, H., and Lee, W. S. (2016b). Should partial hydrolysates be used as starter infant formula? A working group consensus. Journal of Pediatric Gastroenterology and Nutrition 62(1): 22–35.

von Pirquet, C. (1906). Allergie. Mnch Med Wochenschr 53: 1457.

Wahn, U., Lau, S., Bergmann, R., Kulig, M., Forster, J., Bergmann, K., and Guggenmoos-Holzmann, I. (1997). Indoor allergen exposure is a risk factor for sensitization during the first three years of life. The Journal of Allergy and Clinical Immunology 99(6 Pt 1): 763–769.

Weijers, H. A., van de Kamer, J. H., Dicke, W. K., and Ijsseling, J. (1961). Diarrhoea caused by deficiency of sugar splitting enzymes. I. Acta Paediatr 50(1): 55–71.

CHAPTER 2

Food Allergy in Children

Sophia Tsabouri,[1,*] *Gavriela Feketea*[2] and
Nicolaos Nicolaou[3,4]

Introduction

Food Allergy (FA) refers to an immune response directed toward food (Chafen *et al.*, 2010). As defined in the 2010 US National Institutes of Allergy and Infectious Diseases (NIAID)–sponsored guidelines, FA is "an adverse health effect arising from a specific immune response that occurs reproducibly on exposure to a given food" (Boyce *et al.*, 2010a). This definition encompasses immune responses that are IgE-mediated, non-IgE-mediated or a combination of both and is in agreement with other international guidelines (Fiocchi *et al.*, 2010; Sackeyfio *et al.*, 2011; Urisu *et al.*, 2011). Allergic sensitization occurs when food-specific IgE (sIgE) antibodies are produced by plasma cells that have differentiated from allergen-specific B lymphocytes. The sIgE antibodies bind to the surface of tissue mast cells and blood basophils, and on re-exposure to the food, antigenic proteins in the food bind to and cross-link these cell surface–bound sIgE antibodies, which triggers the release of symptom-causing mediators, such as histamine and leukotrienes. Subjects can have allergic sensitization (production of sIgE) to food allergens without having clinical symptoms of an allergic reaction on exposure. Thus, sensitization alone is not sufficient to define food allergy. IgE-mediated food allergy requires both the

[1] Professor of Paediatrics-Paediatric Allergy, Child Health Department, University of Ioannina, Greece.
[2] Consultant in Paediatrics and Paediatric Allergy Paediatric Department, General Hospital of Ilias, Amaliada Hospital Unit.
  Email: gabychri@otenet.gr
[3] The University of Manchester, Institute of Inflammation and Repair, University Hospital of South Manchester NHS Foundation Trust, Manchester, UK.
[4] The University of Nicosia Medical School, Nicosia, Cyprus.
  Email: nic.nicolaou@gmail.com, nicolas@allergycy.com
* Corresponding author: stsabouri@gmail.com, tsabouri@cc.uoi.gr

presence of sensitization and the development of specific signs and symptoms on exposure to that food (Boyce *et al.*, 2010a).

There are numerous adverse reactions to foods that do not involve an immune response and therefore are not considered as a result of FA (Boyce *et al.*, 2010b). These include metabolic disorders, such as lactose and alcohol intolerance, response to pharmacologically active foods components (e.g., caffeine) or illness in response to toxins from microbial contamination (Sicherer and Sampson, 2014). Certain psychological or neurological responses (food aversion or rhinorrhea caused by spicy foods) can also mimic FA but are not considered allergic disorders (Fig. 2.1).

Epidemiology

In the United States, prevalence estimates range from 1 to 10%, and most are derived from self-report or parent report of FA (Sicherer and Sampson, 2014). A recent United State of America (USA) nationally representative population-based study (the National Health and Nutrition Examination Survey [NHANES]) found the prevalence of self-reported FA in children from 2007 to 2010 to be 6.53% (McGowan and Keet, 2013). The most common childhood FA reported were to milk (1.94%), peanut (1.16%) and shellfish (0.87%). A slightly higher estimate of childhood FA prevalence (8%) was reported in another USA population-based study (Gupta *et al.*, 2011). In other developed

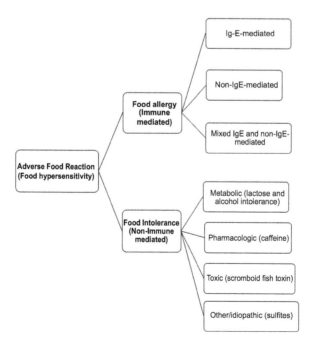

Fig. 2.1: Classification of food reactions [modified from (Sampson *et al.*, 2014)].

countries, the overall prevalence estimates are in line with USA reports. A recent meta-analysis of European FA prevalence from 2000 to 2012 found an overall prevalence of self-reported FA of 5.9%. Although many of the primary studies had at least moderate potential for bias (Nwaru *et al.*, 2014). Estimates relying on self-reports are of course limited in part by the subjective nature of the data. Other, more objective methods include measuring sensitization using food allergen sIgE. Using NHANES data, prevalence estimates for sensitization were 7.6% to peanut, 5.9% to shrimp, 4.8% to milk and 3.4% to egg in the overall population aged 6 and over, and 6.8% to peanut, 21.8% to milk and 14.2% to egg in children aged 1 to 5 years old in the USA. These are certainly an overestimation of true clinical FA prevalence but are valuable because they provide some objectivity (Salo *et al.*, 2014).

Food Allergens

Food allergens, which are usually proteins but sometimes chemical haptens, are recognized by allergen-specific immune cells and elicit specific immunologic reactions, resulting in characteristic symptoms (Boyce *et al.*, 2010a). Most food allergens can cause reactions when ingested either in the raw form or after being cooked, and occasionally after inhalation. Cross-reactivity can occur when a food allergen has structural or sequence similarity with a different food allergen or aeroallergen. The likelihood of having clinical allergic reactions to cross-reactive allergens is highly variable and depends on the type of food. For example, clinical cross-reactivity among legumes is generally uncommon (e.g., most patients with peanut allergy tolerate beans and peas), whereas clinical cross-reactivity among different types of crustacean shellfish is common (Tsabouri *et al.*, 2012). Although any food can potentially trigger an allergic response a minority of foods cause the majority of allergic reactions, namely peanut, tree nuts, egg, milk, fish, crustacean shellfish, wheat and soy (Boyce *et al.*, 2010a). Celery, mustard, sesame, lupine and molluscan shellfish have been identified as significant allergens in European countries, and in Japan buckwheat is also a common allergen (Akiyama *et al.*, 2011). Protein-containing food additives and colouring agents, such as annatto, carmine and gelatine, can induce allergic reactions. Chemical additives, such as artificial flavours (e.g., tartrazine) and preservatives (e.g., glutamates and sulphites), might cause adverse reactions, but an immune mechanism has not been identified, and such reactions are classified as intolerances.

Clinical manifestations of food allergy

Based on the underlining pathophysiological mechanism, FA can be classified as IgE-mediated, non-IgE-mediated and mixed IgE/non-IgE-mediated reactions. According to the time pattern of food-induced allergic reactions, these may be: (i) immediate (occurring within minutes to a few hours of exposure to the offending food and typically involve IgE-mediated mechanisms), or (ii) delayed (occurring within several hours to a few days, usually involving cellular mechanisms) (Boyce *et al.*, 2010a). Clinical manifestations (Table 2.1) vary depending on the systems that are affected. IgE-mediated reactions may present with symptoms affecting the skin, gastrointestinal tract, respiratory system and circulatory system, while non-IgE-mediated and mixed IgE- and non-IgE-mediated reactions present predominantly with gastrointestinal symptoms (vomiting, diarrhoea, abdominal pain, bloody stools) (Burks *et al.*, 2012).

Furthermore, a wide range of disorders is recognized to be secondary to FA (Table 2.2) (Sampson, 2014). The table does not include disorders that are not clinically specific to syndromes associated with FA. Thus infantile colic, constipation and gastrointestinal reflux disease are not listed.

Table 2.1: Symptoms and signs of food-induced allergic reactions [modified from (Boyce *et al.*, 2010b)].

Target system	Systemic, circulatory	Skin	Respiratory	Gastrointestinal
IgE-mediated	anaphylaxis hypotension arrhythmia drowsiness syncope	urticaria angioedema erythema itching	nasal congestion rhinorrhea hoarseness laryngeal oedema stridor cough chest tightness dyspnoea wheezing	nausea vomiting colic-like abdominal pain
Non-IgE-mediated	loss of appetite food aversion failure to thrive		nasal congestion rhinorrhea cough wheezing haemoptysis	nausea vomiting abdominal pain gastroesophageal reflux (GER) hematochezia bloody stools
Mixed IgE and non-IgE-mediated		exacerbation of atopic dermatitis		nausea vomiting-regurgitation abdominal pain gastroesophageal reflux heartburn

Table 2.2: Clinical manifestations secondary to FA [modified from (Sicherer and Sampson, 2014) (Worm *et al.*, 2015)].

Affected system	Generalized	Skin	Respiratory	Gastrointestinal
IgE-mediated (immediate onset -30 min up to 2 hours)	Anaphylaxis	Urticaria	Rhinitis	Oral allergy syndrome (Pollen associated food allergy syndrome)
	Food-depended exercise-induced anaphylaxis (FDEIA)	Angioedema	Asthma	Immediate gastrointestinal hypersensitivity
Non-IgE-mediated (delayed onset - few hours to days)		Contact dermatitis	Food-induced pulmonary hemosiderosis (Heiner's syndrome)	Food protein-induced enterocolitis syndrome (FPIES)
		Dermatitis herpetiformis		Food protein-induced enteropathy
				Food protein-induced proctocolitis
Mixed IgE and non-IgE-mediated (delayed onset)		Atopic dermatitis		Eosinophilic esophagitis
				Eosinophilic gastroenteritis

IgE-mediated reactions

In IgE-mediated reactions, symptoms may present from almost any system (Table 2.1). Skin, oral, gastrointestinal and respiratory symptoms are usually the most frequently observed (Lack, 2008). Food allergic reactions range from mild and often spontaneously resolving events to life-threatening anaphylaxis which unfortunately sometimes becomes fatal (Bock *et al.*, 2007). The clinical course of the Oral Allergy Syndrome (OAS) commonly described in older children and adults allergic to pollens is usually mild; symptoms are limited to the oropharynx and resolve within an hour in the majority of cases (Hofmann and Burks, 2008). Patients with OAS, who are allergic to pollens, cross-react to homologous food proteins (Table 2.3) Anaphylaxis is a severe systemic reaction involving significant respiratory and/or cardiovascular compromise (Muraro *et al.*, 2007). Food-induced anaphylaxis is the leading cause of anaphylactic reactions presented to the Accident and Emergency hospital departments in both children and adults (de Silva *et al.*, 2008; Ross *et al.*, 2008). Peanut and tree nuts are amongst the most common food allergens related to fatal anaphylaxis (Pumphrey, 2000). Food-allergic individuals with asthma (particularly those with uncontrolled asthma) are at higher risk of developing anaphylaxis (Bock *et al.*, 2007).

Table 2.3: Cross-reactivity between pollens and fruits and vegetables in OAS.

Pollens	Fruits and vegetables
Birch pollen	apples, carrots, celery, hazelnuts, almond, nuts, peaches, pears, nectarine, plum, kiwi, raw potatoes
Ragweed pollen	bananas, melons, cucumber, courgette
Grasses	melons, oranges, peanuts, tomatoes, white potato
Mugwort pollen	apples, bell peppers, carrots, celery, garlic, onion, some spices (coriander, anise seeds, fennel seeds)

Food-Dependent Exercise-Induced Anaphylaxis (FDEIA) is a special condition occurring where exercise following allergen ingestion triggers anaphylaxis, although exercise and allergen exposure are independently tolerated (Kleiman and Ben-Shoshan, 2014).

Non-IgE-mediated reactions

Food Protein-Induced Allergic Proctocolitis (FPIAP) is the most common non-IgE mediated FA in the first months of life, characterized by blood-streaked stools in otherwise healthy, thriving infants. Food Protein-Induced Enterocolitis Syndrome (FPIES) is an increasingly recognized disorder affecting young infants. It is typically presents with profuse vomiting and diarrhoea 2 to 4 hours after ingestion of the incriminating food. If untreated, it may lead to life-threatening hypovolemic shock (Caubet *et al.*, 2014). It is often caused by cow's milk, soy and rice. The development of FPIES into secondary IgE-mediated allergy has been described. Food Protein-induced Enteropathy (FPE) manifests with diarrhoea, failure to thrive, vomiting and abdominal distension (Feuille and Nowak-Wegrzyn, 2015). Heiner syndrome (pulmonary hemosiderosis) is a rare food hypersensitivity pulmonary disease mostly caused by cow's milk. It affects infants primarily and is characterized by unexplained chronic pulmonary infiltrates (Moissidis *et al.*, 2005).

IgE and non-IgE-mediated (mixed) reactions

Atopic Dermatitis (AD) is a chronic inflammatory skin disease characterized by intense itching and recurrent eczematous lesions. One in three children with moderate to severe AD has food allergy, where egg and milk being the most common allergens involved (Burks, 2003).

Eosinophilic esophagitis is the most common among the eosinophilic gastrointestinal disorders and represents a chronic, immune/antigen-mediated disease. It is clinically characterized by symptoms related to esophageal dysfunction and histologically by eosinophil-predominant inflammation (Liacouras *et al.*, 2011). It is clinically characterized by dysphagia, regurgitation, abdominal and/or chest pain, poor appetite and failure to thrive (Sampson *et al.*, 2014).

Diagnostic workup in food allergy

Although there is evidence to suggest that the prevalence of FA is increasing, recent studies have demonstrated that many "self-reported" FA cases are not confirmed when objectively assessed, and unnecessary over-restricted diets are often followed (Nwaru *et al.*, 2014). Given the impact of FA on patients, families and healthcare systems, accurate diagnosis is critically important (Bollinger *et al.*, 2006). The diagnosis of suspected FA is generally based on detailed clinical history and physical examination, determination of sensitization (to the food/s in question) by skin tests and/or the measurement of specific IgE (sIgE) antibodies in serum, elimination diets, and the outcome of Oral Food Challenge (OFC) (Boyce *et al.*, 2010a). Endoscopy and biopsy may be required to establish the diagnosis in the case of some non-IgE- or mixed IgE/non-IgE-mediated food-related disorders, e.g. (eosinophilic esophagitis). However, any *in vivo* and/or *in vitro* testing performed in the diagnostic work-up of FA should be guided and interpreted according to the clinical history and the suspected underlying immunologic mechanism. A number of unproved or non-standardized procedures and tests, including allergen-specific IgG measurement, cytotoxicity assays, applied kinesiology, provocation neutralization and hair analysis are not considered useful in the evaluation of food allergy (Sampson *et al.*, 2014).

History and physical examination

As for any other medical condition a detailed history and thorough clinical examination are of paramount importance in the diagnostic process. History taking in suspected FA is complex detective work and requires fastidious attention to detail from the physician as there is considerable overlap of symptoms in the clinical spectrum of adverse reactions to foods (Fig. 2.1). It can provide clues suggestive of the immunologic mechanisms involved and the likely causative food allergens (Burks *et al.*, 2012). Clinicians should consider that culprit food allergens may differ depending on the different epidemiology aspects related to the affected individuals (e.g., age, origin and dietary habits). For example, egg and milk in early life vs. fruits, nuts and seafood in older children and adults, and peach in the Mediterranean area vs. apple in central/northern Europe.

Amongst others, the medical history should capture information on the nature of the suspected allergenic food, the timing of exposure to the initiation of the reaction, the type, duration and severity of symptoms, the treatment received and the patient's response, as well as the presence of allergic and other diseases. Important questions to be precisely answered when obtaining the history from food-allergic individuals, particularly when suspecting IgE-mediated food allergy are summarized in Table 2.4.

Although the physical examination alone cannot be considered diagnostic of FA, it may reveal indicative findings. Signs of anaphylaxis (e.g., generalized

Table 2.4: Key history questions in the evaluation of food allergy.

- When and where? (age of patient, environment)
- What food and how? (list of ingredients, preparation, quantity, route of exposure)
- What symptoms? (timing, onset, duration, severity, reproducibility)
- What associated factors? (exercise, alcohol, drugs)
- What treatment? (medication, response)
- What management plan? (avoidance, re-exposure)
- What other health problems? (atopic dermatitis, asthma, rhino-conjunctivitis)

urticaria and wheezing) in a child presenting to the Accident and Emergency department within minutes of exposure to food is highly suggestive of IgE-mediated food allergy. Growth impairment is often associated with non-IgE-mediate food allergies, whereas the presence of other allergies (e.g., eczema, rhinitis) usually increases the likelihood of IgE-mediated food allergies (Sampson *et al.*, 2014).

Skin tests

Skin Prick Tests (SPTs) are commonly used in the assessment of FA and aid in the identification of the culprit food allergens in IgE-mediated reactions (see Chapter 6). They are generally easy to perform, minimally invasive, safe, relatively inexpensive, and results are available within 15 minutes of application. A number of factors may affect skin test reactivity including the quality of the food allergen extracts (e.g., standardization, stability), the technique followed and area of skin tested (e.g., back response > forearm), the age and ethnicity of the tested individual (e.g., increase with age), and potential effect of medication taken by the patient (e.g., decreased by antihistamines) (Asero *et al.*, 2007). In the investigation of FA to vegetables and fruits the prick to prick method with native fresh foods may provide more accurate results (Rance *et al.*, 1997). Intradermal tests are not recommended for the diagnosis of FA, and the utility of the Atopy Patch Test (APT) in the diagnostic work-up (particularly in eosinophilic esophagitis) remains a controversial issue (Boyce *et al.*, 2010b).

SPT wheal size diameter at least 3 mm greater than the negative control is considered a positive test by the majority of investigators. In general, SPTs have high sensitivity and negative predictive accuracy (~ 95%), but low specificity and positive predictive value (~ 50%) (Cox *et al.*, 2008). Therefore, a negative test is extremely useful and almost rules out the presence of IgE-mediated FA, whereas a positive test does not accurately predict clinical reactivity. The specificity of the SPT test increases with the increasing size of the weal diameter response to the tested food, and cut-off points indicating > 95% probability of clinical reactivity have been estimated for some foods (e.g., 8 mm for milk and peanut, and 7 mm for egg) (Sporik *et al.*, 2000). However, these values may not be applicable to every population (or setting) as they depend on various parameters, including age and the prevalence of the disease in the study population they have derived from.

Serum specific IgE

Tests which determine the presence and quantity of food allergen sIgE circulating unbound in the serum are also useful tools in the evaluation of FA. They are particularly helpful when SPT cannot be reliable such as in the case of patients with extensive skin disease or unable to discontinue antihistamines (Sampson *et al.*, 2014). As with SPTs, serum specific IgE tests have high sensitivity and low specificity. Despite their limitations, positive and negative predictive values are more helpful tools in practice. Clinicians and patients are likely more interested in knowing the probability of reactivity for a given test value rather than in the sensitivity or specificity of a test.

Sampson and Ho were the first to estimate the 95% positive predictive values for a number of common allergenic foods (15 kUa/L for milk, 7 kUa/L for egg, 14 kUa/L for peanut and 20 kUa/L for fish), and suggest for their usefulness in the FA clinic (Sampson and Ho, 1997). Subjects with sIgE values above the proposed predictive values are more than 95% likely to react if exposed to the specific food allergen, thus reducing the need for oral food challenges. However, in patients with sIgE values below the diagnostic decision points, OFC is often required to establish the diagnosis. Over the last years emerging studies (Celik-Bilgili *et al.*, 2005) have generated various 95% diagnostic decision points, therefore questioning the general applicability of the proposed sIgE cut-off points.

It is important to emphasize that both positive SPTs and sIgE tests confirm sensitization to a specific food allergen and not clinical reactivity. IgE antibodies to different food allergens may be present without obvious clinical allergy in many individuals [e.g., children with atopic dermatitis often show sensitization to common food allergens but do not react when exposed to these allergens (Eller *et al.*, 2009)]. In addition, allergic reactions have been observed in patients with negative tests and therefore SPTs, and sIgE results should always be interpreted in the context of clinical history. When allergy test results are not clearly assisting in the diagnosis making process, oral food challenge should be performed to establish allergy or tolerance to the suspected food (Sampson *et al.*, 2014).

Oral food challenge

An oral food challenge is generally performed when the diagnosis of FA is not reached after considering the clinical history in combination with the results of allergy testing (SPTs/sIgE), to determine whether a patient with diagnosed FA (e.g., young child with milk allergy) has outgrown his/her clinical allergy, and in scientific protocols for research purposes (Bindslev-Jensen *et al.*, 2004). There are three different types of OFC: Open, Single-blind, and Double-blind challenge. In all types of OFC, incremental doses of the food challenge material are usually given in 15–30 minutes interval until objective allergic signs are observed or the final dose (generally representing a normal serving for age) is tolerated by the patient. In suspected food-dependent exercise-induced reactions the OFC is followed by exercise.

The Double-Blind Placebo-Controlled Food Challenge (DBPCFC) is considered the gold standard for the diagnosis of FA, as it controls for both patient and health care professionals bias (Nowak-Wegrzyn *et al.*, 2009). It is the challenge of choice for patients reporting subjective symptoms and in research studies. Adequate disguising of the allergenic food in a food matrix tolerated by the patient is essential. A negative DBPCFC may be followed by on Open OFC with the usual edible form of the food to control for possible false-negative results due to the destruction of the allergens during the preparation of the challenge material (Bernhisel-Broadbent *et al.*, 1992). In young children, a physician supervising open OFC is often sufficient to establish tolerance or allergy and is frequently preferred when testing for the reintroduction of food in the diet of an allergic child.

OFC may potentially induce a significant allergic reaction to the subject under investigation. For this reason, OFCs should be performed by experienced personnel in a setting where equipment and medication for resuscitation are readily available (Boyce *et al.*, 2010b). Patients at high risk for severe reactions including those who have experienced a previous life-threatening reaction or those suffering from brittle asthma should preferably not undergo OFC. Patients reacting on OFC should be treated accordingly and observed for a satisfactory period before being discharged with a tailored-measured management plan (Bindslev-Jensen *et al.*, 2004).

Elimination diets

Elimination diets may be extremely useful in the assessment of patients with non-IgE- or mixed IgE/non-mediated FA. Complete avoidance of the suspected food allergen(s) for a period of 2–6 weeks is often required for the achievement of clinical improvement and resolution of symptoms (Burks *et al.*, 2012). Recurrence of symptoms with the reintroduction of the eliminated food(s) points towards the culprit food allergen(s). Involvement of an experienced dietician in the field of FA is essential to avoid nutritional risks associated with prolonged or multiple dietary eliminations (Burks *et al.*, 2012; Sampson *et al.*, 2014).

Component resolved diagnostics

Over the last few years, the huge progress in molecular biology and biochemistry has led to the isolation, characterization and recombinant production of many allergenic proteins, as well as the synthesis of IgE epitope-emulating peptides for individual food allergens (Marsh *et al.*, 2008). These molecules are increasingly used within the concept of Component Resolved Diagnostics (CRD) to facilitate more accurate diagnostic tools for the assessment of FA (Lidholm *et al.*, 2006). Using recombinant components or synthetic epitopes in diagnostic tests a detailed analysis of a patient's sensitization profile can be determined and significant clinically relevant associations established.

So far, a number of studies employing the CRD methodology have shown that the molecular analysis of the allergen sensitization patterns may serve to enhance the diagnostic and predictive power of IgE-based allergy diagnostics. A study assessing the CRD-based *in vitro* diagnosis of cherry allergy across Europe showed that the combination of rPruav 1, 3 and 4 was superior to diagnostic methods based on cherry extract (Reuter *et al.*, 2006). In another study, reactivity to Omega-5 gliadin was associated with wheat-dependent exercise-induced anaphylaxis (Matsuo *et al.*, 2005). Sensitization to Ara h 2 has increasingly been shown to predict clinical reactivity to peanut in several populations in certain geographic regions (Nicolaou and Custovic, 2011). It appears that with the CRD concept and microarray development food allergy diagnostics is entering a promising era. However, inconsistencies exist, and a number of adequately powered clinical trials are required before the introduction of these methods into general clinical practice (Steckelbroeck *et al.*, 2008).

Management of Food Allergy

At present, strict avoidance of the offending food allergen(s) and the early recognition and prompt treatment of inadvertent reactions are the mainstay of management for all types of FA (Sampson *et al.*, 2014). Regular follow-up (6–12 months) of patients is significantly important as many types of food allergies resolve over time.

Food-allergic patients often experience subsequent reactions after consuming meals or snacks that they are unaware contain the allergens to which they are allergic (Uguz *et al.*, 2005). Therefore, careful food label reading and avoidance of foods with an unknown list of ingredients (e.g., from buffets, takeaways) are essential in reducing the likelihood of accidental exposures to the causal food allergens. Involvement of a dietician with experience in FA is crucial particularly for the management of patients with multiple food allergies (Kapoor *et al.*, 2004). Education of the patient and family in avoiding only the relevant food allergens is important in order to avoid unnecessary or over restricted diets often leading to inadequate nutrient intake and adverse effects on general health (e.g., rickets, growth impairment) (Noimark and Cox, 2008).

In addition to the employment of good avoidance strategies, patients, family and caregivers should be made aware of the early symptoms of food-allergic reactions and trained how to administer appropriate treatment. It is important to have a tailor-made action plan and suitable medication readily available for every individual suffering from food allergies. For example, patients with IgE-mediated FA and previous life-threatening reactions or those with unstable asthma should be provided with self-injectable adrenaline. Minor reactions such as those involving only the skin or the oral mucosa are usually managed with oral antihistamines alone, whereas more severe episodes manifesting with significant difficulty in breathing or cardiovascular compromise require early treatment with intramuscular adrenaline. It is acknowledged that intramuscular adrenaline (preferably to the lateral thigh) is the treatment of choice for anaphylaxis and that second-line therapies including volume expanders, nebulized bronchodilators, corticosteroids and antihistamines may also be required. The management of anaphylaxis and the indications for self-injectable adrenaline prescription have recently been reviewed by the World Allergy Organization (WAO) (Simons *et al.*, 2015). Optimal management of asthma and other medical conditions that may increase the risk of life-threatening anaphylaxis in food-allergic patients is also fundamental. Once adrenaline devices have been prescribed, ongoing support and training to patients and families by an allergy care team is essential to warrant safe and effective use (Arkwright and Farragher, 2006).

Over the last few years, a number of experimental therapeutic approaches including oral, sublingual and epicutaneous immunotherapy, treatment with humanized monoclonal anti-IgE antibodies, and a Chinese herbal formula have increased the hope that we may be getting closer to a definite cure for FA (Nowak-Wegrzyn and Sampson, 2011). Recent reports on successful oral allergen-specific immunotherapy in patients allergic to milk, eggs, and peanut are encouraging, but several issues including safety and long-term efficacy need to be clarified before general implementation of these immunotherapy treatments (Sampson *et al.*, 2014).

Avoidance of the offending food(s) from the diet is also the mainstay of management in non-IgE- and mixed IgE/non-IgE-mediated FA. Milk is the most common trigger in allergic proctocolitis and its elimination from the diet up to the age of 12 months often results in resolution of symptoms. In the case of FPIES, volume replacement treatment is essential for the management of the acute episodes. Empirical or targeted food-elimination diets in addition to corticosteroid therapy and collaboration with gastroenterologists may be required for the successful management of EoE.

Natural History and Prevention of Food Allergy

Natural history

The natural history of FA refers to both the acquisition of clinical allergy and its resolution or persistence. The timing of the onset of allergy and likelihood and timing of tolerance development varies depending on the food in question and on the underlying immune mechanism (Savage and Johns, 2015). The proportions of children who will outgrow allergy to a given food vary between studies, but allergy to milk, eggs, soy or wheat is more likely to be outgrown, whereas allergy to peanuts, tree nuts, fish or crustacean shellfish usually persist into adulthood (Host and Halken, 1990; Sicherer, 2003; Sicherer *et al.*, 2004). Resolution of an FA can occur as late as the teenage years (Nicolaou *et al.*, 2014). Levels of immune markers may be helpful in predicting clinical resolution of FA (Pyziak and Kamer, 2011) (Fiocchi *et al.*, 2010; Shek *et al.*, 2004). A high initial sIgE level is associated with a lower rate of resolution. In children, reductions in sIgE levels often precede the onset of tolerance. Changes in immediate SPT responses are less well defined; reductions in the size of an SPT induced wheal might be a marker for the onset of tolerance to food, yet in some cases SPT responses remain positive long after tolerance has developed. Peters *et al.* (2012) extensively reviewed the predictive value of SPTs for challenge-proved food allergy. The predictability of an SPT wheal size cutoff for determining tolerance or allergy appears to be limited to each study population because of differences in sample populations, testing technique and quality of the allergen test materials. The specific proteins within a food extract recognized by the sIgE of an individual patient can also predict the timing or likelihood of tolerance development or the risk of anaphylaxis (Jarvinen *et al.*, 2007). The measurement of ratios of IgE and IgG for specific determinants of an individual food protein (epitopes), may also be useful in the prediction of the clinical course of FA (Kim *et al.*, 2011a; Wang *et al.*, 2010).

Milk allergy

The natural history of Cow's Milk Protein Allergy (CMPA) shows heterogeneity and is closely related to the immunological and clinical phenotype by which CMPA presents. Children with non-IgE-mediated CMPA tend to develop tolerance at an earlier age and at a higher percentage compared to those with the IgE-mediated disease. In subjects with severe symptoms CMPA may persist for longer or ever. Although, the majority of children will outgrow their allergy, the individual timing of tolerance acquisition is largely unknown (Nicolaou and Custovic, 2011; Nicolaou *et al.*, 2014). Recent data suggest that baked milk is tolerated by the majority (75%) of children who are reactive to uncooked milk (Nowak-Wegrzyn *et al.*, 2008) and ingestion of baked milk may accelerate the resolution of milk allergy (Kim *et al.*, 2011b).

Egg allergy

The natural history of egg allergy shows similarities with that of milk allergy and most children will outgrow it. In a more recent prospective study of egg-allergic children recruited from primary care offices, the median age of resolution (defined by OFC and the successful home introduction of a whole egg) was 6 years with a rate of resolution of nearly 50%. Of those children with unresolved allergy, 38.1% were able to tolerate some baked egg products (Sicherer *et al.*, 2014).

Peanut allergy

The most common age for the presentation of peanut allergy is 18 months, although peanut allergy can present later in childhood or adulthood, most often as part of the pollen–food allergy syndrome (Green *et al.*, 2007; Vereda *et al.*, 2011). The timing of peanut allergy resolution is not clearly defined, but cases of resolution in adulthood have been reported (Savage *et al.*, 2007), suggesting that patients can benefit from long-term follow-up for peanut allergy. The largest study to date reported that 21.5% of patients had become peanut-tolerant when patients aged 4 to 20 years with a history of peanut allergy and peanut-specific IgE of less than 20 kUA/L were offered an OFC (Savage and Johns, 2015).

Prevention

Despite the considerable progress towards a permanent therapy, the ideal goal in FA management would be the employment of strategies that would prevent the development of the disease. The early onset of food allergy in childhood and the observed rise in its prevalence have led to a great interest into early-life exposures, in an effort to identify potential risk factors and possible intervention strategies (de Silva *et al.*, 2014; Marrs *et al.*, 2013; Warner and Warner, 2014).

Influence of maternal diet

Prenatal exposures including infections, environmental pollutants, as well as nutrients provided via the mother may act upon the developing foetal immune system, influencing towards the acquisition of tolerance or allergy (Abelius *et al.*, 2014; Miles and Calder, 2015; Wopereis *et al.*, 2014). As an example, a recent large population-based birth cohort study from Finland showed that high maternal consumption of milk products during pregnancy may protect children from developing cow's milk allergy, especially in offspring of non-allergic mothers (Tuokkola *et al.*, 2016). Food allergens have been detected in breast milk under physiologic conditions, but the role of this passage in food allergies is still unclear (Liao *et al.*, 2014). Furthermore, maternal dietary interventions have been questioned in several studies as an effective strategy to prevent allergic diseases in infants, and there is not enough evidence to recommend antigen avoidance to high-risk women during both pregnancy and lactation (Munblit *et al.*, 2015).

Influence of infants' diet

In the last years, some national and international paediatric societies have implemented the use of hydrolysates to prevent FA in their recommendations for children at risk who cannot exclusively breastfeed in the first 4–6 months of life (Agostoni *et al.*, 2008; Fleischer *et al.*, 2013). Many studies were focused on high-risk children: the German Infant Nutritional Intervention (GINI) programme recruited 2252 infants with a heredity risk for atopy and conducted a prospective, double-blind randomized controlled trial to study the effectiveness of hydrolysates for allergy prevention (von Berg, 2013; von Berg *et al.*, 2013). This study showed evidence that hydrolysates play a role in the prevention of Atopic Dermatitis (AD), but not of allergic respiratory diseases, nor of sensitization at school age (von Berg, 2013). Recently, the EAACI (European Academy of Allergy and Clinical Immunology). Food Allergy and Anaphylaxis Guidelines Group concluded that the use of extensively hydrolyzed whey or casein formula in infants at high risk for the first 4 months may have benefits in preventing FA (de Silva *et al.*, 2014). The supplementation with probiotics in infancy is another debated approach to prevent FA and allergic sensitization. Recently, two important evidence-based recommendations were published (Fiocchi *et al.*, 2015; Muraro *et al.*, 2014) with conflicting conclusions. The EAACI Food Allergy and Anaphylaxis Guidelines do not recommend probiotics to prevent FA due to the lack of sufficient evidence (Muraro *et al.*, 2014). On the other hand, the WAO Guideline Panel Recommendation, although recognizing a low level of evidence, suggested a likely net benefit from using probiotics resulting primarily from the prevention of eczema (Fiocchi *et al.*, 2015).

Introduction of complementary foods

Until recently it was generally believed that early exposure to food allergens may promote the development of FA and delayed weaning with potentially high allergenic foods (e.g., eggs, fish, and peanut) was recommended by many international health societies (Sampson *et al.*, 2014).

The current EAACI Guidelines recommend the introduction of complementary foods from 4 to 6 months of age according to the local standard practices and the needs of the infant, irrespective of atopic heredity (Muraro *et al.*, 2014), but the timing to introduce allergenic food is still a matter of controversy. However, new evidence from the LEAP (Learning Early about Peanut Allergy) study which compared the effect of early exposure to peanut with that of complete avoidance in high-risk infants showed that early introduction of peanuts significantly decreased the frequency of the development of peanut allergy and modulated immune responses to peanut (Du Toit *et al.*, 2015). The preventive effect of the early introduction of peanuts was also observed in the Enquiring About Tolerance (EAT) study, which recruited breastfed infants from the general population (Perkin *et al.*, 2016). Similar findings in the EAT study were revealed for eggs, whereas early introduction of milk, wheat, sesame and fish did not show a significant preventive effect.

Conclusion

Ingested food represents the greatest foreign antigenic load confronting the human immune system. In the vast majority of individuals, tolerance develops to food antigens, which are constantly gaining access to the body properly. However, when tolerance fails to develop, the immune system responds with a hypersensitivity reaction. Inadvertent ingestion of food allergens may provoke various gastrointestinal, cutaneous, respiratory symptoms, and/or systemic anaphylaxis with shock. For many years, management of food allergy consisted of allergen avoidance and emergency treatment while waiting for allergies to be outgrown. However, during the last years, food allergy-specific immunotherapy has appeared as an optional treatment, although still confined to an experimental clinical setting, showing high evidence of efficacy but with a lack of studies on safety and long-term follow-up. The future lies in prevention and early recovery by inducing tolerance or prevention by early introduction. Further studies will be helpful to confirm and consolidate our knowledge about these promising preventive and therapeutic approaches to offer a novel perspective in the management and treatment of food allergies.

Keywords: food allergy, clinical manifestations of food allergy, IgE mediated reactions, non IgE-mediated reactions, cross reactions, diagnosis, natural history of food allergy, prevention of food allergy, management of food allergy, children

References

Abelius, M. S., Lempinen, E., Lindblad, K., Ernerudh, J., Berg, G., Matthiesen, L., Nilsson, L. J., and Jenmalm, M. C. (2014). Th2-like chemokine levels are increased in allergic children and influenced by maternal immunity during pregnancy. Pediatric of Allergy Immunology 25(4): 387–393.

Agostoni, C., Decsi, T., Fewtrell, M., Goulet, O., Kolacek, S., Koletzko, B., Michaelsen, K. F., Moreno, L., Puntis, J., Rigo, J., Shamir, R., Szajewska, H., Turck, D., and van Goudoever, J. (2008). Complementary feeding: a commentary by the ESPGHAN committee on nutrition. Journal of Pediatric Gastroenterology and Nutrition 46(1): 99–110.

Akiyama, H., Imai, T., and Ebisawa, M. (2011). Japan food allergen labelling regulation—history and evaluation. Advances in Food and Nutrition Research 62: 139–171.

Arkwright, P. D., and Farragher, A. J. (2006). Factors determining the ability of parents to effectively administer intramuscular adrenaline to food allergic children. Pediatric of Allergy Immunology 17(3): 227–229.

Asero, R., Ballmer-Weber, B. K., Beyer, K., Conti, A., Dubakiene, R., Fernandez-Rivas, M., Hoffmann-Sommergruber, K., Lidholm, J., Mustakov, T., Oude Elberink, J. N., Pumphrey, R. S., Stahl Skov, P., van Ree, R., Vlieg-Boerstra, B. J., Hiller, R., Hourihane, J. O., Kowalski, M., Papadopoulos, N. G., Wal, J. M., Mills, E. N., and Vieths, S. (2007). IgE-mediated food allergy diagnosis: Current status and new perspectives. Molecular Nutrition and Food Research 51(1): 135–147.

Bernhisel-Broadbent, J., Strause, D., and Sampson, H. A. (1992). Fish hypersensitivity. II: Clinical relevance of altered fish allergenicity caused by various preparation methods. The Journal of Allergy and Clinical Immunology 90(4 Pt 1): 622–629.

Bindslev-Jensen, C., Ballmer-Weber, B. K., Bengtsson, U., Blanco, C., Ebner, C., Hourihane, J., Knulst, A. C., Moneret-Vautrin, D. A., Nekam, K., Niggemann, B., Osterballe, M., Ortolani, C., Ring, J., Schnopp, C., and Werfel, T. (2004). Standardization of food challenges in patients with immediate reactions to foods—position paper from the European academy of allergology and clinical immunology. Allergy 59(7): 690–697.

Bock, S. A., Munoz-Furlong, A., and Sampson, H. A. (2007). Further fatalities caused by anaphylactic reactions to food, 2001–2006. The Journal of Allergy and Clinical Immunology 119(4): 1016–1018.

Bollinger, M. E., Dahlquist, L. M., Mudd, K., Sonntag, C., Dillinger, L., and McKenna, K. (2006). The impact of food allergy on the daily activities of children and their families. Annals of Allergy, Asthma & Immunology: Official Publication of the American College of Allergy, Asthma, & Immunology 96(3): 415–421.

Boyce, J. A., Assa'ad, A., Burks, A. W., Jones, S. M., Sampson, H. A., Wood, R. A., Plaut, M., Cooper, S. F., Fenton, M. J., Arshad, S. H., Bahna, S. L., Beck, L. A., Byrd-Bredbenner, C., Camargo, C. A., Jr., Eichenfield, L., Furuta, G. T., Hanifin, J. M., Jones, C., Kraft, M., Levy, B. D., Lieberman, P., Luccioli, S., McCall, K. M., Schneider, L. C., Simon, R. A., Simons, F. E., Teach, S. J., Yawn, B. P., and Schwaninger, J. M. (2010a). Guidelines for the diagnosis and management of food allergy in the United States: Report of the NIAID-sponsored expert panel. The Journal of Allergy and Clinical Immunology 126(6 Suppl): S1–58.

Boyce, J. A., Assa'ad, A., Burks, A. W., Jones, S. M., Sampson, H. A., Wood, R. A., Plaut, M., Cooper, S. F., Fenton, M. J., Arshad, S. H., Bahna, S. L., Beck, L. A., Byrd-Bredbenner, C., Camargo, C. A. Jr., Eichenfield, L., Furuta, G. T., Hanifin, J. M., Jones, C., Kraft, M., Levy, B. D., Lieberman, P., Luccioli, S., McCall, K. M., Schneider, L. C., Simon, R. A., Simons, F. E., Teach, S. J., Yawn, B. P., and Schwaninger, J. M. (2010b). Guidelines for the diagnosis and management of food allergy in the United States: Summary of the NIAID-sponsored expert panel report. The Journal of Allergy and Clinical Immunology 126(6): 1105–1118.

Burks, A. W., Tang, M., Sicherer, S., Muraro, A., Eigenmann, P. A., Ebisawa, M., Fiocchi, A., Chiang, W., Beyer, K., Wood, R., Hourihane, J., Jones, S. M., Lack, G., and Sampson, H. A. (2012). ICON: food allergy. The Journal of Allergy and Clinical Immunology 129(4): 906–920.

Burks, W. (2003). Skin manifestations of food allergy. Pediatrics 111(6 Pt 3): 1617–1624.

Celik-Bilgili, S., Mehl, A., Verstege, A., Staden, U., Nocon, M., Beyer, K., and Niggemann, B. (2005). The predictive value of specific immunoglobulin E levels in serum for the outcome of oral food challenges. Clinical and Experimental Allergy: Journal of the British Society for Allergy and Clinical Immunology 35(3): 268–273.

Chafen, J. J., Newberry, S. J., Riedl, M. A., Bravata, D. M., Maglione, M., Suttorp, M. J., Sundaram, V., Paige, N. M., Towfigh, A., Hulley, B. J., and Shekelle, P. G. (2010). Diagnosing and managing common food allergies: a systematic review. JAMA : The Journal of the American Medical Association 303(18): 1848–1856.

Cox, L., Williams, B., Sicherer, S., Oppenheimer, J., Sher, L., Hamilton, R., and Golden, D. (2008). Pearls and pitfalls of allergy diagnostic testing: report from the American College of Allergy, Asthma and Immunology/American Academy of Allergy, Asthma and Immunology Specific IgE Test Task Force. Annals of Allergy, Asthma & Immunology: Official Publication of the American College of Allergy, Asthma, & Immunology 101(6): 580–592.

de Silva, D., Geromi, M., Halken, S., Host, A., Panesar, S. S., Muraro, A., Werfel, T., Hoffmann-Sommergruber, K., Roberts, G., Cardona, V., Dubois, A. E., Poulsen, L. K., Van Ree, R., Vlieg-Boerstra, B., Agache, I., Grimshaw, K., O'Mahony, L., Venter, C., Arshad, S. H., and Sheikh, A. (2014). Primary prevention of food allergy in children and adults: systematic review. Allergy 69(5): 581–589.

de Silva, I. L., Mehr, S. S., Tey, D., and Tang, M. L. (2008). Paediatric anaphylaxis: a 5 year retrospective review. Allergy 63(8): 1071–1076.

Du Toit, G., Roberts, G., Sayre, P. H., Bahnson, H. T., Radulovic, S., Santos, A. F., Brough, H. A., Phippard, D., Basting, M., Feeney, M., Turcanu, V., Sever, M. L., Gomez Lorenzo, M., Plaut,

M., and Lack, G. (2015). Randomized trial of peanut consumption in infants at risk for peanut allergy. The New England Journal of Medicine 372(9): 803–813.

Eller, E., Kjaer, H. F., Host, A., Andersen, K. E., and Bindslev-Jensen, C. (2009). Food allergy and food sensitization in early childhood: results from the DARC cohort. Allergy 64(7): 1023–1029.

Feuille, E., and Nowak-Wegrzyn, A. (2015). Food protein-induced enterocolitis syndrome, allergic proctocolitis, and enteropathy. Current Allergy and Asthma Reports 15(8): 50.

Fiocchi, A., Schunemann, H. J., Brozek, J., Restani, P., Beyer, K., Troncone, R., Martelli, A., Terracciano, L., Bahna, S. L., Rance, F., Ebisawa, M., Heine, R. G., Assa'ad, A., Sampson, H., Verduci, E., Bouygue, G. R., Baena-Cagnani, C., Canonica, W., and Lockey, R. F. (2010). Diagnosis and Rationale for Action Against Cow's Milk Allergy (DRACMA): a summary report. The Journal of Allergy and Clinical Immunology 126(6): 1119–1128.e1112.

Fiocchi, A., Pawankar, R., Cuello-Garcia, C., Ahn, K., Al-Hammadi, S., Agarwal, A., Beyer, K., Burks, W., Canonica, G. W., Ebisawa, M., Gandhi, S., Kamenwa, R., Lee, B. W., Li, H., Prescott, S., Riva, J. J., Rosenwasser, L., Sampson, H., Spigler, M., Terracciano, L., Vereda-Ortiz, A., Waserman, S., Yepes-Nunez, J. J., Brozek, J. L., and Schunemann, H. J. (2015). World Allergy Organization-McMaster University Guidelines for Allergic Disease Prevention (GLAD-P): Probiotics. The World Allergy Organization Journal 8(1): 4.

Fleischer, D. M., Spergel, J. M., Assa'ad, A. H., and Pongracic, J. A. (2013). Primary prevention of allergic disease through nutritional interventions. The Journal of Allergy and Clinical Immunology. In Practice. 1(1): 29–36.

Green, T. D., LaBelle, V. S., Steele, P. H., Kim, E. H., Lee, L. A., Mankad, V. S., Williams, L. W., Anstrom, K. J., and Burks, A. W. (2007). Clinical characteristics of peanut-allergic children: recent changes. Pediatrics 120(6): 1304–1310.

Gupta, R. S., Springston, E. E., Warrier, M. R., Smith, B., Kumar, R., Pongracic, J., and Holl, J. L. (2011). The prevalence, severity, and distribution of childhood food allergy in the United States. Pediatrics 128(1): e9–17.

Hofmann, A., and Burks, A. W. (2008). Pollen food syndrome: update on the allergens. Current Allergy and Asthma Reports 8(5): 413–417.

Host, A., and Halken, S. (1990). A prospective study of cow milk allergy in Danish infants during the first 3 years of life. Clinical course in relation to clinical and immunological type of hypersensitivity reaction. Allergy 45(8): 587–596.

Jarvinen, K. M., Beyer, K., Vila, L., Bardina, L., Mishoe, M., and Sampson, H. A. (2007). Specificity of IgE antibodies to sequential epitopes of hen's egg ovomucoid as a marker for persistence of egg allergy. Allergy 62(7): 758–765.

Kapoor, S., Roberts, G., Bynoe, Y., Gaughan, M., Habibi, P., and Lack, G. (2004). Influence of a multidisciplinary paediatric allergy clinic on parental knowledge and rate of subsequent allergic reactions. Allergy 59(2): 185–191.

Kim, E. H., Bird, J. A., Kulis, M., Laubach, S., Pons, L., Shreffler, W., Steele, P., Kamilaris, J., Vickery, B., and Burks, A. W. (2011a). Sublingual immunotherapy for peanut allergy: clinical and immunologic evidence of desensitization. The Journal of Allergy and Clinical Immunology 127(3): 640–646.e641.

Kim, J. S., Nowak-Wegrzyn, A., Sicherer, S. H., Noone, S., Moshier, E. L., and Sampson, H. A. (2011b). Dietary baked milk accelerates the resolution of cow's milk allergy in children. The Journal of Allergy and Clinical Immunology 128(1): 125–131.e122.

Kleiman, J., and Ben-Shoshan, M. (2014). Food-dependent exercise-induced anaphylaxis with negative allergy testing. BMJ Case Reports [Electronic Resource] 2014.

Lack, G. (2008). Clinical practice. Food allergy. The New England Journal of Medicine 359(12): 1252–1260.

Liacouras, C. A., Furuta, G. T., Hirano, I., Atkins, D., Attwood, S. E., Bonis, P. A., Burks, A. W., Chehade, M., Collins, M. H., Dellon, E. S., Dohil, R., Falk, G. W., Gonsalves, N., Gupta, S. K., Katzka, D. A., Lucendo, A. J., Markowitz, J. E., Noel, R. J., Odze, R. D., Putnam, P. E., Richter, J. E., Romero, Y., Ruchelli, E., Sampson, H. A., Schoepfer, A., Shaheen, N. J., Sicherer, S. H., Spechler, S., Spergel, J. M., Straumann, A., Wershil, B. K., Rothenberg, M. E., and Aceves, S. S. (2011). Eosinophilic esophagitis: updated consensus recommendations for children and adults. The Journal of Allergy and Clinical Immunology 128(1): 3–20.e26; quiz 21-22.

Liao, S. L., Lai, S. H., Yeh, K. W., Huang, Y. L., Yao, T. C., Tsai, M. H., Hua, M. C., and Huang, J. L. (2014). Exclusive breastfeeding is associated with reduced cow's milk sensitization in early childhood. Pediatric of Allergy Immunology 25(5): 456–461.

Lidholm, J., Ballmer-Weber, B. K., Mari, A., and Vieths, S. (2006). Component-resolved diagnostics in food allergy. Current Opinion in Allergy and Clinical Immunology 6(3): 234–240.

Marrs, T., Bruce, K. D., Logan, K., Rivett, D. W., Perkin, M. R., Lack, G., and Flohr, C. (2013). Is there an association between microbial exposure and food allergy? A systematic review. Pediatric of Allergy Immunology 24(4): 311–320.e318.

Marsh, J., Rigby, N., Wellner, K., Reese, G., Knulst, A., Akkerdaas, J., van Ree, R., Radauer, C., Lovegrove, A., Sancho, A., Mills, C., Vieths, S., Hoffmann-Sommergruber, K., and Shewry, P. R. (2008). Purification and characterisation of a panel of peanut allergens suitable for use in allergy diagnosis. Molecular Nutrition and Food Research 52 Suppl 2: S272–285.

Matsuo, H., Kohno, K., Niihara, H., and Morita, E. (2005). Specific IgE determination to epitope peptides of omega-5 gliadin and high molecular weight glutenin subunit is a useful tool for diagnosis of wheat-dependent exercise-induced anaphylaxis. Journal of Immunology (Baltimore, Md.: 1950) 175(12): 8116–8122.

McGowan, E. C., and Keet, C. A. (2013). Prevalence of self-reported food allergy in the National Health and Nutrition Examination Survey (NHANES) 2007–2010. The Journal of Allergy and Clinical Immunology 132(5): 1216–1219.e1215.

Miles, E. A., and Calder, P. C. (2015). Maternal diet and its influence on the development of allergic disease. Clinical and Experimental Allergy: Journal of the British Society for Allergy and Clinical Immunology 45(1): 63–74.

Moissidis, I., Chaidaroon, D., Vichyanond, P., and Bahna, S. L. (2005). Milk-induced pulmonary disease in infants (Heiner syndrome). Pediatric of Allergy Immunology 16(6): 545–552.

Munblit, D., Boyle, R. J., and Warner, J. O. (2015). Factors affecting breast milk composition and potential consequences for development of the allergic phenotype. Clinical and Experimental Allergy: Journal of the British Society for Allergy and Clinical Immunology 45(3): 583–601.

Muraro, A., Roberts, G., Clark, A., Eigenmann, P. A., Halken, S., Lack, G., Moneret-Vautrin, A., Niggemann, B., and Rance, F. (2007). The management of anaphylaxis in childhood: position paper of the European academy of allergology and clinical immunology. Allergy 62(8): 857–871.

Muraro, A., Halken, S., Arshad, S. H., Beyer, K., Dubois, A. E., Du Toit, G., Eigenmann, P. A., Grimshaw, K. E., Hoest, A., Lack, G., O'Mahony, L., Papadopoulos, N. G., Panesar, S., Prescott, S., Roberts, G., de Silva, D., Venter, C., Verhasselt, V., Akdis, A. C., and Sheikh, A. (2014). EAACI food allergy and anaphylaxis guidelines. Primary prevention of food allergy. Allergy 69(5): 590–601.

Nicolaou, N., and Custovic, A. (2011). Molecular diagnosis of peanut and legume allergy. Current Opinion in Allergy and Clinical Immunology 11(3): 222–228.

Nicolaou, N., Tsabouri, S., and Priftis, K. N. (2014). Reintroduction of cow's milk in milk-allergic children. Endocrine, Metabolic & Immune Disorders Drug Targets 14(1): 54–62.

Noimark, L., and Cox, H. E. (2008). Nutritional problems related to food allergy in childhood. Pediatric of Allergy Immunology 19(2): 188–195.

Nowak-Wegrzyn, A., Bloom, K. A., Sicherer, S. H., Shreffler, W. G., Noone, S., Wanich, N., and Sampson, H. A. (2008). Tolerance to extensively heated milk in children with cow's milk allergy. The Journal of Allergy and Clinical Immunology 122(2): 342–347, 347.e341-342.

Nowak-Wegrzyn, A., Assa'ad, A. H., Bahna, S. L., Bock, S. A., Sicherer, S. H., and Teuber, S. S. (2009). Work Group report: oral food challenge testing. The Journal of Allergy and Clinical Immunology 123(6 Suppl): S365–383.

Nowak-Wegrzyn, A., and Sampson, H. A. (2011). Future therapies for food allergies. The Journal of Allergy and Clinical Immunology 127(3): 558–573; quiz 574-555.

Nwaru, B. I., Hickstein, L., Panesar, S. S., Muraro, A., Werfel, T., Cardona, V., Dubois, A. E., Halken, S., Hoffmann-Sommergruber, K., Poulsen, L. K., Roberts, G., Van Ree, R., Vlieg-Boerstra, B. J., and Sheikh, A. (2014). The epidemiology of food allergy in Europe: a systematic review and meta-analysis. Allergy 69(1): 62–75.

Perkin, M. R., Logan, K., Tseng, A., Raji, B., Ayis, S., Peacock, J., Brough, H., Marrs, T., Radulovic, S., Craven, J., Flohr, C., and Lack, G. (2016). Randomized trial of introduction of allergenic foods in breast-fed infants. The New England Journal of Medicine 374(18): 1733–1743.

Peters, R. L., Gurrin, L. C., and Allen, K. J. (2012). The predictive value of skin prick testing for challenge-proven food allergy: a systematic review. Pediatric of Allergy Immunology 23(4): 347–352.

Pumphrey, R. S. (2000). Lessons for management of anaphylaxis from a study of fatal reactions. Clinical and Experimental Allergy: Journal of the British Society for Allergy and Clinical Immunology 30(8): 1144–1150.

Pyziak, K., and Kamer, B. (2011). Natural history of IgE-dependent food allergy diagnosed in children during the first three years of life. Advances in Medical Sciences 56(1): 48–55.

Rance, F., Juchet, A., Bremont, F., and Dutau, G. (1997). Correlations between skin prick tests using commercial extracts and fresh foods, specific IgE, and food challenges. Allergy 52(10): 1031–1035.

Reuter, A., Lidholm, J., Andersson, K., Ostling, J., Lundberg, M., Scheurer, S., Enrique, E., Cistero-Bahima, A., San Miguel-Moncin, M., Ballmer-Weber, B. K., and Vieths, S. (2006). A critical assessment of allergen component-based *in vitro* diagnosis in cherry allergy across Europe. Clinical and Experimental Allergy: Journal of the British Society for Allergy and Clinical Immunology 36(6): 815–823.

Ross, M. P., Ferguson, M., Street, D., Klontz, K., Schroeder, T., and Luccioli, S. (2008). Analysis of food-allergic and anaphylactic events in the National Electronic Injury Surveillance System. The Journal of Allergy and Clinical Immunology 121(1): 166–171.

Sackeyfio, A., Senthinathan, A., Kandaswamy, P., Barry, P. W., Shaw, B., and Baker, M. (2011). Diagnosis and assessment of food allergy in children and young people: summary of NICE guidance. BMJ: British Medical Journal/British Medical Association 342: d747.

Salo, P. M., Arbes, S. J., Jr., Jaramillo, R., Calatroni, A., Weir, C. H., Sever, M. L., Hoppin, J. A., Rose, K. M., Liu, A. H., Gergen, P. J., Mitchell, H. E., and Zeldin, D. C. (2014). Prevalence of allergic sensitization in the United States: results from the National Health and Nutrition Examination Survey (NHANES) 2005–2006. The Journal of Allergy and Clinical Immunology 134(2): 350–359.

Sampson, H. A., and Ho, D. G. (1997). Relationship between food-specific IgE concentrations and the risk of positive food challenges in children and adolescents. The Journal of Allergy and Clinical Immunology 100(4): 444–451.

Sampson, H. A., Aceves, S., Bock, S. A., James, J., Jones, S., Lang, D., Nadeau, K., Nowak-Wegrzyn, A., Oppenheimer, J., Perry, T. T., Randolph, C., Sicherer, S. H., Simon, R. A., Vickery, B. P., Wood, R., Bernstein, D., Blessing-Moore, J., Khan, D., Lang, D., Nicklas, R., Oppenheimer, J., Portnoy, J., Randolph, C., Schuller, D., Spector, S., Tilles, S. A., Wallace, D., Sampson, H. A., Aceves, S., Bock, S. A., James, J., Jones, S., Lang, D., Nadeau, K., Nowak-Wegrzyn, A., Oppenheimer, J., Perry, T. T., Randolph, C., Sicherer, S. H., Simon, R. A., Vickery, B. P., and Wood, R. (2014). Food allergy: a practice parameter update-2014. The Journal of Allergy and Clinical Immunology 134(5): 1016–1025.e1043.

Savage, J., and Johns, C. B. (2015). Food allergy: epidemiology and natural history. Immunology and Allergy Clinics of North America 35(1): 45–59.

Savage, J. H., Limb, S. L., Brereton, N. H., and Wood, R. A. (2007). The natural history of peanut allergy: Extending our knowledge beyond childhood. The Journal of Allergy and Clinical Immunology 120(3): 717–719.

Shek, L. P., Soderstrom, L., Ahlstedt, S., Beyer, K., and Sampson, H. A. (2004). Determination of food specific IgE levels over time can predict the development of tolerance in cow's milk and hen's egg allergy. The Journal of Allergy and Clinical Immunology 114(2): 387–391.

Sicherer, S. H. (2003). Clinical aspects of gastrointestinal food allergy in childhood. Pediatrics 111(6 Pt 3): 1609–1616.

Sicherer, S. H., Munoz-Furlong, A., and Sampson, H. A. (2004). Prevalence of seafood allergy in the United States determined by a random telephone survey. The Journal of Allergy and Clinical Immunology 114(1): 159–165.

Sicherer, S. H., and Sampson, H. A. (2014). Food allergy: Epidemiology, pathogenesis, diagnosis, and treatment. The Journal of Allergy and Clinical Immunology 133(2): 291–307; quiz 308.

Sicherer, S. H., Wood, R. A., Vickery, B. P., Jones, S. M., Liu, A. H., Fleischer, D. M., Dawson, P., Mayer, L., Burks, A. W., Grishin, A., Stablein, D., and Sampson, H. A. (2014). The natural history of egg allergy in an observational cohort. The Journal of Allergy and Clinical Immunology 133(2): 492–499.

Simons, F. E., Ebisawa, M., Sanchez-Borges, M., Thong, B. Y., Worm, M., Tanno, L. K., Lockey, R. F., El-Gamal, Y. M., Brown, S. G., Park, H. S., and Sheikh, A. (2015). 2015 update of the evidence base: World Allergy Organization anaphylaxis guidelines. The World Allergy Organization Journal 8(1): 32.

Sporik, R., Hill, D. J., and Hosking, C. S. (2000). Specificity of allergen skin testing in predicting positive open food challenges to milk, egg and peanut in children. Clinical and Experimental Allergy: Journal of the British Society for Allergy and Clinical Immunology 30(11): 1540–1546.

Steckelbroeck, S., Ballmer-Weber, B. K., and Vieths, S. (2008). Potential, pitfalls, and prospects of food allergy diagnostics with recombinant allergens or synthetic sequential epitopes. The Journal of Allergy and Clinical Immunology 121(6): 1323–1330.

Tsabouri, S., Triga, M., Makris, M., Kalogeromitros, D., Church, M. K., and Priftis, K. N. (2012). Fish and shellfish allergy in children: review of a persistent food allergy. Pediatric of Allergy Immunology 23(7): 608–615.

Tuokkola, J., Luukkainen, P., Tapanainen, H., Kaila, M., Vaarala, O., Kenward, M. G., Virta, L. J., Veijola, R., Simell, O., Ilonen, J., Knip, M., and Virtanen, S. M. (2016). Maternal diet during pregnancy and lactation and cow's milk allergy in offspring. European Journal of Clinical Nutrition 70(5): 554–559.

Uguz, A., Lack, G., Pumphrey, R., Ewan, P., Warner, J., Dick, J., Briggs, D., Clarke, S., Reading, D., and Hourihane, J. (2005). Allergic reactions in the community: a questionnaire survey of members of the anaphylaxis campaign. Clinical and Experimental Allergy: Journal of the British Society for Allergy and Clinical Immunology 35(6): 746–750.

Urisu, A., Ebisawa, M., Mukoyama, T., Morikawa, A., and Kondo, N. (2011). Japanese guideline for food allergy. Allergology International: Official Journal of the Japanese Society of Allergology 60(2): 221–236.

Vereda, A., van Hage, M., Ahlstedt, S., Ibanez, M. D., Cuesta-Herranz, J., van Odijk, J., Wickman, M., and Sampson, H. A. (2011). Peanut allergy: Clinical and immunologic differences among patients from 3 different geographic regions. The Journal of Allergy and Clinical Immunology 127(3): 603–607.

von Berg, A. (2013). The role of hydrolysates for allergy prevention—pro. Pediatric of Allergy Immunology 24(8): 720–723.

von Berg, A., Filipiak-Pittroff, B., Kramer, U., Hoffmann, B., Link, E., Beckmann, C., Hoffmann, U., Reinhardt, D., Grubl, A., Heinrich, J., Wichmann, H. E., Bauer, C. P., Koletzko, S., and Berdel, D. (2013). Allergies in high-risk schoolchildren after early intervention with cow's milk protein hydrolysates: 10-year results from the German Infant Nutritional Intervention (GINI) study. The Journal of Allergy and Clinical Immunology 131(6): 1565–1573.

Wang, J., Lin, J., Bardina, L., Goldis, M., Nowak-Wegrzyn, A., Shreffler, W. G., and Sampson, H. A. (2010). Correlation of IgE/IgG4 milk epitopes and affinity of milk-specific IgE antibodies with different phenotypes of clinical milk allergy. The Journal of Allergy and Clinical Immunology 125(3): 695–702, 702.e691-702.e696.

Warner, J. O., and Warner, J. A. (2014). Fetal and early-life origins of allergy. Pediatric of Allergy Immunology 25(1): 7–8.

Wopereis, H., Oozeer, R., Knipping, K., Belzer, C., and Knol, J. (2014). The first thousand days—intestinal microbiology of early life: establishing a symbiosis. Pediatric of Allergy Immunology 25(5): 428–438.

CHAPTER 3

Peanut Allergy
Clinical Relevance and Allergen Characterisation

Joana Costa, Caterina Villa, Telmo J.R. Fernandes,
M. Beatriz P.P. Oliveira and *Isabel Mafra**

Introduction

Peanuts (*Arachis hypogaea*) are the edible seeds of a legume that belongs to the Fabaceae family (frequently termed as Leguminosae or pea family). Peanuts or groundnuts are their most common designation, although they are also known by less usual names (earth nuts, goober peas, monkey nuts, pygmy nuts and pig nuts). *Arachis hypogaea* is an allotetraploid species that contains two complete genomes of its wild ancestors: *Arachis duranensis* and *Arachis ipaensis*. Peanuts were originated and first domesticated in South America, but today they are widely cultivated throughout tropical and subtropical areas (PeanutBase, 2016). In 2014, China, India and USA were their main producers, accounting for more than 58% of the global peanut production (FAOSTAT, 2016).

With a total fat content of 49%, they present a high proportion of mono- and polyunsaturated fatty acids (40%), thus representing an important oil source for the food industry. Additionally, peanuts have a high protein content (25%) (USDA-NNDSR, 2016), making them matrices of great technological interest, namely as extenders in processed meat products (Arya *et al.*, 2016). Peanuts are most appreciated for their flavour, which is similar to different species of the tree nuts. Likewise, peanuts are commonly consumed as snacks and are present in a wide variety of processed foods, namely peanut butter, chocolates, soups and desserts among others.

REQUIMTE-LAQV, Faculdade de Farmácia, Universidade do Porto, Rua de Jorge Viterbo Ferreira, 228, 4050-313 Porto, Portugal.
* Corresponding author: isabel.mafra@ff.up.pt

Peanuts have been highlighted as functional foods owing to their content of bioactive compounds (e.g., antioxidants, vitamins). Their consumption has been related to health benefits, such as reducing the relative risk of coronary heart disease, protective effect on cancer risk, cholesterol-lowering effect, inflammation and vascular reactivity. Additionally, beneficial effects on blood pressure, visceral adiposity and metabolic syndrome have also been correlated with peanut and other nut consumption (Ros, 2010). However, peanuts are well-known as allergenic foods, representing one of the eight groups responsible for the majority (> 90%) of the reported adverse immunological responses in sensitised/allergic individuals.

In this chapter, it is intended to provide a broad overview on peanut allergy. Topics such as the prevalence of peanut allergy and the molecular characterisation of identified allergens will be focused here. Additionally, related subjects concerning clinical relevance, the definition of threshold levels and insight on the available diagnosis and immunotherapies for peanut allergy will also be addressed.

Prevalence of Peanut Allergy

Most of the available studies concerning the prevalence of food allergies are based on self-reported reactions to foods through surveys and questionnaires, which tend to overrate their actual prevalence. Contrarily, objective assessments, such as Open Food Challenges (OFC), Double-Blind, Placebo-Controlled Food Challenge (DBPCFC) tests, or determined sensitisation to foods by serum Immunoglobulin E (IgE), and Skin Prick Tests (SPT) are considered more accurate, but also more demanding in terms of study design (Zuidmeer et al., 2008). Despite the quantity of studies estimating the prevalence of food allergies based on questionnaires and surveys, only a few determine the sensitisation to foods using serum IgE reactivity and SPT, OFC or DBPCFC. Additionally, the number of studies providing global indicators for the prevalence of food allergies is scarce, since most reports are restricted to one geographical region (e.g., country).

Accordingly, in a study involving numerous centres from 11 countries in Europe, as well as USA and Australia, sensitisation to peanut was estimated to an overall prevalence of 2.6 and 1.8% when excluding the birch-positive individuals (Burney et al., 2010). Similar indices for peanut allergy were reported by Mackenzie et al. (2014) with 2.8 or 2.9% of maximum prevalence in European or non-European countries, respectively. Among children, the prevalence of peanut allergy seems to be increasing in the past years (1.4–3.0%), being higher in children (< 18 years) than in adult population (Venter et al., 2010). Umasunthar et al. (2015) performed a systematic review and meta-analysis, using the inverse variance method and including data from 34 studies reporting serious food allergic reactions (anaphylaxis). In the referred report global prevalences of 3 and 3.9% were estimated for food allergy in adults and children, respectively, and an overall prevalence of 1% for peanut allergy.

Clinical threshold levels for peanut allergy

Peanut allergy has been related to most fatal food-allergic reactions, both in adults and children and whose prevalence seems to be increasing in recent years (EFSA, 2013; Venter *et al.*, 2010).

For a better management of peanut allergy, both at individual (patients, caretakers, health professionals) or at population (food industry, regulatory entities) levels, the definition of clinical thresholds for peanuts constitutes a critical piece of information (Crevel *et al.*, 2008; Santos *et al.*, 2015). The clinical threshold is most commonly defined as the highest dose without inducing any objective effect (No Observed Adverse Effect Level—NOAEL) or as the lowest dose eliciting an observed adverse effect level (LOAEL), although the "true" threshold level should lie between the two doses (Taylor *et al.*, 2009).

The determination of peanut threshold doses depends on OFC and/or DBPCFC studies performed in peanut-allergic patients, which carry out some potential health risks for these individuals. Despite the difficulties on study design and cooperation of the test population, some clinical thresholds have been advanced for peanut allergy. Based on a DBPCFC study conducted on 268 peanut-allergic individuals (adults and children), Taylor *et al.* (2010) reported eliciting doses (ED) of 14.4 mg and 7.3 mg of whole groundnut, respectively at which 10% (ED_{10}) and 5% (ED_{05}) of the test population evidenced objective clinical symptoms. Considering that peanut contains 25% of proteins (USDA-NNDSR, 2016), those levels corresponded to 3.6 mg and 1.8 mg of peanut proteins for the respective ED_{10} and ED_{05}. In the same study, Taylor *et al.* (2010) also verified that there were no significant differences between the ED_{10} for non-severe (10.2 mg protein) or severe (10.4 mg protein) allergic reactions. In a different study (Blom *et al.*, 2013), using a test population of 135 peanut-allergic patients (children < 18 years), similar threshold values for objective clinical symptoms were described for ED_{10} (4.4 mg of protein) and ED_{05} (1.6 mg of protein). When considering any symptom, the ED_{10} and ED_{05} were 10-times lower, being 0.52 and 0.14 mg of peanut protein, respectively (Blom *et al.*, 2013). Using a modified OFC with dose increments every 2 hours on a test population of 63 children (< 18 years), Blumchen *et al.* (2014) reported an ED_{05} of 1.95 mg of peanut protein. Ballmer-Weber *et al.* (2015a) described an ED_{10} of 2.8 mg of protein in a total of 191 patients (participants of the pan-European EuroPrevall project), presenting objective clinical symptoms to peanut. The ED_{10} associated with any symptom was approximately 100-fold lower (0.03 mg of peanut protein) (Ballmer-Weber *et al.*, 2015a). Based on the individual threshold levels using OFC and DBPCFC studies, some mathematical models have been generated to estimate population thresholds for different allergenic foods. In the case of peanut, reference doses or minimum eliciting doses ranging from 0.2 to 0.4 mg of protein have been advanced as threshold levels for all peanut-allergic patients (Taylor *et al.*, 2014; Zhu *et al.*, 2015).

Diagnostic, therapeutic and immunotherapy

Peanut allergy is a classical immunological disease mediated by IgE mechanisms (Fig. 3.1). Typically, clinical symptoms can occur within few minutes up to 2 hours after peanut ingestion. Sensitisation often happens through skin or air, but near-fatal symptoms are normally consequences of peanut oral ingestion (Burks, 2008). Diagnosis of peanut allergy is common in children at an early age (~ 14 months), with approximately 74% of those requiring clinical treatment at the first known ingestion of peanut (Sicherer *et al.*, 2001).

The diagnosis of peanut allergy starts with clear definition of a medical history that normally includes the temporal association between ingestion and appearance of the first observable symptoms, the amount of ingested peanut, the type of symptoms and target organs/systems (skin, gastrointestinal or respiratory), and the symptoms after eating similar foods (Burks, 2008). When classical signs and symptoms (e.g., urticaria, repetitive vomiting or angioedema) of IgE-mediated response are evidenced up to 2 hours after peanut ingestion, diagnostic testing methods are required for measuring the specific IgE to peanut, namely skin prick test and the *in vitro* serum-specific IgE test (ImmunoCAP FEIA test) (Lee and Burks, 2009). Although the sensitivity of peanut SPT is high, the specificity is low, so the results from SPT must be

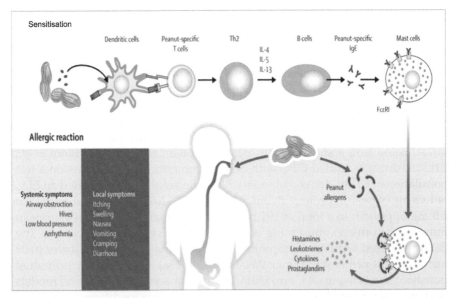

Fig. 3.1: Schematic representation of peanut allergic reaction. Reprinted with permission from Burks (2008). Copyright©2016, Elsevier.

carefully evaluated. While a positive SPT indicates that the patient has been sensitised (but not necessarily allergic), a negative result does not confirm the absence of peanut allergy. ImmunoCAP FEIA test is considered a more specific quantitative method, enabling to correlate the diagnostic levels for peanut with the results from OFC. In this sense, a result of peanut-specific IgE level > 14 kU/L by ImmunoCAP FEIA test along with a convincing medical history supports the diagnosis of peanut allergy (Lee and Burks, 2009).

There is no effective treatment for peanut allergy rather than the prophylactic measure of its total avoidance. However, peanut-allergic patients are still at risk of suffering severe immunological episodes upon accidental exposure to peanut. At this level, corrective treatments are indicated, such as injecting epinephrine for patients experiencing respiratory, cardiovascular or neurologic compromise (or at risk of an anaphylactic shock) (Fleischer et al., 2013; Lee and Burks, 2009).

Peanut allergy is typically classified as a life-persisting syndrome since children with clinical diagnosis of peanut allergy tend to suffer from those through their adulthood. However, recent data also seem to suggest that as many as 20% of children can develop peanut tolerance. In children with newly-diagnosed allergy, if peanut-specific IgE levels decrease to < 2 kUA/L upon annual evaluation, children (≥ 4 years) are estimated to outgrow their sensitivity to peanut (Perry et al., 2004). In this case, children are advised to consume peanut on a regular basis during 1 year, while maintaining vigilance for any potential severe reaction. Contrarily, if children (> 5 years) present peanut-specific IgE level remains > 15 kUA/L or fail OFC at a lower level, they are less likely to develop natural tolerance (Lee and Burks, 2009).

So far, different forms of immunotherapy are currently being exploited for patients with persistent food allergy, namely subcutaneous immunotherapy (SCIT), sublingual immunotherapy (SLIT) or oral immunotherapy (OIT). SCIT protocols have successfully been used to treat allergic rhinitis and asthma allergies, but after the report of severe allergic reactions to peanut injections (Nelson et al., 1997), this treatment was discontinued (Khoriaty and Umetsu, 2013).

In SLIT, small amounts (micrograms-milligrams) of allergen preparation are delivered to the sublingual region and expelled or swallowed after 2–5 minutes. So far, some SLIT trials have been carried out with successful desensitisation to peanut after 12 months of treatment (Burks et al., 2015; Fleischer et al., 2013; Kim et al., 2011). Despite evidencing a long-term safety profile, patients from most SLIT protocols have difficulty in maintaining a daily dosing and several of them drop the programme (Burks et al., 2015). Contrarily to SLIT, OIT consists of orally providing the offending allergenic ingredient mixed with a food vehicle, starting with small amounts and increasing the doses at variable rates (Khoriaty and Umetsu, 2013). OIT is the most investigated approach for persistent peanut allergy. Different studies state the reduction of peanut-specific T_H2 cytokine production, while increasing the peanut thresholds after OIT protocol. Additionally, OIT induces basophil and mast cell desensitisation and long-term tolerance in some children (Anagnostou *et al.*, 2014; Blumchen *et al.*, 2010; Clark *et al.*, 2009; Narisety *et al.*, 2015; Varshney *et al.*, 2011).

Allergen Characterisation and Clinical Relevance

So far, 17 groups of allergenic proteins have been identified and characterised in peanut (Table 3.1). Excluding the Ara h agglutinin that is only classified as an allergen by the ALLERGOME database (ALLERGOME, 2016), all the remaining molecules have already been included in the World Health Organisation-International Union of Immunological Societies (WHO-IUIS) official list of allergens (ALLERGEN, 2016). However, some of those are still at a provisional state of classification since pertinent information supporting biochemical or immunoreactivity data (e.g., Ara h 16 and Ara h 17) is still waiting for confirmation. Peanut allergens belong to different families of proteins with distinct biological functions.

Cupin superfamily

Ara h 1 and Ara h 3

Included in the cupin superfamily, Ara h 1 (vicilin) and Ara h 3 (legumin) are classified as dicupins (Table 3.1), presenting two beta-barrel motifs in their conformation (Radauer and Breiteneder, 2007). The vicilins (trimeric 7S globulins) and the legumins (hexameric 11S globulins) are globular seed storage proteins, which represent major protein components of several plant foods, namely of peanut (Breiteneder and Radauer, 2004). Both vicilins and legumins are thermostable proteins, suffering partial unfolding of their conformational structures at temperatures above 70°C and 94°C, respectively. In general, legumins refold even after submitted to high temperatures, while vicilins can suffer some conformational disruptions or covalent modifications as a result of glycation processes or Maillard rearrangements during food processing (Mills *et al.*, 2007). Previous classification of peanut allergens included another legumin (Ara h 4), but owing to its great similarity in molecular size, identical biological function and 67% or more, of amino acid identity (Radauer *et al.*, 2014) with Ara h 3.01, its designation was revised to Ara h 3.02 (isoallergen of Ara h 3).

Ara h 1 and Ara h 3 are considered major and minor allergens, respectively, according to the current allergen nomenclature (Radauer *et al.*, 2014). Ara h 1 maintain IgE-binding capacity even after submitted to harsh wet or dry-heat conditions, which indicate that its reactivity might be related to linear epitopes rather than to conformational ones (Koppelman *et al.*, 1999). Additionally, Ara h 1 and Ara h 3 undergo glycation, leading to the formation of advanced

Table 3.1: Identification of peanut allergens according to their biochemical characterisation, biological function and clinical relevance.

Allergen	Isoallergens	Isoforms or variants	MW/ length	Biochemical classification	Biological Function	Clinical relevance	Nucleotide (NCBI)	Protein (NCBI)	Protein (UniProt)	RCSB-PDB
Ara h 1	Ara h 1.01	Ara h 1.0101	71.3 kDa (626 aa)	Vicilin (7S globulin) (Cupin superfamily)	Storage of nutrients for plant growth	Major allergen. Severe and systemic allergic reactions	L34402	AAB00861	P43238	3SMH, 3S7I, 3S7E
Ara h 2	Ara h 2.01	Ara h 2.0101	18.7 kDa (158 aa)	Conglutin (2S albumin) (Prolamin superfamily)	Storage of nutrients for plant growth	Major allergen. Severe and systemic allergic reactions	AY007229	AAK96887	Q6PSU2-2	–
	Ara h 2.02	Ara h 2.0201	20.1 kDa (172 aa)	Conglutin (2S albumin) (Prolamin superfamily)			AY158467	AAN77576	Q6PSU2	–
Ara h 3	Ara h 3.01	Ara h 3.0101	58.4 kDa (507 aa)	Legumin (11S globulin) (Cupin superfamily)	Storage of nutrients for plant growth	Minor allergen. Severe and systemic allergic reactions	AF093541	AAC63045	O82580	–
	Ara h 3.02	Ara h 3.0201	61.0 kDa (530 aa)				AF086821	AAD47382	Q9SQH7	–
Ara h 5	Ara h 5.01	Ara h 5.0101	14.1 kDa (131 aa)	Profilin (Profilin family)	Binds to actin and affects the structure of the cytoskeleton	Minor allergen. Mild allergic reactions	AF059616	AAD55587	Q9SQI9	–
Ara h 6	Ara h 6.01	Ara h 6.0101	16.9 kDa (145 aa)	Conglutin (2S albumin) (Prolamin superfamily)	Same function as Ara h 1	Minor allergen (suggested revision) Severe and systemic allergic reactions	AF092846	AAD56337	Q647G9	1W2Q

Table 3.1 contd. ...

Table 3.1 contd.

Allergen	Isoallergens	Isoforms or variants	MW/ length	Biochemical classification	Biological Function	Clinical relevance	Nucleotide (NCBI)	Protein (NCBI)	Protein (UniProt)	RCSB-PDB
Ara h 7	Ara h 7.01	Ara h 7.0101	18.4 kDa (160 aa)	Conglutin (2S albumin) (Prolamin superfamily)	Same function as Ara h 1	Minor allergen. Severe and systemic allergic reactions	AF091737	AAD56719	Q9SQH1	–
	Ara h 7.02	Ara h 7.0201	19.3 kDa (164 aa)				EU046325	ABW17159	B4XID4	–
Ara h 8	Ara h 8.01	Ara h 8.0101	17.0 kDa (157 aa)	PR-10 (Bet v 1 - homologous) (Pathogenesis-related protein family)	Involved in mechanisms of defence and biotic stimulus responses	Major allergen. Mild to potentially severe allergic reactions	AY328088	AAQ91847	Q6VT83	–
	Ara h 8.02	Ara h 8.0201	16.4 kDa (153 aa)				EF436550	ABP97433	B0YIU5	4M9B, 4M9W, 4MA6, 4MAP
Ara h 9	Ara h 9.01	Ara h 9.0101	11.7 kDa (116 aa)	nsLTP 1 (PR-14 proteins) (Prolamin superfamily)	Transference of phospholipids and galactolipids across membranes. Antimicrobial activity	Minor/major allergen classification depending on geographical region. Potential severe and systemic allergic reactions	EU159429	ABX56711	B6CEX8	–
	Ara h 9.02	Ara h 9.0201	9.1 kDa (92 aa)				EU161278	ABX75045	B6CG41	–

Ara h 10	Ara h 10.0101	17.8 kDa (169 aa)	Oleosin (oleosin family)	Cellular component. Intervene in lipid metabolism and storage, regulation of intracellular trafficking and signal transduction	Suggested minor allergen classification.	AY722694	AAU21499	Q647G5	—
	Ara h 10.0102	15.5 kDa (150 aa)			Potential severe and systemic allergic reactions	AY722695	AAU21500	Q647G4	—
Ara h 11	Ara h 11.0101	14.3 kDa (137 aa)	Oleosin (oleosin family)	Same function as Ara h 10	Suggested minor allergen classification.	DQ097716	AAZ20276	Q45W87	—
	Ara h 11.0102	14.3 kDa (137 aa)			Potential severe and systemic allergic reactions	DQ097717	AAZ20277	Q45W86	—
Ara h 12	Ara h 12.0101	5.1 kDa[b] (46 aa)	Defensin (Defensin/myotoxin-like superfamily)	Antifungal activity	Suggested minor allergen classification. Potential severe and systemic allergic reactions	EY396089	—	—	—
Ara h 13	Ara h 13.0101	5.5 kDa[b] (47 aa)	Defensin (Defensin/myotoxin-like superfamily)	Antifungal activity	Suggested minor allergen classification.	EY396019	—	—	—
	Ara h 13.0102	5.5 kDa[b] (47 aa)			Potential severe and systemic allergic reactions	EE124955	—	—	—

Table 3.1 contd. ...

Table 3.1 contd.

Allergen	Isoallergens	Isoforms or variants	MW/length	Biochemical classification	Biological Function	Clinical relevance	Nucleotide (NCBI)	Protein (NCBI)	Protein (UniProt)	RCSB-PDB
Ara h 14	Ara h 14.01	Ara h 14.0101	18.4 kDa (176 aa)	Oleosin (oleosin family)	Same function as Ara h 10	Suggested minor allergen classification.	AF325917	AAK13449	Q9AXI1	–
		Ara h 14.0102	18.4 kDa (176 aa)			Potential severe and systemic allergic reactions	AF325918	AAK13450	Q9AXI0	–
		Ara h 14.0103	18.4 kDa (176 aa)				AY605694	AAT11925	Q6J1J8	–
Ara h 15		Ara h 15.0101	16.9 kDa (166 aa)	Oleosin (oleosin family)	Same function as Ara h 10	Suggested minor allergen classification. Potential severe and systemic allergic reactions	AY722696	AAU21501	Q647G3	–
Ara h 16[a]		Ara h 16.0101	7.0 kDa	nsLTP 2 (Prolamin superfamily)		Suggested minor allergen classification.	–	–	–	–
Ara h 17[a]		Ara h 17.0101	9.4 kDa	nsLTP 1 (PR-14 proteins) (Prolamin superfamily)	Same function as Ara h 9	Suggested minor allergen classification.	–	–	–	–

			Molecular mass	Family	Classification				PDB
Ara h agglutinin	–	–	29.3 kDa (273 aa)	Galactose-binding lectin (leguminous lectin family)	Suggested major allergen classification. Mild allergic reactions	S42352	AAB22817	P02872	1BZW, 1CR7, 1CIW, 1CQ9, 1QF3, 1RIR, 1RIT, 1V6I, 1V6J, 1V6K, 1V6L, 1V6M, 1V6N, 1V6O, 2DH1, 2DV9, 2DVA, 2DVB, 2DVD, 2DVF, 2DVG, 2PEL, 2TEP
			29.1 kDa (271 aa)			U22471	AAA74574	Q38711	
			29.6 kDa (276 aa)			U22468	AAA74571	Q43373	
			26.2 kDa (248 aa)			U22470	AAA74573	Q43375	
			26.2 kDa (246 aa)			AJ311170	CAC85156	Q8W0P8	

[a] provisional classification as food allergens in the WHO-IUIS official list of allergens.
[b] molecular mass yet to confirm, although the referred proteins are estimated to present higher molecular mass (~ 8 kDa).

glycation end-products that bind specific receptors in dendritic cells and consequently eliciting immunological responses. When the sensitisation to peanut allergens happens through the interaction of Maillard products with the respective dendritic cells' receptors, those are likely to bind modified Ara h 1 and Ara h 3 (Mueller *et al.*, 2013). Clinical symptoms related to these proteins are commonly classified as severe, similarly to the other seed storage proteins in peanut, namely Ara h 2, Ara h 6 and Ara h 7 (Ballmer-Weber *et al.*, 2015b).

Prolamin superfamily

Ara h 2, Ara h 6 and Ara h 7

The prolamin superfamily encompasses important groups of allergenic proteins, namely the 2S albumins, the non-specific Lipid Transfer Proteins (nsLTP) and the cereal alpha-amylase/trypsin inhibitors (Breiteneder and Radauer, 2004). Rich in residues of proline, glutamine (source of its designation) and cysteine, the members of this superfamily share low molecular weight, similar conformational structures with high content in alpha-helices and great stability to thermal processing/proteolysis (Kumar *et al.*, 2012). Like the cupins, many of the allergens belonging to prolamins are considered important class I food allergens, which are responsible for triggering severe and systemic allergic reactions (e.g., anaphylaxis) in sensitised individuals (Egger *et al.*, 2010).

   Included in the 2S albumins, the Ara h 2, Ara h 6 and Ara h 7 allergens (Table 3.1) are seed storage proteins with a major role in plant germination, acting as important donors of nitrogen and sulphur (Breiteneder and Ebner, 2000; Hauser *et al.*, 2008). Ara h 2 is considered a major allergen in peanut, being responsible for inducing adverse immunological responses in more than 85% of allergic individuals (Kleber-Janke *et al.*, 1999). In Europe, the sensitisation pattern to Ara h 2 is the highest (56%) when compared to other peanut allergens. Ara h 6 and Ara h 7 are classified as minor allergens, although recent data seem to indicate strong sensitisation of Ara h 6 with Ara h 2 (Ballmer-Weber *et al.*, 2015b). Therefore, the classification of Ara h 6 should be revised to major allergen. The clinical symptoms associated with Ara h 2 and Ara h 6 are severe, with the target in multiple systems (respiratory and gastrointestinal), which often result in life-threatening episodes (Ballmer-Weber *et al.*, 2015b; Kukkonen *et al.*, 2015).

Ara h 9, Ara h 16 and Ara h 17

Also included in the prolamin superfamily, the nsLTP are small, but highly conserved proteins that are widely distributed in the plant kingdom (Hauser *et al.*, 2010). These types of proteins are mainly involved in the transport of different lipids (fatty acids, phospholipids, glycolipids and sterols) across membranes. Although they are known to intervene in mechanisms of plant defence (antifungal and antibacterial activities) (Ebner *et al.*, 2001) or plant growth/development (embryogenesis, germination) (Salcedo *et al.*, 2007). Due to these apparent secondary roles in plant defence, the nsLTP are also included in the Pathogenesis-Related (PR) protein family with the designation of PR-14. The nsLTP are divided into two subfamilies of 9 kDa proteins (nsLTP 1) or 7 kDa proteins (nsLTP 2) (Hauser *et al.*, 2010), whereas the majority of the allergenic nsLTP belong to nsLTP 1. Owing to its high sequence and structural similarity with other allergenic proteins from distantly related species, they are classified as panallergens (Hauser *et al.*, 2010). In spite of being classified as minor allergens, panallergens are considered important airborne and food allergens, with special impact on the allergic population of the Mediterranean area (Salcedo *et al.*, 2007). nsLTP are normally resistant to gastrointestinal digestion, to thermal processing and to pH alterations (Breiteneder and Mills, 2005), which contribute to the observable severity of the induced allergic reactions.

In peanut, there are three allergenic proteins classified as minor allergens, two belonging to the nsLTP 1 (Ara h 9 and Ara h 17) and one to the nsLTP 2 (Ara h 16) (Table 3.1). Ara h 16 and Ara h 17 were only reported as food allergens very recently (ALLERGEN, 2016), thus little information has been made available regarding these two proteins. Like the case of other panallergens (e.g., Pru p 3 in peach, Cor a 8 in hazelnut), the pattern of sensitisation to Ara h 9 is greatly dependent on the geographical region (Ballmer-Weber *et al.*, 2015b; Scala *et al.*, 2015). Supporting this fact, recent data suggest a higher sensitisation to Ara h 9 in the South of Europe (67%), in contrast with North, West/Central or East European regions (12–33%). Additionally, sensitisation to Ara h 9 seems to occur as a consequence of a primary sensitisation to Pru p 3 (peach) due to their high cross reactivity (Ballmer-Weber *et al.*, 2015b). Clinical symptoms related to Ara h 9 can vary from mild and restricted to oral allergy syndrome (OAS) (Garcia-Blanca *et al.*, 2015), to severe and systemic (e.g., bronchospasm, anaphylaxis), especially among the population of the Mediterranean area (Arkwright *et al.*, 2013; Scala *et al.*, 2015).

Pathogenesis-related protein family

Ara h 8

Ara h 8 belong to the PR-10 family (Table 3.1), which is one of the 14 groups comprised of the pathogenesis-related proteins that are engaged in responses to pathogen infection, to environmental stress and/or antibiotic stimuli. This group of proteins is commonly designated as Bet v 1-related proteins due to their great sequence and structural homology. PR-10 proteins are characterised by small size, stability at low pH and resistance to proteolysis, being considered excellent candidates for triggering allergic reactions in sensitised individuals (Hauser *et al.*, 2008). When submitted to harsh processing conditions, these proteins tend to suffer conformational unfolding, leading to the destruction of conformational epitopes. Conversely, the thermostability of the bet v 1-homologous proteins is variable according to distinct plant sources (Mills *et al.*, 2007).

Under the WHO/IUIS official list of allergens, Ara h 8 is classified as a major allergen in peanut, being associated with birch-pollen allergy via the sequential and/or conformational similarity of molecules (Mittag *et al.*, 2004). However, recent data suggest that the overall sensitisation to Ara h 8 is about 34%, presenting its higher incidence among West/Central European regions (52%). In opposition, no sensitisation towards Ara h 8 was found among allergic individuals in the South of Europe (Ballmer-Weber *et al.*, 2015b). As in the case of Ara h 9, the clinical symptoms related to Ara h 8 vary from mild (OAS) to severe (flush, rhinitis, conjunctivitis, throat tightness, urticaria, nausea and/ or vomiting) (Mittag *et al.*, 2004).

Profilin family

Ara h 5

Profilins are small cytosolic molecules (12–15 kDa) that exhibit highly conserved sequence identities (> 75%) with proteins from distantly related organisms (Hauser *et al.*, 2010). They play structural biological functions, being involved in mechanisms related to cell-motility through the regulation of actin microfilament polymerisation dynamics (Hauser *et al.*, 2008). Additionally, profilins are known to bind different ligands (phosphoinositides and poly-L-proline stretches), suggesting their contribution in other mechanisms, such as signalling pathways or membrane trafficking/organisation (Hauser *et al.*, 2010). As a consequence of their essential participation is several cellular processes, they are commonly found in most of the eukaryotic organisms. Along with nsLTP, the profilins are also considered as panallergens.

Ara h 5 is a profilin classified as a minor allergen in peanut (Table 3.1) (Kleber-Janke *et al.*, 1999). It presents high sequence and/or structural similarities with other profilins, namely Bet v 2 and Phl p 2, being suggested as a potential marker for profilin allergy (Cabanos *et al.*, 2010; Wang *et al.*, 2013). The route of sensitisation to profilins is via inhalation of cross-reactive pollen, which is common to class II food allergy (Asero *et al.*, 2003). Since these proteins are heat-labile and susceptive to gastrointestinal digestion, most of the reported cases of allergic reactions are limited to mild symptoms (OAS) as a result of their consumption as raw or minimally processed (Asero *et al.*, 2003). Nonetheless, the clinical relevance of profilins is still unclear because other reports also suggest that they can induce severe adverse immunological responses in sensitised individuals (Asero *et al.*, 2008).

Oleosin family

Ara h 10, Ara h 11, Ara h 14 and Ara h 15

In the cytosol of plant cells, the triacylglycerols are hydrophobic compounds that have to be stored in oleosomes (oil bodies), which are spherical structures surrounded by a monolayer of phospholipids containing embedded proteins that stabilise their structures (Huang, 1992; Napier *et al.*, 1996). The main proteins in oleosomes are oleosins, whose biological functions are mainly centred in stabilizing lipid bodies (oil bodies), by preventing their coalescence during the desiccation of seeds. Presenting molecular sizes of 16–24 kDa, oleosins are composed by three domains: a N-terminal hydrophilic region of variable length (30–60 residues); a highly conserved central hydrophobic antiparallel/β-strand domain (~ 70 residues); and a C-terminal amphipathic region of variable length (60–100 residues), containing an alpha-helix that is conserved in several oleosins (Hauser *et al.*, 2008; Tzen *et al.*, 1992). Since each oil body is composed by 1–4% of oleosins, seeds and nuts presenting high content of lipids contain high amounts of oleosins in their protein fraction (Huang, 1992).

So far, only eight oleosins have been identified and classified as food allergens in the WHO/IUIS official list of allergens (ALLERGEN, 2016). From those, two allergenic proteins were identified in hazelnut (Cor a 12 and Cor a 13), two in sesame (Ses i 4 and Ses i 5) and four in peanut (Ara h 10, Ara h 11, Ara h 14 and Ara h 15) (Table 3.1). According to allergen nomenclature (ALLERGEN, 2016), Ara h 14 and Ara h 15 are two oleosins from peanut presenting positive reactivity with the sera of 15 out of 33 peanut allergic patients, thus suggesting a possible classification as minor allergens. Additionally, sequence similarity of Ara h 15 with Ara h 10/Ara h 11 or Ara h 14 is below 48 and 30%, respectively, thus confirming the identity of this new allergenic protein. Only one report was available in literature describing IgE reactivity of Ara h 10, Ara h 11, Ara h 14 and Ara h 15 with sera of three, out of four, peanut allergic patients with clinical diagnostic of severe allergic reactions to peanut (anaphylactic shock, cardiac problems, generalized urticaria, dyspnea, hypotonia, angioedema and laryngeal edema) (Schwager *et al.*, 2015).

Defensin/myotoxin-like superfamily

Ara h 12 and Ara h 13

Plant defensins are a family of proteins widely spread throughout the plant kingdom. They share similar structures and biological functions with different animal and insect defensins. Mature defensins are small cationic peptides comprised of 45–55 residues with a molecular mass between 5 and 7 kDa

(Thomma *et al.*, 2002). In spite of exhibiting variable primary sequences, plant defensins share a small and globular tri-dimensional structure composed by three antiparallel beta-sheets and one alpha-helix that is stabilized by a conserved pattern of eight cysteine residues involved in four disulphide bridges (Carvalho and Gomes, 2009). Their main biological function is the antifungal activity. Defensins are also involved in other functions, such as protein translation inhibitors, α-amylase inhibitors, microbial inhibitors, zinc tolerance mediators, enzymatic activity, ion channel blockers, protease inhibitors and self-compatibility, among others (Carvalho and Gomes, 2009; Thomma *et al.*, 2002).

So far, five defensins have been included in the WHO/IUIS official list of allergens, but only Ara h 12 and Ara h 13 from peanut were classified as food allergens (Table 3.1) (ALLERGEN, 2016). Due to its recent discovery, little information regarding Ara h 12 and Ara h 13 is still available. Based on the report of Petersen *et al.* (2015), Ara h 12 presents a molecular mass of 12 kDa, while Ara h 13 is composed by two isoforms, namely Ara h 13.01010 and Ara h 13.0102 with 11 and 10 kDa, respectively. From a test panel of 25 individuals, three sera of patients with clear diagnostic of severe allergic reactions (vomiting, urticaria, tussive irritation, swelling of mucosa of mouth-throat-larynx, swallowing problems, dyspnea, hypotonia and tremor) were strongly positive to all peanut defensins (Petersen *et al.*, 2015). Serum from one patient with moderate peanut allergic reactions (OAS to peanut and seasonal rhinoconjunctivitis) was weakly reactive to all three defensins. Additionally, two sera of individuals presenting severe clinical symptoms after peanut contact or ingestion (urticaria with subsequent OAS, laryngeal edema, maximal fatigue, dyspnea, cardiac symptoms and anaphylaxis) were IgE positive to the 12 kDa defensin (Ara h 12). Under reduction conditions, only one serum was weakly IgE reactive to peanut defensins, indicating that their allergenicity might be related to their conformational structure. In that case, denaturing conditions might be sufficient to reduce defensin allergenicity (Petersen *et al.*, 2015). Based on this study, Ara h 12 and Ara h 13 could be categorised as minor allergens, but to validate this classification a large test population must be used.

Leguminous lectin family

Ara h agglutinin

These molecules belong to the leguminous lectin family, being composed of two or four subunits with 25–30 kDa, each one containing a carbohydrate-binding site (Sharon and Lis, 1990). Lectins can bind monosaccharides (glucose, mannose, galactose) or polysaccharides depending on their specificity, being the interaction carbohydrate-lectin regulated by calcium and manganese ions (or other transition metal ion). They also share similar conformational structures, despite presenting variable primary sequences (Sharon and Lis, 1990). The biological activity of lectins is mainly correlated with an active role as mediators in the symbiosis of nitrogen-fixing organisms and leguminous plants. Other functions in plant defence mechanisms against pathogens or in seed maturation and cell wall assembly are also attributed to lectins (Roopashree *et al.*, 2006).

Ara h agglutinin was identified as food allergen in the ALLERGOME database and is a galactose-binding lectin, also known as PNA or agglutinin (Table 3.1). For Ara h agglutinin, there are five protein and respective nucleotide sequences available at NCBI (2016) and UniProt (2016) databases, and about 20 entries of peanut agglutinin for the experimental tri-dimensional structures in the PDB (2016) database. Information regarding clinical reactivity of this allergen is still unclear. Preliminary data reporting the use of sera from 16 peanut-allergic patients with clinical symptoms associated with asthma, eczema, pollinic rhinitis and rhinoconjunctivitis were all IgE reactive to peanut agglutinin (Rougé *et al.*, 2010). A major allergen classification could be suggested for this allergen, although an inclusion in the official list of allergens is still pending.

Management and Traceability

The management of food allergies has been faced as a multidisciplinary task, involving regulatory authorities, stakeholders (food industry, clinicians, caretakers) and sensitised/allergic consumers. Regulatory authorities are responsible for the protection of public health, while the food industry is accountable for providing safe foods for all intended consumers (e.g., comply with legislation) (Regulation (EU) No. 1169/2011). The ultimate responsibility lies on the allergic patients, who have to strictly avoid any contact/ingestion of the offending food (and cross-reactive ones). In spite of presenting different perspectives, all entities target the common feature of protecting the health of allergic patients (Crevel *et al.*, 2008). However, those individuals are still at risk of suffering allergic reactions as a consequence of accidental exposure to hidden allergens in foods owing to mislabelling or cross-contaminations during food processing (e.g., shared production lines) (Costa *et al.*, 2012; Costa *et al.*, 2014; Costa *et al.*, 2016). Correct and adequate labelling information is one of the most important measures to ensure allergic consumer's safety. Thus, the development of proper and highly sensitive analytical methodologies represents an essential asset to help the industrial management of allergenic foods.

Presently, a wide spectrum of analytical methods has become available to assess the presence/quantification of different allergenic foods, either targeting proteins or DNA. Particularly for peanut, a great number of methodologies has been proposed based on the classical immunochemical assays, quantitative real-time polymerase chain reaction and the latest cutting-edge technologies (mass spectrometry and biosensors) (Prado *et al.*, 2016). The lack of available testing/reference materials and official methods for their detection represent main constrains in the management of food allergens. Moreover, the absence of harmonisation towards the best methodology for allergen detection is still a matter of extensive debate among researchers. The choice of a method should follow specific criteria, such as target analyte (proteins or DNA), cross-reactivity, basis of detection (e.g., chemical), cost analysis, setup cost, the need for expertise knowledge and possibility of multi-target detection (Costa *et al.*, 2014; Costa *et al.*, 2016).

Final Remarks

Owing to its relevance as food, peanuts are an integral part of daily diets in many countries (e.g., USA). Allied with the global commercialisation of processed foods, peanuts can be found in all sort of processed foods, even in regions where peanut is not so commonly consumed. Classified as one of the eight groups of foods known to be responsible for more than 90% of the reported allergic reactions, peanut has been pointed out as an important allergenic food, not only in developed countries but also in developing ones. So far, 17 groups of proteins have been identified as IgE reactive with sera from peanut-allergic individuals, being already included in the WHO/IUIS official list of allergens. Most of those have been related to severe and systemic clinical symptoms (anaphylaxis) in sensitised/allergic patients, requiring hospital treatments and often resulting in fatal outcomes. Children are the most affected group of individuals, which are often the target of accidental exposures to peanut.

Currently, peanut allergy seems to be growing in prevalence, particularly in Europe and USA. Until now, no known cure is yet available for peanut allergy, rather than the total elimination of the offending food from the diet. In this sense, the management of allergenic foods has a crucial role to avoid the presence of hidden allergens, together with the assessment of labelling compliance that should rely on specific and sensitive analytical tools. In the last years, some immunotherapies have been successfully proposed to induce tolerance to peanut in peanut-allergic individuals. However, the difficulty in maintaining peanut daily doses routinely and the high rate of dropout patients are considered major drawbacks in this type of studies.

In spite of the impressive number of available reports concerning peanut allergy, much research is still necessary in this field, and new advances are expected in near future.

Acknowledgments

This work has been supported by Fundação para a Ciência e a Tecnologia (FCT) through grants no. UID/QUI/50006/2013, by the project NORTE-

01-0145-FEDER-000011 and COST Action FA1402 "Improving Allergy Risk Assessment Strategy for new food proteins (ImpARAS)". Joana Costa, Caterina Villa and Telmo J.R. Fernandes are grateful to FCT Post-doc grant (SFRH/BPD/102404/2014) and PhD grants (PD/BD/114576/2016 and SFRH/BD/93711/2013), respectively, financed by POPH-QREN (subsidised by FSE and MCTES).

Keywords: food allergy, peanut, prevalence, clinical thresholds, diagnostic, immunotherapy, allergen characterisation, allergen management

References

ALLERGEN. (2016). Allergen Nomenclature, WHO/IUIS Allergen Nomenclature Sub-Committee. Available at: http://www.allergen.org/ (last accessed on January 2016).

ALLERGOME. (2016). Allergome—a database of allergenic molecules, Allergy Data Laboratories, Latina, Italy. Available at: http://www.allergome.org/ (last accessed on January 2016).

Anagnostou, K., Islam, S., King, Y., Foley, L., Pasea, L., Bond, S. *et al.* (2014). Assessing the efficacy of oral immunotherapy for the desensitisation of peanut allergy in children (STOP II): a phase 2 randomised controlled trial. The Lancet 383: 1297–1304.

Arkwright, P. D., Summers, C. W., Riley, B. J., Alsediq, N., and Pumphrey, R. S. H. (2013). IgE sensitization to the nonspecific lipid-transfer protein Ara h 9 and peanut-associated bronchospasm. BioMed Research International.

Arya, S. S., Salve, A. R., and Chauhan, S. (2016). Peanuts as functional food: a review. Journal of Food Science and Technology 53: 31–41.

Asero, R., Mistrello, G., Roncarolo, D., Amato, S., Zanoni, D., Barocci, F. *et al.* (2003). Detection of clinical markers of sensitization to profilin in patients allergic to plant-derived foods. Journal of Allergy and Clinical Immunology 112: 427–432.

Asero, R., Monsalve, R., and Barber, D. (2008). Profilin sensitization detected in the office by skin prick test: a study of prevalence and clinical relevance of profilin as a plant food allergen. Clinical and Experimental Allergy 38: 1033–1037.

Ballmer-Weber, B. K., Fernandez-Rivas, M., Beyer, K., Defernez, M., Sperrin, M., Mackie, A.R. *et al.* (2015a). How much is too much? Threshold dose distributions for 5 food allergens. Journal of Allergy and Clinical Immunology 135: 964–971.

Ballmer-Weber, B. K., Lidholm, J., Fernández-Rivas, M., Seneviratne, S., Hanschmann, K. M., Vogel, L. *et al.* (2015b). IgE recognition patterns in peanut allergy are age dependent: perspectives of the EuroPrevall study. Allergy 70: 391–407.

Blom, W. M., Vlieg-Boerstra, B. J., Kruizinga, A. G., van der Heide, S., Houben, G. F., and Dubois, A. E. J. (2013). Threshold dose distributions for 5 major allergenic foods in children. Journal of Allergy and Clinical Immunology 131: 172–179.

Blumchen, K., Ulbricht, H., Staden, U., Dobberstein, K., Beschorner, J., de Oliveira, L. C. L. *et al.* (2010). Oral peanut immunotherapy in children with peanut anaphylaxis. Journal of Allergy and Clinical Immunology 126: 83–91.e1.

Blumchen, K., Beder, A., Beschorner, J., Ahrens, F., Gruebl, A., Hamelmann, E. *et al.* (2014). Modified oral food challenge used with sensitization biomarkers provides more real-life clinical thresholds for peanut allergy. Journal of Allergy and Clinical Immunology 134: 390–398.e4.

Breiteneder, H., and Ebner, C. (2000). Molecular and biochemical classification of plant-derived food allergens. Journal of Allergy and Clinical Immunology 106: 27–36.

Breiteneder, H., and Radauer, C. (2004). A classification of plant food allergens. Journal of Allergy and Clinical Immunology 113: 821–830.

Breiteneder, H., and Mills, C. (2005). Nonspecific lipid-transfer proteins in plant foods and pollens: an important allergen class. Current Opinion in Allergy and Clinical Immunology 5: 275–279.

Burks, A. W. (2008). Peanut allergy. The Lancet 371: 1538–1546.

Burks, A. W., Wood, R. A., Jones, S. M., Sicherer, S. H., Fleischer, D. M., Scurlock, A. M. *et al.* (2015). Sublingual immunotherapy for peanut allergy: Long-term follow-up of a randomized multicenter trial. Journal of Allergy and Clinical Immunology 135: 1240–1248.e3.

Burney, P., Summers, C., Chinn, S., Hooper, R., Van Ree, R., and Lidholm, J. (2010). Prevalence and distribution of sensitization to foods in the European Community Respiratory Health Survey: a EuroPrevall analysis. Allergy 65: 1182–1188.

Cabanos, C., Tandang-Silvas, M. R., Odijk, V., Brostedt, P., Tanaka, A., Utsumi, S. *et al.* (2010). Expression, purification, cross-reactivity and homology modeling of peanut profilin. Protein Expression and Purification 73: 36–45.

Carvalho, A. d. O., and Gomes, V. M. (2009). Plant defensins—Prospects for the biological functions and biotechnological properties. Peptides 30: 1007–1020.

Clark, A. T., Islam, S., King, Y., Deighton, J., Anagnostou, K., and Ewan, P. W. (2009). Successful oral tolerance induction in severe peanut allergy. Allergy 64: 1218–1220.

Costa, J., Mafra, I., Carrapatoso, I., and Oliveira, M. B. P. P. (2012). Almond allergens: molecular characterization, detection, and clinical relevance. Journal of Agricultural and Food Chemistry 60: 1337–1349.

Costa, J., Carrapatoso, I., Oliveira, M. B. P. P., and Mafra, I. (2014). Walnut allergens: molecular characterization, detection and clinical relevance. Clinical and Experimental Allergy 44: 319–341.

Costa, J., Mafra, I., Carrapatoso, I., and Oliveira, M. B. P. P. (2016). Hazelnut allergens: molecular characterisation, detection and clinical relevance. Critical Reviews in Food Science and Nutrition 56: 2579–2605.

Crevel, R. W. R., Ballmer-Weber, B. K., Holzhauser, T., Hourihane, J. O. B., Knulst, A. C., Mackie, A. R. *et al.* (2008). Thresholds for food allergens and their value to different stakeholders. Allergy 63: 597–609.

Ebner, C., Hoffmann-Sommergruber, K. and Breiteneder, H. (2001). Plant food allergens homologous to pathogenesis-related proteins. Allergy 56: 43–44.

EFSA. (2013). Literature searches and reviews related to the prevalence of food allergy in Europe. EFSA-Q-2012-00376. University of Portsmouth, EN-506: 343. Available at: http://www.efsa.europa.eu/sites/default/files/scientific_output/files/main_documents/506e.pdf (last accessed on January 2016).

Egger, M., Hauser, M., Mari, A., Ferreira, F., and Gadermaier, G. (2010). The role of lipid transfer proteins in allergic diseases. Current Allergy and Asthma Reports 10: 326–335.

FAOSTAT. (2016). at: http://faostat3.fao.org/home/E (last accessed on January 2016).

Fleischer, D. M., Burks, A. W., Vickery, B. P., Scurlock, A. M., Wood, R. A., Jones, S. M. *et al.* (2013). Sublingual immunotherapy for peanut allergy: A randomized, double-blind, placebo-controlled multicenter trial. Journal of Allergy and Clinical Immunology 131: 119–127.e7.

Garcia-Blanca, A., Aranda, A., Blanca-Lopez, N., Perez, D., Gomez, F., Mayorga, C. *et al.* (2015). Influence of age on IgE response in peanut-allergic children and adolescents from the Mediterranean area. Pediatric Allergy and Immunology 26: 497–502.

Hauser, M., Egger, M., Wallner, M., Wopfner, N., Schmidt, G., and Ferreira, F. (2008). Molecular properties of plant food allergens: a current classification into protein families. The Open Immunology Journal 1: 1–12.

Hauser, M., Roulias, A., Ferreira, F., and Egger, M. (2010). Panallergens and their impact on the allergic patient. Allergy, Asthma & Clinical Immunology 6: 1–14.

Huang, A. H. C. (1992). Oil bodies and Oleosins in seeds. Annual Review of Plant Physiology and Plant Molecular Biology 43: 177–200.

Khoriaty, E., and Umetsu, D. T. (2013). Oral immunotherapy for food allergy: towards a new horizon. Allergy, Asthma & Immunology Research 5: 3–15.

Kim, E. H., Bird, J. A., Kulis, M., Laubach, S., Pons, L., Shreffler, W. *et al.* (2011). Sublingual immunotherapy for peanut allergy: clinical and immunologic evidence of desensitization. Journal of Allergy and Clinical Immunology 127: 640–646.e1.

Kleber-Janke, T., Crameri, R., Appenzeller, U., Schlaak, M., and Becker, W. M. (1999). Selective cloning of peanut allergens, including profilin and 2S albumins, by phage display technology. International Archives of Allergy and Immunology 119: 265–274.

Koppelman, S. J., Bruijnzeel-Koomen, C. A. F. M., Hessing, M., and de Jongh, H. H. J. (1999). Heat-induced conformational changes of Ara h 1, a major peanut allergen, do not affect its allergenic properties. The Journal of Biological Chemistry 274: 4770–4777.

Kukkonen, A. K., Pelkonen, A. S., Mäkinen-Kiljunen, S., Voutilainen, H., and Mäkelä, M. J. (2015). Ara h 2 and Ara h 6 are the best predictors of severe peanut allergy: a double-blind placebo-controlled study. Allergy 70: 1239–1245.

Kumar, S., Verma, A. K., Das, M., and Dwivedi, P. D. (2012). Allergenic diversity among plant and animal food proteins. Food Reviews International 28: 277–298.

Lee, L. A., and Burks, A. W. (2009). New insights into diagnosis and treatment of peanut food allergy. Frontiers in Biosciences 14: 3361–71.

Mackenzie, H., Venter, C., Kilburn, S., Moonesinghe, H. R., Lee, K., and Dean, T. (2014). Prevalence of peanut allergy: a systematic review. Journal of Allergy and Clinical Immunology 133: AB202.

Mills, C. E., Sancho, A. I., Moreno, J., and Kostyra, H. (2007). The effects of food processing on allergens. pp. 117–133. In: C. Mills, H. Wichers and K. Hoffmann-Sommergruber (eds.). Managing Allergens in Food. CRC Press, Boca Raton, FL, USA.

Mittag, D., Akkerdaas, J., Ballmer-Weber, B. K., Vogel, L., Wensing, M., Becker, W. -M. et al. (2004). Ara h 8, a Bet v 1–homologous allergen from peanut, is a major allergen in patients with combined birch pollen and peanut allergy. Journal of Allergy and Clinical Immunology 114: 1410–1417.

Mueller, G. A., Maleki, S. J., Johnson, K., Hurlburt, B. K., Cheng, H., Ruan, S. et al. (2013). Identification of Maillard reaction products on peanut allergens that influence binding to the receptor for advanced glycation end products. Allergy 68: 1546–1554.

Napier, J., Stobart, A. K., and Shewry, P. (1996). The structure and biogenesis of plant oil bodies: the role of the ER membrane and the oleosin class of proteins. Plant Mol. Biol. 31: 945–956.

Narisety, S. D., Frischmeyer-Guerrerio, P. A., Keet, C. A., Gorelik, M., Schroeder, J., Hamilton, R. G. et al. (2015). A randomized, double-blind, placebo-controlled pilot study of sublingual versus oral immunotherapy for the treatment of peanut allergy. Journal of Allergy and Clinical Immunology 135: 1275–1282.e6.

NCBI. (2016). National Center for Biotechnology Information, U.S. National Library of Medicine, Bethesda, MD, USA. Available at: http://www.ncbi.nlm.nih.gov/ (last accessed on January 2016).

Nelson, H. S., Lahr, J., Rule, R., Bock, A., and Leung, D. (1997). Treatment of anaphylactic sensitivity to peanuts by immunotherapy with injections of aqueous peanut extract. Journal of Allergy and Clinical Immunology 99: 744–51.

PDB. (2016). RCSB PDB Research Collaboratory for Structural Bioinformatics - Protein Data Bank, San Diego, USA. Available at: http://www.rcsb.org/pdb/home/home.do (last accessed on January 2016).

PeanutBase. (2016). Peanut Genomics Initiative, USDA-ARS SoyBase and Legume Clade Database group, Ames, IA, USA. Available at: http://peanutbase.org/ (last accessed on January 2016).

Perry, T. T., Matsui, E. C., Kay Conover-Walker, M., and Wood, R. A. (2004). The relationship of allergen-specific IgE levels and oral food challenge outcome. Journal of Allergy and Clinical Immunology 114: 144–149.

Petersen, A., Kull, S., Rennert, S., Becker, W. -M., Krause, S., Ernst, M. et al. (2015). Peanut defensins: Novel allergens isolated from lipophilic peanut extract. Journal of Allergy and Clinical Immunology 136: 1295–1301.e5.

Prado, M., Ortea, I., Vial, S., Rivas, J., Calo-Mata, P., and Barros-Velázquez, J. (2016). Advanced DNA- and protein-based methods for the detection and investigation of food allergens. Critical Reviews in Food Science and Nutrition 56: 2511–2542.

Radauer, C., and Breiteneder, H. (2007). Evolutionary biology of plant food allergens. Journal of Allergy and Clinical Immunology 120: 518–525.

Radauer, C., Nandy, A., Ferreira, F., Goodman, R. E., Larsen, J. N., Lidholm, J. et al. (2014). Update of the WHO/IUIS Allergen Nomenclature Database based on analysis of allergen sequences. Allergy 69: 413–419.

Regulation (EU) No 1169/2011 of 25 October 2011 on the provision of food information to consumers, amending Regulations (EC) No. 1924/2006 and (EC) No. 1925/2006 of the

European Parliament and of the Council, and repealing Commission Directive 87/250/EEC, Council Directive 90/496/EEC, Commission Directive 1999/10/EC, Directive 2000/13/EC of the European Parliament and of the Council, Commission Directives 2002/67/EC and 2008/5/EC and Commission Regulation (EC) No. 608/2004. Off. J. Eur. Union, L 304: 18–63.

Roopashree, S., Singh, S. A., Gowda, L. R., and Rao, A. G. A. (2006). Dual-function protein in plant defence: seed lectin from *Dolichos biflorus* (horse gram) exhibits lipoxygenase activity. Biochemical Journal 395: 629–639.

Ros, E. (2010). Health benefits of nut consumption. Nutrients 2: 652–682.

Rougé, P., Culerrier, R., Granier, C., Rancé, F., and Barre, A. (2010). Characterization of IgE-binding epitopes of peanut (*Arachis hypogaea*) PNA lectin allergen cross-reacting with other structurally related legume lectins. Molecular of Immunology 47: 2359–2366.

Salcedo, G., Sanchez-Monge, R., Barber, D., and Diaz-Perales, A. (2007). Plant non-specific lipid transfer proteins: an interface between plant defence and human allergy. BBA Molecular and Cell Biology of Lipids 1771: 781–791.

Santos, A. F., Du Toit, G., Douiri, A., Radulovic, S., Stephens, A., Turcanu, V. *et al.* (2015). Distinct parameters of the basophil activation test reflect the severity and threshold of allergic reactions to peanut. Journal of Allergy and Clinical Immunology 135: 179–186.

Scala, E., Till, S. J., Asero, R., Abeni, D., Guerra, E. C., Pirrotta, L. *et al.* (2015). Lipid transfer protein sensitization: reactivity profiles and clinical risk assessment in an Italian cohort. Allergy 70: 933–943.

Schwager, C., Kull, S., Krause, S., Schocker, F., Petersen, A., Becker, W. -M. *et al.* (2015). Development of a novel strategy to isolate lipophilic allergens (oleosins) from peanuts. PLoS ONE 10: e0123419.

Sharon, N., and Lis, H. (1990). Legume lectins—a large family of homologous proteins. The FASEB Journal 4: 3198–208.

Sicherer, S. H., Furlong, T. J., Muñoz-Furlong, A., Burks, A. W., and Sampson, H. A. (2001). A voluntary registry for peanut and tree nut allergy: Characteristics of the first 5149 registrants. Journal of Allergy and Clinical Immunology 108: 128–132.

Taylor, S. L., Crevel, R. W. R., Sheffield, D., Kabourek, J., and Baumert, J. (2009). Threshold dose for peanut: Risk characterization based upon published results from challenges of peanut-allergic individuals. Food and Chemical Toxicology 47: 1198–1204.

Taylor, S. L., Moneret-Vautrin, D. A., Crevel, R. W. R., Sheffield, D., Morisset, M., Dumont, P. *et al.* (2010). Threshold dose for peanut: Risk characterization based upon diagnostic oral challenge of a series of 286 peanut-allergic individuals. Food and Chemical Toxicology 48: 814–819.

Taylor, S. L., Baumert, J. L., Kruizinga, A. G., Remington, B. C., Crevel, R. W. R., Brooke-Taylor, S. *et al.* (2014). Establishment of reference doses for residues of allergenic foods: report of the VITAL Expert Panel. Food and Chemical Toxicology 63: 9–17.

Thomma, B. P., Cammue, B. P., and Thevissen, K. (2002). Plant defensins. Planta 216: 193–202.

Tzen, J. T., Lie, G. C., and Huang, A. H. (1992). Characterization of the charged components and their topology on the surface of plant seed oil bodies. The Journal of Biological Chemistry 267: 15626–15634.

Umasunthar, T., Leonardi-Bee, J., Turner, P. J., Hodes, M., Gore, C., Warner, J. O. *et al.* (2015). Incidence of food anaphylaxis in people with food allergy: a systematic review and meta-analysis. Clinical and Experimental Allergy 45: 1621–1636.

UniProt. (2016). UniProt (Universal Protein Resource) Consortium. Available at: http://www.uniprot.org/ (last accessed on January 2016).

USDA-NNDSR. (2016). National Nutrient Database for Standard Reference. Available at: http://ndb.nal.usda.gov/ (last accessed on January 2016).

Varshney, P., Jones, S. M., Scurlock, A. M., Perry, T. T., Kemper, A., Steele, P. *et al.* (2011). A randomized controlled study of peanut oral immunotherapy (OIT): clinical desensitization and modulation of the allergic response. Journal of Allergy and Clinical Immunology 127: 654–660.

Venter, C., Hasan Arshad, S., Grundy, J., Pereira, B., Bernie Clayton, C., Voigt, K. *et al.* (2010). Time trends in the prevalence of peanut allergy: three cohorts of children from the same geographical location in the UK. Allergy 65: 103–108.

Wang, Y., Fu, T. -J., Howard, A., Kothary, M. H., McHugh, T. H., and Zhang, Y. (2013). Crystal structure of peanut (*Arachis hypogaea*) allergen Ara h 5. Journal of Agricultural and Food Chemistry 61: 1573–1578.

Zhu, J., Pouillot, R., Kwegyir-Afful, E. K., Luccioli, S., and Gendel, S. M. (2015). A retrospective analysis of allergic reaction severities and minimal eliciting doses for peanut, milk, egg, and soy oral food challenges. Food Chemical and Toxicology 80: 92–100.

Zuidmeer, L., Goldhahn, K., Rona, R. J., Gislason, D., Madsen, C., Summers, C. *et al.* (2008). The prevalence of plant food allergies: A systematic review. Journal of Allergy and Clinical Immunology 121: 1210–1218.e4.

CHAPTER 4

The Pollen-Food Syndrome

An Update on Diagnostic and Therapeutic Approaches

Sara Huber, Claudia Asam, Anargyros Roulias, Fatima Ferreira and *Lorenz Aglas**

Introduction

In Europe, the current prevalence of IgE sensitization to foods in adults fluctuates between 6.6 to 23.6% of which, 60% of allergic symptoms caused by food consumption are associated with an inhalant allergy. Allergic reactions that are triggered by the consumption of various foods and linked with sensitization to pollen allergens are summarized within the expression "pollen-food syndrome". Such allergic reactions include local reactions restricted to the oral mucosa as well as systemic reactions like anaphylaxis. The major socio-economic impact of pollen-related food allergies should not be downplayed; the associated symptoms negatively affect the quality of life and thereby represent a burden for each patient (Burney *et al.*, 2014; Kashyap and Kashyap, 2015; Popescu, 2015).

Pollen-food syndrome diagnosis is a complex issue, not only because of the huge panel of involved cross-reacting inhalant and food allergens but up until now a diagnostic assay clearly discriminating class 1 food allergy and the pollen-food syndrome is unavailable, despite being urgently required. During the current diagnosis, discrepancies between the clinical and immunological findings often appear. The mechanism that leads from sensitization of an

Department of Molecular Biology, University of Salzburg, Hellbrunnerstrasse 34 5020 Salzburg, Austria.
Emails: Sara.Huber@sbg.ac.at; Claudia.Asam@sbg.ac.at; Anargyros.Roulias@sbg.ac.at; Fatima.Ferreira@sbg.ac.at
* Corresponding author: Lorenz.Aglas@sbg.ac.at

inhaled allergen to a clinically relevant allergic reaction against an ingested cross-reactive food allergen is not fully understood. This often complicates the evaluation of diagnosis data, further highlighting the need for more elaborate techniques for both diagnosis and therapy (Carrard *et al.*, 2015).

In this chapter, we are discussing class II food allergens involved in the clinical manifestation of the syndrome, and thus dealing with the molecular mechanism responsible for the occurrence of a pollen-food syndrome. Herewith we present a precise update on diagnostic and therapeutic approaches that are available for clinicians to handle pollen-food syndromes. Furthermore, within this chapter we highlight new prospective therapeutic approaches for allergen-specific, as well as allergen-non-specific immunotherapy, to treat pollen-related food allergy conditions with a focus on a novel and more experimental point of view.

How to Diagnose a Pollen-Food Syndrome

Diagnosis of food allergies, in general, is a complex issue due to the large panel of varying clinical manifestations and allergens involved. Cross-reactions and co-sensitization to pollen allergens, as is the case in the pollen-food syndrome, pose even greater difficulty in food allergy diagnosis. At first, it is important to identify the particular food(s) causing the symptoms. In this respect, the diagnostic effort is subdivided into four levels of diagnostic methods. In clinical practice, these guidelines should ideally be followed in chronological order (Macchia *et al.*, 2015).

First-level methods

The first level of diagnosis consists of a precise description of the patient´s medical history followed by the performance of well-standardized diagnostic skin tests such as skin prick tests, prick-to-prick tests and atopy patch tests.

In suspected food allergies, obtaining an accurate patients' clinical history is essential for a correct diagnosis and comprises of standard parameters including physiological condition and genetic predisposition as well as all allergy relevant data and information. This includes a report of the type of symptoms, the food ingested up to 4 hours before the onset of symptoms, the processing of the involved food and the suspicion of a cross-reaction or co-sensitization to pollen.

The *in vivo* Skin Prick Test (SPT) is the first-line diagnostic method to detect potential allergens and is performed routinely by allergologists. Heinzerling *et al.* reported a recommended procedure of how to perform a European standardized SPT in clinical practice. For this inexpensive and rapid procedure (results are available within 20 minutes), allergenic extracts, fresh plant food preparations or recombinant proteins in comparison with control substances (e.g., histamine) are applied to the patient's skin. A positive SPT only provides information about the availability of specific IgE antibodies in the skin and it neither reflects the presence of allergic symptoms nor the level of symptom severity (Heinzerling *et al.*, 2013).

If a pollen-food syndrome is suspected, it is mandatory to test the patient additionally to the food allergen preparations as well as inhalant allergens. Food extracts are commercially available, but in contrast to inhalant allergen extracts, they are not standardized and differ highly from batch to batch due to varying protein content and the lability of the allergens. The sensitivity of SPTs performed with plant food extracts, as obtained from celery, carrots, cherries or hazelnuts, can vary between 20 and 65% and thus are relatively low (Ballmer-Weber, 2014; Henzgen *et al.*, 2008). Compared to thermolabile allergenic molecules, extracts that contain stable food allergens present higher sensitivity and specificity in SPTs (Erdmann *et al.*, 2003). In this respect and because of the thereby resulting false-negative outcome, a definitive diagnosis from an SPT result cannot be concluded, and the use of further diagnostic applications is recommended.

If an SPT with food extracts is negative, but clinical history supports a contrary opinion, it is advisable to perform a prick + prick test (P + P). This modified version of the SPT can be performed with almost any food such as fruits, vegetables or nuts, first punctured with a lancet and consequently pricked into the patient's skin. Although false positive results can occur due to a high histamine and/or lectin-rich content, the P + P results are more reliable than the conventional SPT and the predictive negative values are higher (O'Keefe *et al.*, 2014).

All *in vivo* diagnostic procedures, including the SPT, carry a risk of provoking a systemic allergic reaction especially in patients with a high-grade sensitization to foods associated with the onset of severe anaphylaxis. Therefore, it is recommended to perform the diagnostic method if the emergency equipment is available and under the surveillance of appropriately trained health care professionals.

In the daily clinical routine, SPTs are not yet performed with purified natural or recombinantly produced allergens, although promising data towards natural peach nsLTP (Pru p 3), date profilin (Pho d 2) and recombinant apple Mal d 1 and Mal d 4 are available (Goikoetxea *et al.*, 2015).

Second-level methods

On the second diagnostic level, ambiguous first-level diagnoses are reviewed by *in vitro* assays for measurement of total serum IgE and specific IgE (sIgE) levels to putative sensitizing and cross-reacting allergens. The determination of total serum IgE alone is, in respect of allergy diagnosis and its clinical manifestation, of minor significance. Therefore, a dissection of the involved molecular components is used to detect specific sensitizing molecules within previously identified allergen sources (e.g., food extracts). *In vitro* Molecular-

Based Diagnosis (MBD), also called Component Resolved Diagnosis (CRD), uses allergenic proteins, either isolated and purified from a natural source or generated by recombinant protein expression, to quantify the amount of circulating allergen-specific IgE antibodies. The use of recombinant allergens for sIgE detection provides a higher standardization than purified natural proteins, which vary from batch to batch, while molecules like rBet v 1, rMal d 1, rMal d 3, rMal d 4 and rPru p 3 show good results in terms of specificity and sensitivity (Gamboa *et al.*, 2009; Rance *et al.*, 1997).

MBD is an effective method to improve the diagnostic outcome and its accuracy by providing complex sensitization profiles and information on involved cross-reacting allergens. The field of application for MBD is clearly defined, although it is not recommended for clinicians and health personnel to use this method in the daily routine since a precise interpretation of experimental results requires comprehensive background knowledge.

In food allergy diagnosis, the major diagnostic value of MBD is providing sensitizing molecule information, i.e., identification of primary sensitizers. Especially in the context of the pollen-food syndrome, MBD is pivotal for the differentiation between a genuine sensitization towards food allergens and multiple sensitizations to aeroallergens and food allergens. The protein-specific sensitization profiles are not only useful to determine the probability of allergic reactions to other food sources, but also to grade allergic symptoms according to their levels of severity. This makes it easier for clinicians to distinguish between relatively moderate local (mild oral reactions caused by PR-10 and profilins) and severe systemic reactions, facilitating the treatment choice and vaccine prescription such as auto-injectable adrenaline and permanent allergen avoidance in case of a reasonable suspicion of life-threatening anaphylaxis (e.g., caused by nsLTPs). In this context, MBD can define the candidates for allergen-specific immunotherapy (AIT) as well as the specific allergenic molecules to be administered (Luengo and Cardona, 2014).

Most commercially available therapeutic extracts have been established for "major allergens" and not for "minor allergens", such as profilins, that play an important role in pollen-related food allergies (described above). In addition to the adjustment of AIT, by selecting the appropriate patients and molecules, MBD can also be used to evaluate treatment efficacy during therapy. The most commonly used commercially available tool for *in vitro* MBD is the ImmunoCAP® (Phadia AB, Uppsala, Schweden) Immuno-Sorbent Allergen Chip (ISAC), which is a multiplexed allergen microarray used for detecting and quantifying the reactivity of specific IgE antibodies towards more than 100 allergens and allergen components (Syed *et al.*, 2013).

The disadvantages of MBD are, on the one hand, that the technique is much more expensive compared to other diagnostic methods, like the SPT, and depends on appropriate equipment and technology for analysis. On the other hand, a crucial step is the correct interpretation of the obtained data which, without a proper background knowledge and expertise, could be a challenging burden. For instance, the results of patients' sIgE profiles are varying significantly depending on geographic region and allergen source (Ebo *et al.*, 2012; Vereda *et al.*, 2011).

MBD performed with molecules from the PR-10 protein family, due to extensive cross-reactivity, cannot be used to discriminate between mono-sensitization towards a specific allergen, such as Mal d 1 from apple, Bet v 1 from birch pollen, Ara h 8 from peanut or Cor a 1.04 from hazelnut, and a case of co-sensitization, where the patient is sensitized to at least two PR-10 proteins (Van Gasse *et al.*, 2015). In patients allergic to peanut, Ara h 8 is a known marker that indicates cross-reactivity to Fagales tree pollen, whereas the peanut profilin Ara h 5 is cross-reacting with the pollen profilins from birch (Bet v 2) and timothy grass (Phl p 12). Sensitization to Ara h 1, Ara h 2 and Ara h 3, all storage proteins, characterizes a genuine class 1 food allergy. Thus MBD facilitates the discrimination between a class 1 food allergy and the pollen-food syndrome (Becker and Jappe, 2014; Cabanos *et al.*, 2010; Mittag *et al.*, 2004). In the case of nsLTPs, if significant associations to food nsLTPs, such as Pru p 3 or Ara h 8, are reported together with the presence of IgE against pollen nsLTPs, like plane tree Pla a 3 and mugwort Art v 3, pollen-food syndrome should be considered as a possible scenario. Furthermore, as a sensitization to nsLTPs can lead to (local) mild but also systemic reactions, the ISU-E values (ISAC Standardized Units for specific IgE) can be used to grade the level of severity of the symptoms. Regarding the prediction of potential food-induced systemic reactions, it should be noted that patients are reacting to more than 5 nsLTPs in microarray assays, without a co-sensitization to profilin/PR-10 proteins, are at high risk of developing severe reactions (Pastorello *et al.*, 2011; Scala *et al.*, 2015).

Clearly standardized guidelines and defined exclusion criteria to interpret the outcome of microarray assays are not yet available, although MBD possesses the potential to reduce the number of necessary application of oral provocation tests which is up to now still considered to be the gold standard for food allergy diagnosis (Hoffmann-Sommergruber *et al.*, 2015).

Third-level method

Neither SPTs nor assays quantifying patients' IgE represent an accurate diagnosis since their results merely reflect sensitization rates and do not inevitably correlate with clinical manifestations. The Oral Provocation Test (OPT)—also termed Oral Food Challenge (OFC)—is the only available *in vivo* test able to confirm that a certain suspected food is associated with the eliciting of symptoms. The patient is fed with increasing doses of the tested food and thus, observed clinical reactions provide a higher resolution of the final diagnosis. An OPT is recommended if the patients' clinical history is unconvincing and SPT and sIgE testing results are not conclusive. Therefore, due to the potential risk of provoking severe reactions, in the majority of patients, an OPT is not necessary. However, it is rather useful to perform OPT during a follow-up study of AIT to investigate the onset of oral tolerance for a specific food (O'Keefe *et al.*, 2014; Syed *et al.*, 2013). The Double-Blind Placebo-Controlled Food Challenge (DBPCFC) test is the standard method to diagnose food allergies, although there is a great need for standardization of materials and administered food or allergen preparations. Kinaciyan *et al.* identified a sufficient dose of 50 µg of recombinant Mal d 1 for sublingual challenge tests to diagnose Birch Pollen-Related Food Allergy (BPRFA). The authors also suggested that their concept can be adopted for other PR-10 proteins, such as Gly m 4 from soybeans, to improve security and reproducibility of diagnosis of pollen-associated food allergies (Kinaciyan *et al.*, 2015; Kopac *et al.*, 2012).

Fourth-level method

The Basophil Activation Test (BAT) is a cellular *ex vivo* provocation test used to study IgE-mediated allergic reactions. The basophil activation is assessed by the determination of mediator release (e.g., histamine) or the expression of surface markers, such as CD63 and CD203c (Hoffmann-Sommergruber *et al.*, 2015). The BAT can either be performed with allergen extracts, with freshly prepared food extracts showing higher specificity and sensitivity than commercial extracts, or with purified recombinant allergens. Nowadays it is getting more and more common to carry out BATs with recombinant proteins instead of food extracts, increasing the low specificity of conventional extracts. Erdmann *et al.* compared the diagnostic value of basophil activation with sIgE testing and concluded that the use of recombinant Bet v 1, Bet v 2, Api g 1, Dau c 1 and Mal d 1 in both methods resulted in similar values of sensitivity and specificity (Erdmann *et al.*, 2005). Other studies dealing with such comparisons support these findings or even revealed a higher sensitivity and specificity in BATs, especially when using native extracts over commercial ones (Ebo *et al.*, 2005; Erdmann *et al.*, 2003). Apart from this, the BAT is the ideal method to enhance diagnostic resolution by differentiating between allergic and non-allergic individuals, since its results are correlating with DBPCFC severity scores (Song *et al.*, 2015).

For monitoring the effect of immunotherapy and the induction of oral tolerance, a BAT is not the appropriate choice. Inuo *et al.* investigated the influence of pollen allergen-specific subcutaneous immunotherapy (SCIT) on patients suffering from pollen-food allergy syndrome and found out that no significant changes in basophil activation before and after treatment were observable, in contrast to sensitized individuals who did not display Oral Allergy Syndrome (OAS) symptoms (Inuo *et al.*, 2015). Similar findings reported by Kopac *et al.* showed that there was no significant difference in basophil activation before and after oral immunotherapy (OIT) highlighting the absence of BAT results correlation with the induction of oral tolerance (Kopac *et al.*, 2012).

Pollen-food syndrome diagnosis can be a little bit tricky, mostly due to the lack of standardization and availability of a simple, inexpensive, easily interpretable and safe functional assay that could clearly differentiate a class 1 food allergy from the pollen-food syndrome. These guidelines underline the most common diagnostic methods that should be followed for an accurate pollen-food syndrome diagnosis and therapy.

Therapeutic Approaches (Treatment Strategies for Birch-Pollen Related Food Allergy)

Pollen-related food allergies are a steadily increasing health problem with the number of affected people rising each year. Such allergies and their associated symptoms impair the patient quality of life as well as affect their families, social interactions but also school and work attendance (Popescu, 2015). Therefore, the need for an effective therapy of pollen-related food allergies to induce desensitization and a long-lasting immunologic tolerance in the patients is growing (Kamdar and Bryce, 2010).

Currently, the only effective treatment for pollen allergies is the allergen-specific immunotherapy (AIT) which acts by targeting the underlying immune mechanisms. During AIT high levels of allergen-specific IgG antibodies, especially IgG4, are induced. These antibodies, also known as "blocking antibodies," act in competing with IgE for allergen-binding which in turn prevents the activation of basophils and mast cells as well as the allergen uptake and presentation to T-cells. Furthermore, the cytokine production and proliferation of allergen-specific effector T-cells is reduced and a skewing from Th2 to Th1 immune responses is observed (Brinda Subbarayal, 2012; Larche *et al.*, 2006).

Pollen-Food Syndrome (PFS) is a hypersensitivity reaction to specific foods triggered by prior sensitization to plant inhalant allergens and occurs due to the structural relationship between the sensitizing pollen proteins and their homologs from food. However, the use of pollen-specific immunotherapies to remedy associated food allergies is controversially discussed. Some studies have shown beneficial effects using subcutaneous immunotherapy (SCIT) in patients suffering from birch pollen OAS. Subjects presented a decrease of clinical sensitivity and skin reactivity to apple as well as an increase of the tolerated quantity of apple and hazelnut (Asero, 1998, 2003, 2004; Katelaris, 2010; Yang and Chiang, 2014). Other studies, however, reported on limited curative effects or even the development of adverse reactions to food during the course of therapy (Bucher *et al.*, 2004; Herrmann *et al.*, 1995; Modrzynski *et al.*, 2002; Nowak-Wegrzyn and Sampson, 2011; van Hoffen *et al.*, 2011). Kinaciyan *et al.* investigated the effects of birch pollen extract sublingual immunotherapy (SLIT) on associated apple allergy when directly applied at the site of food-induced allergic symptoms. Their findings indicated that pollen-associated food allergy is not ameliorated by pollen immunotherapy even if respiratory symptoms significantly improved (Kinaciyan *et al.*, 2007). In contrast, Bergmann *et al.* observed a reduction of more than 50% of apple OAS in 33/37 patients after 12 months of SLIT with birch pollen extract (Bergmann *et al.*, 2008). Additionally, Worm *et al.* reported that daily dosing of sublingual birch pollen extract solution improved pollen-induced allergic rhinitis and symptoms of OAS in birch-allergic patients (Worm *et al.*, 2014).

A study about SLIT for profilin-sensitized patients with OAS to apple using increasing amounts of a palm profilin solution was recently published by Nucera *et al.* The selected method seems to be as promising as nsLTP sublingual desensitization which was investigated by Fernandez-Rivas *et al.* and Pereira *et al.* including the administration of peach extract. In both cases, immunotherapy was performed with the primary sensitizer triggering the hypersensitivity reaction. Tolerance was assessed with a careful recording of every adverse event which is especially important for the administration of nsLTPs as they can cause severe and life-threatening reactions (Fernandez-Rivas *et al.*, 2009; Nucera *et al.*, 2015; Pereira *et al.*, 2009).

Oral immunotherapy (OIT) by gradually increasing consumption of apple outside the pollen season was performed in a study of Kopac *et al.* where they could transiently induce tolerance in birch pollen allergic patients suffering from OAS to apple (Kopac *et al.*, 2012).

The current treatment options are limited to strict dietary avoidance, nutritional counseling, and emergency treatment with auto-injectable epinephrine and antihistamines for milder reactions to relieve symptoms evoked upon accidental ingestion, which occurs even in the most careful patients.

The intake of antihistamines before eating raw fruits and vegetables can be used to suppress allergic symptoms (Bindslev-Jensen *et al.*, 1991). Thus far, medicines to eradicate allergic reactions based on altering the immune system do not exist and hence complete avoidance of the offending allergen is a common measure for allergic patients. This prevents patients from consuming a great variety of fresh fruits and vegetables which contain vitamins and are considered to be healthy; this indicates that avoidance, in turn, can also lead to collateral health problems in the patients. Hereby, it has also to be kept in mind that the list of the symptom-causing cross-reactants to be avoided can be very long. Peeling off the foods, particularly fruits, is not an adequate protection, as one can get contaminated during handling. Moreover, the flesh could also contain the stimulatory allergen.

A diet using extensively heated fruits can be an option to improve patients' quality of life. Cooked fruits and pasteurised juice containing PR-10 and profilins can generally be consumed, as these proteins are labile and heat sensitive. Their tertiary structure is destroyed after cooking which in turn leads to the loss of their IgE binding capacity as most IgE epitopes are conformational epitopes (Mittag *et al.*, 2006; Neudecker *et al.*, 2003; Scheurer *et al.*, 1999). However, it was shown that heating does not necessarily destroy linear epitopes which are recognized by T-cells and, despite the reduced IgE binding capacity caused by the loss of conformational IgE epitopes, could lead to late T-cell mediated symptoms (Bohle *et al.*, 2006). Additionally, non-specific lipid transfer proteins are more stable, and heating or processing does not prevent reactions in allergic people. Without proper monitoring and previous evaluation of heat-treated protein tolerance, this treatment method can be extremely dangerous; especially as many foods contain both heat-stable LTPs and heat-labile PR-10 proteins, which means that in these cases heating is ineffective for prophylaxis.

In general food allergy is still a highly stressful condition with elevated anxiety not only in patients but also in their families. The limited treatment options existing so far indicate that there is an essential need for an effective treatment for pollen-related food allergies.

Novel Aspects/Future Trends in the Treatment of Pollen-Related Food Allergies

While there is no current curative treatment for pollen-related food allergies, several promising therapeutic strategies are under investigation aiming to improve current treatment options and/or the method of administration. Moreover, completely new treatment strategies are being developed. Treatment approaches can be classified as pollen/food allergen-specific and non-specific.

Allergen-specific immunotherapy

The use of pollen-specific immunotherapies to cure associated food allergies is a matter of debate. One reason for this might be that crude pollen extracts contain a heterogeneous mixture of various proteins, glycoproteins and polysaccharides which are highly influenced by the production process, the source material, as well as the manufacturers (Curin *et al.*, 2011). Although progress has been made to standardize protein extracts and to improve their quality, it is still difficult to predetermine the exact content of the different allergens in this complex mixture since some allergens in the extract are extremely labile and can be degraded during the extract production process. Another disadvantage of extract-based AIT is the potential contamination of other allergen sources or bacterial components (Marth *et al.*, 2014).

Novel aspects including the use of recombinant allergens should open the possibility for a standardized, safe and efficacious allergen-specific immunotherapy to treat pollen-related food allergies. Advantages of recombinant allergens include not only the possibility of unlimited production of a particular allergen but also its full validation regarding identity, quantity, homogeneity, purity, structure, aggregation, solubility and stability. Concerning the treatment of birch pollinosis, recombinant Bet v 1 has already been shown to be as effective as birch pollen extract in injection therapy, thus leading to a significant reduction in rhinoconjunctivitis symptoms, skin sensitivity as well as reduced intake of medication (Pauli *et al.*, 2008). The use of recombinant Bet v 1 in sublingual immunotherapy was also found out to be compatible (Gronlund and Gafvelin, 2010; Winther *et al.*, 2009). For grass pollen immunotherapy a mixture of five recombinant grass pollen allergens turned out to have positive effects on ameliorating allergic rhinitis symptoms (Jutel *et al.*, 2005). These studies raise hope for positive effects in the treatment of pollen-related food allergies by the use of recombinant pollen allergens.

As mentioned above, trials with the disease-eliciting foods could only transiently induce tolerance thus far. However, the use of recombinant food allergens seems to be a promising tool, especially as recombinant DNA technology offers the possibility to easily and selectively modify allergenic molecules (fragmentation or oligomerization, site-directed mutagenesis) altering certain of their properties and functions. By using molecular approaches and genetic engineering, the IgE binding capacity can be reduced, resulting in the generation of so-called hypoallergens. Additionally, multimers of single allergens or hybrids consisting of different allergens can be produced (Mutschlechner *et al.*, 2009).

Clinical trials with recombinant Bet v 1 hypo-allergens have already been shown to be safe and effective in ameliorating symptoms of birch pollen allergy (Kahlert *et al.*, 2008; Vrtala *et al.*, 2001). Furthermore, it has already been demonstrated that the hypoallergen concept provides an elegant alternative for the generation of safe vaccine candidates for pollen-related food allergies where the wild-type allergen causes life-threatening side effects (e.g., for the nsLTPs). In this context Zuidmeer-Jongejan *et al.* evaluated two approaches for achieving hypoallergenicity for the peach LTP Pru p 3, site-directed mutagenesis as well as chemical modification (Zuidmeer-Jongejan *et al.*, 2012). A novel approach using a genetically engineered multi-allergen chimera to treat birch pollen-related food allergies was tested by the group of Ursula Wiedermann. The chimera was composed of immunodominant T cell epitopes of Api g 1 (celery) and Dau c 1 (carrot) linked to the whole Bet v 1 allergen. Intranasal application to the mucosa of mice was followed by decreased Th2 immune responses against Bet v 1 and its homologous food allergens Api g 1 and Dau c 1. Hence, it was suggested that mucosal treatment with a multi-allergen vaccine could be a promising treatment strategy to prevent birch pollen-related food allergy (Hoflehner *et al.*, 2012).

Peptide immunotherapy is another promising tool for the treatment of pollen-related food allergies where the application of the wild-type allergen could lead to severe systemic reactions. It involves the administration of small allergen fragments based on the concept that by disrupting the allergen sequence into short fragments and destroying the IgE binding epitopes, the cross-linking of IgE on basophils and mast cells is abrogated. Therefore, peptides administered during AIT will not be able to induce cross-linking, which in turn should lead to T cell tolerance (Moldaver and Larche, 2011). The possibility to create a stable combination of multiple peptides in one vaccine might be a further major advantage in this context.

Moreover, the modified food allergens can be genetically fused with proteins that promote immune responses and counter-regulate the disease-eliciting T-helper type 2-dominated immune response in allergic individuals, and therefore improving the general efficacy of AIT (Mutschlechner *et al.*, 2009). Such proteins can be bacterial adjuvants or sugar moieties added to the allergen. Both lead to a shift of the immune system to a T-helper type 1-dominated immune response and potentially increase the safety, efficacy and feasibility of the therapy also for pollen-related food allergies.

A recently developed approach for a safe allergy vaccine is the hapten-carrier principle, comprising covalent coupling of non-IgE-reactive allergen-derived peptides to carrier proteins, like viral proteins. Immunization of rabbits with an alum-adsorbed fusion-protein focused IgG responses mainly towards peptides derived from the major IgE-binding area of Bet v 1 but it also induced IgG antibodies against Bet v 1-homologous allergens, like alder (rAln g 1), hazel (rCor a 1), and apple (rMal d 1) (Marth *et al.*, 2013).

Besides SCIT, SLIT and OIT, the currently most frequently used routes of allergen immunotherapy, other approaches such as epicutaneous and intralymphatic treatment options have been explored to improve current treatment strategies for pollen-related food allergens. Both are suggested to ameliorate patient compliance and safety with only mild side effects in comparison to subcutaneous allergen-specific immunotherapy which is an effective treatment of IgE-mediated allergies but requires repeated allergen injections and is accompanied by a high risk of systemic allergic reactions. Epicutaneous immunotherapy involves the delivery of an allergen patch containing solubilized allergen which has been proved for effectiveness in a study by Senti *et al.* on grass pollen allergic patients (Senti *et al.*, 2009). In contrast to that, in intralymphatic immunotherapy the allergen is directly applied to the lymph node via injection. Just like in epicutaneous immunotherapy, it was demonstrated that the lymphatic alternative is a time-saving and cost-effective method (Hylander *et al.*, 2013).

Allergen-non-specific immunotherapies

Beside the specific immunotherapies, which target the symptom-triggering allergens, non-specific therapies can also be of value for class 2 food allergic patients such as anti-IgE therapy, helminth therapy and the induction of a Th2- to Th1-immune response shift by a bacterial strain.

Anti-IgE therapy, for instance, uses a recombinant humanized monoclonal anti-IgE antibody called Omalizumab (IgG1) to reduce the degranulation of basophils and mast cells by preventing IgE from binding to the high-affinity FcεRI receptor. Therefore, Omalizumab possesses the potential to be an effective tool for treating multiple allergies (Nowak-Wegrzyn and Sampson, 2011; Syed *et al.*, 2013), including the pollen-food syndrome.

Another non-specific therapeutic approach is based on the induction of a switch from a Th2- to a Th1-immune response via the expression of the cytokines IL-10 and IL-12 by the bacterial strain *Lactococcus lactis* (Lieberman and Wang, 2012). Helminth therapy is also aiming to alter the immune response by introducing parasitic helminths in humans that protect against IgE sensitization and reduce allergic symptoms by stimulating IL-10 production and secretion (Bashir *et al.*, 2002). A suitable non-specific immunotherapy for food allergy represents agonists of Toll-like receptor 9 (TLR9) to prevent systemic as well as mucosal Th1-type immune responses (Kandimalla *et al.*, 2003; Nowak-Wegrzyn and Sampson, 2011; Wang *et al.*, 2005; Zhu *et al.*, 2004). Other non-specific immunotherapies like food allergy herbal formula from Traditional Chinese Medicine and the use of probiotics are known to have beneficial health effects in allergic individuals (Ozdemir, 2010; Syed *et al.*, 2013; Wang and Li, 2012). However, more studies proving these theories have to be performed to gain better knowledge on their mechanisms of action.

Modern trends are leading in the direction of prophylactic vaccination, and personalized immunotherapy according to the patients' sensitization profile based on an accurate diagnosis (Marth *et al.*, 2014). Therefore, establishing a suitable future treatment strategy for pollen-related food allergies, that combines the optimal allergen-specific and allergen non-specific approaches, should be taken into consideration. Thus, the best of both worlds could be attained (Klunker *et al.*, 2007).

Conclusion

The pollen-food syndrome is a very complex condition on the molecular level (Fig. 4.1). Primary sensitization to inhalant allergens from pollen is eliciting an allergic reaction and its grade of symptomatic severity depends on the

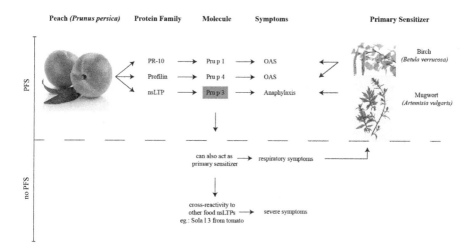

Fig. 4.1: Peach (*Prunus percisa*) allergens involved in pollen-food syndrome and clinical manifestations.

involved molecule. Cross-reactions between the allergens from different plant food origins that are part of the same protein family, and respiratory symptoms caused by pollen as a consequence of primary sensitization to food allergens are not included in the pollen-food syndrome condition. However, this fact is expanding the complexity of the clinical picture and should be considered whenever making a diagnostic decision. Furthermore, it is worth mentioning that a lot of cases of cross-reactions between pollen and plant foods have been reported where the actual causal allergenic molecule has not yet been identified (Table 4.1). This lack of knowledge makes proper diagnosis and treatment extremely difficult.

Current diagnosis of the pollen-food syndrome is significantly dependent on the patient's medical history. To date diagnosis is mainly based on sensitization rates but also on the determination of the involved, cross-reacting allergenic sources from food and pollen as well as the quantification of patients' sIgE towards any associated molecules. If the patients' clinical history is unconvincing and previous diagnostic results are questionable, an oral provocation test is indispensable to definitely confirm the associations of a suspected food with the eliciting symptoms. Nevertheless, it seems that molecular-based diagnosis—in one way or another—is revolutionizing traditional methods and thus permitting a more accurate level of diagnosis.

Improving current treatment options could either be achieved by making different routes of vaccination (i.e., oral, nasal, sublingual, subcutaneous, epicutaneous, intralymphatic) accessible, the use of recombinant allergens (single application or a mixture) with reduced IgE binding capacity but preserved T cell reactivity, or allergen peptides which stimulate allergen-specific T cells.

Modern trends are leading in the direction of combining allergen-specific immunotherapies with allergen-non-specific immunotherapies, prophylactic vaccination and personalized immunotherapy according to the patients' sensitization profile.

Over the last years plenty of new methods and techniques are flooding customers, clinicians and researchers alike with data about sensitization rates that need to be interpreted in a correct manner, and therefore data analysis requires a certain level of expertise. The overwhelming amount of information can result in misdiagnosis as well as over-intervention and can thus subsequently cause an unnecessary reduction of the patient's quality of life. At the same time, special precautions have to be taken for patients with confirmed sensitizations/symptoms to proteins highly prone to cause severe and life-threatening reactions. For improved prevention, diagnosis and treatment there is still an essential need for basic and clinical studies in order to investigate the pathomechanism of PFS in detail that eventually leads to a better understanding of the disease.

Table 4.1: Pollen-food association without identified molecules.

Food causing symptoms	Tree			Weed		Grass	References
	Birch	Olive	Cypress	Ragweed	Mugwort		
Almond *Prunus dulcis*	•					•	(Sloane and Sheffer, 2001; Tawde et al., 2006)
Anise *Pimpinella anisum*	•				•		(Jensen-Jarolim et al., 1997; Sloane and Sheffer, 2001)
Avocado *Persea americana*					•		(Ortega et al., 1999)
Bell pepper *Capsicum annuum*	•				•		(Leitner et al., 1998)
Black pepper *Piper nigrum*					•		(Leitner et al., 1998)
Caraway seed *Carum carvi*					•		(Egger et al., 2006)
Chamomile *Matricaria chamomilla*				•	•	•	(Sloane and Sheffer, 2001)
Chicory *Cichorium intybus*	•						(Cadot et al., 2003)
Coriander *Coriandrum sativum*	•			•	•		(Egger et al., 2006; Ortolani et al., 1988; Price et al., 2015; Sloane and Sheffer, 2001)
Cucumber *Cucumis sativus*				•			(Asero, 2000; Enberg et al., 1987)
Cumin *Cuminum cyminum*	•						(Jensen-Jarolim et al., 1997)
Currant *Ribes sylvestre*						•	(Perez-Ezquerra et al., 2007)
Date fruit *Phoenix dactylifera*	•					•	(Asturias et al., 2005; Kwaasi et al., 2002)
Fennel *Foeniculum vulgare*	•				•		(Jensen-Jarolim et al., 1997; Pastorello et al., 2013)
Fig *Ficus carica*	•					•	(Antico et al., 2003; Hemmer et al., 2010)
Garlic *Allium sativum*					•	•	(Boccafogli et al., 1994; Moneret-Vautrin et al., 2002)

Table 4.1 contd. ...

... Table 4.1 contd.

Food causing symptoms	Tree			Weed		Grass	References
	Birch	Olive	Cypress	Ragweed	Mugwort		
Green/French Bean *Phaseolus vulgaris*		•					(Ibanez *et al.*, 2003)
Jackfruit *Artocarpus integrifolia*	•						(Hemmer *et al.*, 2010)
Lettuce *Lactuca sativa*			•		•		(Garcia Ortiz *et al.*, 1996; Sanchez-Lopez *et al.*, 2011)
Maize *Zea mays*						•	(Oldenburg *et al.*, 2011)
Mango *Mangifera indica*	•				•		(Paschke *et al.*, 2001)
Melon/Honeydew *Cucumis melo*	•	•		•		•	(Asakura *et al.*, 2006; Enberg *et al.*, 1987; Florido Lopez *et al.*, 2002; Sloane and Sheffer, 2001; Tordesillas *et al.*, 2010)
Onion *Allium cepa*					•	•	(Boccafogli *et al.*, 1994; Moneret-Vautrin *et al.*, 2002)
Parsnip *Pastinaca sativa*	•						(Hannuksela and Lahti, 1977)
Pea *Pisum sativum*						•	(de Martino *et al.*, 1988)
Pistachio *Pistacia vera*					•	•	(Egger *et al.*, 2006; Garcia Ortiz *et al.*, 1996; Liccardi *et al.*, 1996; Liccardi *et al.*, 1999)
Potato *Solanum tuberosum*	•						(Ebner *et al.*, 1995)
Pumpkin/Zucchini *Cucurbita pepo*				•		•	(Enberg *et al.*, 1987; La Shell *et al.*, 2010)
Sunflower seeds *Helianthus annuus*					•		(Garcia Ortiz *et al.*, 1996)
Watermelon *Citrullus lanatus*				•		•	(de Martino *et al.*, 1988; Enberg *et al.*, 1987)
Yellow Mustard *Sinapis alba*		•			•		(Figueroa *et al.*, 2005)

Acknowledgements

The work of Lorenz Aglas was supported by the BM4SIT project of the European Union 7th Framework program (FP7-HEALTH-2013-INNOVATION-1; GA number: 601763) and by the Austrian Science Funds (FWF) project 23417. Sara Huber was supported by the FWF project 26125. Claudia Asam and Anargyros Roulias were supported by FWF project 27589. All authors acknowledge the University of Salzburg's priority program "Allergy-Cancer-BioNano Research Centre" for supporting this work.

Keywords: Pollen-food syndrome, diagnosis, treatment, PR-10, Profilin, nsLTP, cross-reactive IgE, pollen allergen sensitization, plant food allergy

References

Antico, A., Zoccatelli, G., Marcotulli, C., and Curioni, A. (2003). Oral allergy syndrome to fig. International Archives of Allergy and Immunology 131(2): 138–142.

Asakura, K., Honma, T., Yamazaki, N., and Ishikawa, T. (2006). Relationships between oral allergy syndrome and sensitization to pollen antigen, especially to mugwort. Arerugi 55(10): 1321–1326.

Asero, R. (1998). Effects of birch pollen-specific immunotherapy on apple allergy in birch pollen-hypersensitive patients. Clinical and Experimental Allergy 28(11): 1368–1373.

Asero, R. (2000). Fennel, cucumber, and melon allergy successfully treated with pollen-specific injection immunotherapy. Annals of Allergy Asthma and Immunology 84(4): 460–462.

Asero, R. (2003). How long does the effect of birch pollen injection SIT on apple allergy last? Allergy 58(5): 435–438.

Asero, R. (2004). Effects of birch pollen SIT on apple allergy: a matter of dosage? Allergy 59(12): 1269–1271.

Asturias, J. A., Ibarrola, I., Fernandez, J., Arilla, M. C., Gonzalez-Rioja, R., and Martinez, A. (2005). Pho d 2, a major allergen from date palm pollen, is a profilin: cloning, sequencing, and immunoglobulin E cross-reactivity with other profilins. Clinical and Experimental Allergy 35(3): 374–381.

Ballmer-Weber, B. K. (2014). Value of allergy tests for the diagnosis of food allergy. Digestive Diseases 32(1-2): 84–88.

Bashir, M. E., Andersen, P., Fuss, I. J., Shi, H. N., and Nagler-Anderson, C. (2002). An enteric helminth infection protects against an allergic response to dietary antigen. Journal of Immunology 169(6): 3284–3292.

Becker, W. M., and Jappe, U. (2014). Peanut allergens. Chemical Immunology and Allergy 100: 256–267.

Bergmann, K. C., Wolf, H., and Schnitker, J. (2008). Effect of pollen-specific sublingual immunotherapy on oral allergy syndrome: an observational study. World Allergy Organ Journal 1(5): 79–84.

Bindslev-Jensen, C., Vibits, A., Stahl Skov, P., and Weeke, B. (1991). Oral allergy syndrome: the effect of astemizole. Allergy 46(8): 610–613.

Boccafogli, A., Vicentini, L., Camerani, A., Cogliati, P., D'Ambrosi, A., and Scolozzi, R. (1994). Adverse food reactions in patients with grass pollen allergic respiratory disease. Annals of Allergy 73(4): 301–308.

Bohle, B., Zwolfer, B., Heratizadeh, A., Jahn-Schmid, B., Antonia, Y. D., Alter, M., Keller, W., Zuidmeer, L., van Ree, R., Werfel, T., and Ebner, C. (2006). Cooking birch pollen-related food: divergent consequences for IgE- and T cell-mediated reactivity *in vitro* and *in vivo*. The Journal of Allergy and Clinical Immunology 118(1): 242–249.

Brinda Subbarayal, M. G. -S., Barbara Bohle. (2012). Birch pollen-related food allergy: an excellent disease 2012. *In*: C. Pereira (ed.). Allergic Diseases—Highlights in the Clinic, Mechanisms and Treatment: In Tech.

Bucher, X., Pichler, W. J., Dahinden, C. A., and Helbling, A. (2004). Effect of tree pollen specific, subcutaneous immunotherapy on the oral allergy syndrome to apple and hazelnut. Allergy 59(12): 1272–1276.

Burney, P. G., Potts, J., Kummeling, I., Mills, E. N., Clausen, M., Dubakiene, R., Barreales, L., Fernandez-Perez, C., Fernandez-Rivas, M., Le, T. M., Knulst, A. C., Kowalski, M. L., Lidholm, J., Ballmer-Weber, B. K., Braun-Fahlander, C., Mustakov, T., Kralimarkova, T., Popov, T., Sakellariou, A., Papadopoulos, N. G., Versteeg, S. A., Zuidmeer, L., Akkerdaas, J. H., Hoffmann-Sommergruber, K., and van Ree, R. (2014). The prevalence and distribution of food sensitization in European adults. Allergy 69(3): 365–371.

Cabanos, C., Tandang-Silvas, M. R., Odijk, V., Brostedt, P., Tanaka, A., Utsumi, S., and Maruyama, N. (2010). Expression, purification, cross-reactivity and homology modeling of peanut profilin. Protein Expression and Purification 73(1): 36–45.

Cadot, P., Kochuyt, A. M., van Ree, R., and Ceuppens, J. L. (2003). Oral allergy syndrome to chicory associated with birch pollen allergy. International Archives of Allergy and Immunology 131(1): 19–24.

Carrard, A., Rizzuti, D., and Sokollik, C. (2015). Update on food allergy. Allergy.

Curin, M., Reininger, R., Swoboda, I., Focke, M., Valenta, R., and Spitzauer, S. (2011). Skin prick test extracts for dog allergy diagnosis show considerable variations regarding the content of major and minor dog allergens. International Archives of Allergy and Immunology 154(3): 258–263.

de Martino, M., Novembre, E., Cozza, G., de Marco, A., Bonazza, P., and Vierucci, A. (1988). Sensitivity to tomato and peanut allergens in children monosensitized to grass pollen. Allergy 43(3): 206–213.

Ebner, C., Hirschwehr, R., Bauer, L., Breiteneder, H., Valenta, R., Ebner, H., Kraft, D., and Scheiner, O. (1995). Identification of allergens in fruits and vegetables: IgE cross-reactivities with the important birch pollen allergens Bet v 1 and Bet v 2 (birch profilin). The Journal of Allergy and Clinical Immunology 95(5 Pt 1): 962–969.

Ebo, D. G., Hagendorens, M. M., Bridts, C. H., Schuerwegh, A. J., De Clerck, L. S., and Stevens, W. J. (2005). Flow cytometric analysis of *in vitro* activated basophils, specific IgE and skin tests in the diagnosis of pollen-associated food allergy. Cytometry Part B: Clinical Cytometry 64(1): 28–33.

Ebo, D. G., Verweij, M. M., Sabato, V., Hagendorens, M. M., Bridts, C. H., and De Clerck, L. S. (2012). Hazelnut allergy: a multi-faced condition with demographic and geographic characteristics. Acta clinica Belgica 67(5): 317–321.

Egger, M., Mutschlechner, S., Wopfner, N., Gadermaier, G., Briza, P., and Ferreira, F. (2006). Pollen-food syndromes associated with weed pollinosis: an update from the molecular point of view. Allergy 61(4): 461–476.

Enberg, R. N., Leickly, F. E., McCullough, J., Bailey, J., and Ownby, D. R. (1987). Watermelon and ragweed share allergens. The Journal of Allergy and Clinical Immunology 79(6): 867–875.

Erdmann, S. M., Heussen, N., Moll-Slodowy, S., Merk, H. F., and Sachs, B. (2003). CD63 expression on basophils as a tool for the diagnosis of pollen-associated food allergy: sensitivity and specificity. Clinical and Experimental Allergy 33(5): 607–614.

Erdmann, S. M., Sachs, B., Schmidt, A., Merk, H. F., Scheiner, O., Moll-Slodowy, S., Sauer, I., Kwiecien, R., Maderegger, B., and Hoffmann-Sommergruber, K. (2005). *In vitro* analysis of birch-pollen-associated food allergy by use of recombinant allergens in the basophil activation test. International Archives of Allergy and Immunology 136(3): 230–238.

Fernandez-Rivas, M., Garrido Fernandez, S., Nadal, J. A., Diaz de Durana, M. D., Garcia, B. E., Gonzalez-Mancebo, E., Martin, S., Barber, D., Rico, P., and Tabar, A. I. (2009). Randomized double-blind, placebo-controlled trial of sublingual immunotherapy with a Pru p 3 quantified peach extract. Allergy 64(6): 876–883.

Figueroa, J., Blanco, C., Dumpierrez, A. G., Almeida, L., Ortega, N., Castillo, R., Navarro, L., Perez, E., Gallego, M. D., and Carrillo, T. (2005). Mustard allergy confirmed by double-blind placebo-controlled food challenges: clinical features and cross-reactivity with mugwort pollen and plant-derived foods. Allergy 60(1): 48–55.

Florido Lopez, J. F., Quiralte Enriquez, J., Arias de Saavedra Alias, J. M., Saenz de San Pedro, B., and Martin Casanez, E. (2002). An allergen from Olea europaea pollen (Ole e 7) is associated with plant-derived food anaphylaxis. Allergy 57 Suppl 71: 53–59.

Gamboa, P. M., Sanz, M. L., Lombardero, M., Barber, D., Sanchez-Monje, R., Goikoetxea, M. J., Antepara, I., Ferrer, M., and Salcedo, G. (2009). Component-resolved *in vitro* diagnosis in peach-allergic patients. Journal of Investigational Allergology and Clinical Immunology 19(1): 13–20.

Garcia Ortiz, J. C., Cosmes, P. M., and Lopez-Asunsolo, A. (1996). Allergy to foods in patients monosensitized to Artemisia pollen. Allergy 51(12): 927–931.

Goikoetxea, M. J., Berroa, F., Cabrera-Freitag, P., Ferrer, M., Nunez-Cordoba, J. M., Sanz, M. L., and Gastaminza, G. (2015). Do skin prick test and *in vitro* techniques diagnose sensitization to peach lipid transfer protein and profilin equally well in allergy to plant food and pollen? Journal of Investigational Allergology and Clinical Immunology 25(4): 283–287.

Gronlund, H., and Gafvelin, G. (2010). Recombinant Bet v 1 vaccine for treatment of allergy to birch pollen. Human Vaccines 6(12): 970–977.

Hannuksela, M., and Lahti, A. (1977). Immediate reactions to fruits and vegetables. Contact Dermatitis 3(2): 79–84.

Heinzerling, L., Mari, A., Bergmann, K. C., Bresciani, M., Burbach, G., Darsow, U., Durham, S., Fokkens, W., Gjomarkaj, M., Haahtela, T., Bom, A. T., Wohrl, S., Maibach, H., and Lockey, R. (2013). The skin prick test—European standards. Clinical and Translational Allergy 3(1): 3.

Hemmer, W., Focke, M., Marzban, G., Swoboda, I., Jarisch, R., and Laimer, M. (2010). Identification of Bet v 1-related allergens in fig and other Moraceae fruits. Clinical and Experimental Allergy 40(4): 679–687.

Henzgen, M., Ballmer-Weber, B. K., Erdmann, S., Fuchs, T., Kleine-Tebbe, J., Lepp, U., Niggemann, B., Raithel, M., Reese, I., Saloga, J., Vieths, S., Zuberbier, T., and Werfel, T. (2008). Skin testing with food allergens. Guideline of the German Society of Allergology and Clinical Immunology (DGAKI), the Physicians' Association of German Allergologists (ADA) and the Society of Pediatric Allergology (GPA) together with the Swiss Society of Allergology. Journal der Deutschen Dermatologischen Gesellschaft 6(11): 983–988.

Herrmann, D., Henzgen, M., Frank, E., Rudeschko, O., and Jager, L. (1995). Effect of Hyposensitization for Tree Pollinosis on Associated Apple Allergy. Journal of Investigational Allergology and Clinical Immunology 5(5): 259–267.

Hoffmann-Sommergruber, K., Pfeifer, S., and Bublin, M. (2015). Applications of Molecular Diagnostic Testing in Food Allergy. Current Allergy and Asthma Reports 15(9): 56.

Hoflehner, E., Hufnagl, K., Schabussova, I., Jasinska, J., Hoffmann-Sommergruber, K., Bohle, B., Maizels, R. M., and Wiedermann, U. (2012). Prevention of birch pollen-related food allergy by mucosal treatment with multi-allergen-chimers in mice. PLoS One 7(6): e39409.

Hylander, T., Latif, L., Petersson-Westin, U., and Cardell, L. O. (2013). Intralymphatic allergen-specific immunotherapy: An effective and safe alternative treatment route for pollen-induced allergic rhinitis. Journal of Allergy and Clinical Immunology 131(2): 412–420.

Ibanez, M. D., Martinez, M., Sanchez, J. J., and Fernandez-Caldas, E. (2003). [Legume cross-reactivity]. Allergologia et Immunopathologia (Madr) 31(3): 151–161.

Inuo, C., Kondo, Y., Tanaka, K., Nakajima, Y., Nomura, T., Ando, H., Suzuki, S., Tsuge, I., Yoshikawa, T., and Urisu, A. (2015). Japanese cedar pollen-based subcutaneous immunotherapy decreases tomato fruit-specific basophil activation. International Archives of Allergy and Immunology 167(2): 137–145.

Jensen-Jarolim, E., Leitner, A., Hirschwehr, R., Kraft, D., Wuthrich, B., Scheiner, O., Graf, J., and Ebner, C. (1997). Characterization of allergens in Apiaceae spices: anise, fennel, coriander and cumin. Clinical and Experimental Allergy 27(11): 1299–1306.

Jutel, M., Jaeger, L., Suck, R., Meyer, H., Fiebig, H., and Cromwell, O. (2005). Allergen-specific immunotherapy with recombinant grass pollen allergens. Journal of Allergy and Clinical Immunology 116(3): 608–613.

Kahlert, H., Suck, R., Weber, B., Nandy, A., Wald, M., Keller, W., Cromwell, O., and Fiebig, H. (2008). Characterization of a hypoallergenic recombinant Bet v 1 variant as a candidate for allergen-specific immunotherapy. International Archives of Allergy and Immunology 145(3): 193–206.

Kamdar, T., and Bryce, P. J. (2010). Immunotherapy in food allergy. Immunotherapy 2(3): 329–338.

Kandimalla, E. R., Bhagat, L., Wang, D., Yu, D., Zhu, F. G., Tang, J., Wang, H., Huang, P., Zhang, R., and Agrawal, S. (2003). Divergent synthetic nucleotide motif recognition pattern: design and development of potent immunomodulatory oligodeoxyribonucleotide agents with distinct cytokine induction profiles. Nucleic Acids Research 31(9): 2393–2400.

Kashyap, R. R., and Kashyap, R. S. (2015). Oral allergy syndrome: An update for stomatologists. Journal of Allergy (Cairo) 2015: 543928.

Katelaris, C. H. (2010). Food allergy and oral allergy or pollen-food syndrome. Current Opinion in Allergy and Clinical Immunology 10(3): 246–251.

Kinaciyan, T., Jahn-Schmid, B., Radakovics, A., Zwolfer, B., Schreiber, C., Francis, J. N., Ebner, C., and Bohle, B. (2007). Successful sublingual immunotherapy with birch pollen has limited effects on concomitant food allergy to apple and the immune response to the Bet v 1 homolog Mal d 1. Journal of Allergy and Clinical Immunology 119(4): 937–943.

Kinaciyan, T., Nagl, B., Faustmann, S., Kopp, S., Wolkersdorfer, M., and Bohle, B. (2015). Recombinant Mal d 1 facilitates sublingual challenge tests of birch pollen-allergic patients with apple allergy. Allergy.

Klunker, S., Saggar, L. R., Seyfert-Margolis, V., Asare, A. L., Casale, T. B., Durham, S. R., and Francis, J. N. (2007). Combination treatment with omalizumab and rush immunotherapy for ragweed-induced allergic rhinitis: Inhibition of IgE-facilitated allergen binding. Journal of Allergy and Clinical Immunology 120(3): 688–695.

Kopac, P., Rudin, M., Gentinetta, T., Gerber, R., Pichler, C., Hausmann, O., Schnyder, B., and Pichler, W. J. (2012). Continuous apple consumption induces oral tolerance in birch-pollen-associated apple allergy. Allergy 67(2): 280–285.

Kwaasi, A. A., Harfi, H. A., Parhar, R. S., Saleh, S., Collison, K. S., Panzani, R. C., Al-Sedairy, S. T., and Al-Mohanna, F. A. (2002). Cross-reactivities between date palm (Phoenix dactylifera L.) polypeptides and foods implicated in the oral allergy syndrome. Allergy 57(6): 508–518.

La Shell, M. S., Otto, H. F., Whisman, B. A., Waibel, K. H., White, A. A., and Calabria, C. W. (2010). Allergy to pumpkin and crossreactivity to pollens and other foods. Annals of Allergy Asthma and Immunology 104(2): 178–180.

Larche, M., Akdis, C. A., and Valenta, R. (2006). Immunological mechanisms of allergen-specific immunotherapy. Nature Reviews Immunology 6(10): 761–771.

Leitner, A., Jensen-Jarolim, E., Grimm, R., Wuthrich, B., Ebner, H., Scheiner, O., Kraft, D., and Ebner, C. (1998). Allergens in pepper and paprika. Immunologic investigation of the celery-birch-mugwort-spice syndrome. Allergy 53(1): 36–41.

Liccardi, G., Mistrello, G., Noschese, P., Falagiani, P., D'Amato, M., and D'Amato, G. (1996). Oral allergy syndrome (OAS) in pollinosis patients after eating pistachio nuts: two cases with two different patterns of onset. Allergy 51(12): 919–922.

Liccardi, G., Russo, M., Mistrello, G., Falagiani, P., D'Amato, M., and D'Amato, G. (1999). Sensitization to pistachio is common in Parietaria allergy. Allergy 54(6): 643–645.

Lieberman, J. A., and Wang, J. (2012). Nonallergen-specific treatments for food allergy. Current Opinion in Allergy and Clinical Immunology 12(3): 293–301.

Luengo, O., and Cardona, V. (2014). Component resolved diagnosis: when should it be used? Clinical and Translational Allergy 4: 28.

Macchia, D., Melioli, G., Pravettoni, V., Nucera, E., Piantanida, M., Caminati, M., Campochiaro, C., Yacoub, M. R., Schiavino, D., Paganelli, R., and Di Gioacchino, M. (2015). Guidelines for the use and interpretation of diagnostic methods in adult food allergy. Clinical of Molecular Allergy 13: 27.

Marth, K., Breyer, I., Focke-Tejkl, M., Blatt, K., Shamji, M. H., Layhadi, J., Gieras, A., Swoboda, I., Zafred, D., Keller, W., Valent, P., Durham, S. R., and Valenta, R. (2013). A nonallergenic birch pollen allergy vaccine consisting of hepatitis PreS-fused Bet v 1 peptides focuses blocking IgG toward IgE epitopes and shifts immune responses to a tolerogenic and Th1 phenotype. Journal of Immunology 190(7): 3068–3078.

Marth, K., Focke-Tejkl, M., Lupinek, C., Valenta, R., and Niederberger, V. (2014). Allergen peptides, recombinant allergens and hypoallergens for allergen-specific immunotherapy. Current Treatment Options in Allergy 1: 91–106.

Mittag, D., Akkerdaas, J., Ballmer-Weber, B. K., Vogel, L., Wensing, M., Becker, W. M., Koppelman, S. J., Knulst, A. C., Helbling, A., Hefle, S. L., Van Ree, R., and Vieths, S. (2004). Ara h 8, a Bet v 1-homologous allergen from peanut, is a major allergen in patients with combined birch pollen and peanut allergy. The Journal of Allergy and Clinical Immunology 114(6): 1410–1417.

Mittag, D., Batori, V., Neudecker, P., Wiche, R., Friis, E. P., Ballmer-Weber, B. K., Vieths, S., and Roggen, E. L. (2006). A novel approach for investigation of specific and cross-reactive IgE epitopes on Bet v 1 and homologous food allergens in individual patients. Molecular Immunology 43(3): 268–278.

Modrzynski, M., Zawisza, E., Rapiejko, P., and Przybylski, G. (2002). [Specific-pollen immunotherapy in the treatment of oral allergy syndrome in patients with tree pollen hypersensitivity]. Przeglad Lekarski 59(12): 1007–1010.

Moldaver, D., and Larche, M. (2011). Immunotherapy with peptides. Allergy 66(6): 784–791.

Moneret-Vautrin, D. A., Morisset, M., Lemerdy, P., Croizier, A., and Kanny, G. (2002). Food allergy and IgE sensitization caused by spices: CICBAA data (based on 589 cases of food allergy). Allergy Immunology (Paris) 34(4): 135–140.

Mutschlechner, S., Deifl, S., and Bohle, B. (2009). Genetic allergen modification in the development of novel approaches to specific immunotherapy. Clinical and Experimental Allergy 39(11): 1635–1642.

Neudecker, P., Lehmann, K., Nerkamp, J., Haase, T., Wangorsch, A., Fotisch, K., Hoffmann, S., Rosch, P., Vieths, S., and Scheurer, S. (2003). Mutational epitope analysis of Pru av 1 and Api g 1, the major allergens of cherry (Prunus avium) and celery (Apium graveolens): correlating IgE reactivity with three-dimensional structure. Biochemical Journal 376(Pt 1): 97–107.

Nowak-Wegrzyn, A., and Sampson, H. A. (2011). Future therapies for food allergies. Journal of Allergy and Clinical Immunology 127(3): 558–575.

Nucera, E., Aruanno, A., Rizzi, A., Pecora, V., Patriarca, G., Buonomo, A., Mezzacappa, S., and Schiavino, D. (2015). Profilin desensitization: A case series. International Journal of Immunopathology and Pharmacology.

O'Keefe, A. W., De Schryver, S., Mill, J., Mill, C., Dery, A., and Ben-Shoshan, M. (2014). Diagnosis and management of food allergies: new and emerging options: a systematic review. Journal of Asthma Allergy 7: 141–164.

Oldenburg, M., Petersen, A., and Baur, X. (2011). Maize pollen is an important allergen in occupationally exposed workers. Journal of Occupational Medicine and Toxicology 6.

Ortega, N., Quiralte, J., Blanco, C., Castillo, R., Alvarez, M. J., and Carrillo, T. (1999). Tobacco allergy: demonstration of cross-reactivity with other members of Solanaceae family and mugwort pollen. Annals of Allergy Asthma and Immunology 82(2): 194–197.

Ortolani, C., Ispano, M., Pastorello, E., Bigi, A., and Ansaloni, R. (1988). The oral allergy syndrome. Annals of Allergy 61(6 Pt 2): 47–52.

Ozdemir, O. (2010). Various effects of different probiotic strains in allergic disorders: an update from laboratory and clinical data. Clinical and Experimental Immunology 160(3): 295–304.

Paschke, A., Kinder, H., Zunker, K., Wigotzki, M., Steinhart, H., Wessbecher, R., and Vieluf, I. (2001). Characterization of cross-reacting allergens in mango fruit. Allergy 56(3): 237–242.

Pastorello, E. A., Farioli, L., Pravettoni, V., Scibilia, J., Mascheri, A., Borgonovo, L., Piantanida, M., Primavesi, L., Stafylaraki, C., Pasqualetti, S., Schroeder, J., Nichelatti, M., and Marocchi, A. (2011). Pru p 3-sensitised Italian peach-allergic patients are less likely to develop severe symptoms when also presenting IgE antibodies to Pru p 1 and Pru p 4. International Archives of Allergy and Immunology 156(4): 362–372.

Pastorello, E. A., Farioli, L., Stafylaraki, C., Scibilia, J., Giuffrida, M. G., Mascheri, A., Piantanida, M., Baro, C., Primavesi, L., Nichelatti, M., Schroeder, J. W., and Pravettoni, V. (2013). Fennel allergy is a lipid-transfer protein (LTP)-related food hypersensitivity associated with peach allergy. Journal of Agricultural and Food Chemistry 61(3): 740–746.

Pauli, G., Larsen, T. H., Rak, S., Horak, F., Pastorello, E., Valenta, R., Purohit, A., Arvidsson, M., Kavina, A., Schroeder, J. W., Mothes, N., Spitzauer, S., Montagut, A., Galvain, S., Melac, M., Andre, C., Poulsen, L. K., and Malling, H. J. (2008). Efficacy of recombinant birch pollen vaccine for the treatment of birch-allergic rhinoconjunctivitis. Journal of Allergy and Clinical Immunology 122(5): 951–960.

Pereira, C., Bartolome, B., Asturias, J. A., Ibarrola, I., Tavares, B., Loureiro, G., Machado, D., and Chieira, C. (2009). Specific sublingual immunotherapy with peach LTP (Pru p 3). One year treatment: a case report. Cases Journal 2: 6553.

Perez-Ezquerra, P. R., de la Gaspar, M. V., de Fernandez, M. B., Flores, V. T., Alvarez-Santullano, A. V., and de Ocariz, M. L. (2007). Currant allergy and the Rosaceae-grass pollen allergy syndrome: a case report. Annals of Allergy Asthma and Immunology 98(5): 480–482.

Popescu, F. D. (2015). Cross-reactivity between aeroallergens and food allergens. World Journal of Methodology 5(2): 31–50.

Price, A., Ramachandran, S., Smith, G. P., Stevenson, M. L., Pomeranz, M. K., and Cohen, D. E. (2015). Oral allergy syndrome (pollen-food allergy syndrome). Dermatitis 26(2): 78–88.

Rance, F., Juchet, A., Bremont, F., and Dutau, G. (1997). Correlations between skin prick tests using commercial extracts and fresh foods, specific IgE, and food challenges. Allergy 52(10): 1031–1035.

Sanchez-Lopez, J., Asturias, J. A., Enrique, E., Suarez-Cervera, M., and Bartra, J. (2011). Cupressus arizonica pollen: a new pollen involved in the lipid transfer protein syndrome? Journal of Investigational Allergology and Clinical Immunology 21(7): 522–526.

Scala, E., Till, S. J., Asero, R., Abeni, D., Guerra, E. C., Pirrotta, L., Paganelli, R., Pomponi, D., Giani, M., De Pita, O., and Cecchi, L. (2015). Lipid transfer protein sensitization: reactivity profiles and clinical risk assessment in an Italian cohort. Allergy 70(8): 933–943.

Scheurer, S., Son, D. Y., Boehm, M., Karamloo, F., Franke, S., Hoffmann, A., Haustein, D., and Vieths, S. (1999). Cross-reactivity and epitope analysis of Pru a 1, the major cherry allergen. Molecular Immunology 36(3): 155–167.

Senti, G., Graf, N., Haug, S., Ruedi, N., von Moos, S., Sonderegger, T., Johansen, P., and Kundig, T. M. (2009). Epicutaneous allergen administration as a novel method of allergen-specific immunotherapy. Journal of Allergy and Clinical Immunology 124(5): 997–1002.

Sloane, D., and Sheffer, A. (2001). Oral allergy syndrome. Allergy Asthma Proc 22(5): 321–325.

Song, Y., Wang, J., Leung, N., Wang, L. X., Lisann, L., Sicherer, S. H., Scurlock, A. M., Pesek, R., Perry, T. T., Jones, S. M., and Li, X. M. (2015). Correlations between basophil activation, allergen-specific IgE with outcome and severity of oral food challenges. Annals of Allergy Asthma and Immunology 114(4): 319–326.

Syed, A., Kohli, A., and Nadeau, K. C. (2013). Food allergy diagnosis and therapy: where are we now? Immunotherapy 5(9): 931–944.

Tawde, P., Venkatesh, Y. P., Wang, F., Teuber, S. S., Sathe, S. K., and Roux, K. H. (2006). Cloning and characterization of profilin (Pru du 4), a cross-reactive almond (Prunus dulcis) allergen. The Journal of Allergy and Clinical Immunology 118(4): 915–922.

Tordesillas, L., Pacios, L. F., Palacin, A., Cuesta-Herranz, J., Madero, M., and Diaz-Perales, A. (2010). Characterization of IgE epitopes of Cuc m 2, the major melon allergen, and their role in cross-reactivity with pollen profilins. Clinical and Experimental Allergy 40(1): 174–181.

Van Gasse, A. L., Mangodt, E. A., Faber, M., Sabato, V., Bridts, C. H., and Ebo, D. G. (2015). Molecular allergy diagnosis: status anno 2015. Clinica Chimica Acta 444: 54–61.

van Hoffen, E., Peeters, K. A. B. M., van Neerven, R. J. J., van der Tas, C. W. H., Zuidmeer, L., van Ieperen-van Dijk, A. G., Bruijnzeel-Koomen, C. A. F. M., Knol, E. F., van Ree, R., and Knulst, A. C. (2011). Effect of birch pollen-specific immunotherapy on birch pollen-related hazelnut allergy. Journal of Allergy and Clinical Immunology 127(1): 100–U176.

Vereda, A., van Hage, M., Ahlstedt, S., Ibanez, M. D., Cuesta-Herranz, J., van Odijk, J., Wickman, M., and Sampson, H. A. (2011). Peanut allergy: Clinical and immunologic differences among patients from 3 different geographic regions. The Journal of Allergy and Clinical Immunology 127(3): 603–607.

Vrtala, S., Hirtenlehner, K., Susani, M., Akdis, M., Kussebi, F., Akdis, C. A., Blaser, K., Hufnagl, P., Binder, B. R., Politou, A., Pastore, A., Vangelista, L., Sperr, W. R., Semper, H., Valent, P., Ebner, C., Kraft, D., and Valenta, R. (2001). Genetic engineering of a hypoallergenic trimer of the major birch pollen allergen Bet v 1. The FASEB Journal 15(11): 2045–2047.

Wang, D., Kandimalla, E. R., Yu, D., Tang, J. X., and Agrawal, S. (2005). Oral administration of second-generation immunomodulatory oligonucleotides induces mucosal Th1 immune responses and adjuvant activity. Vaccine 23(20): 2614–2622.

Wang, J., and Li, X. M. (2012). Chinese herbal therapy for the treatment of food allergy. Current Allergy and Asthma Reports 12(4): 332–338.

Winther, L., Poulsen, L. K., Robin, B., Melac, M., and Malling, H. (2009). Safety and Tolerability of Recombinant Bet v 1 (rBet v 1) Tablets in Sublingual Immunotherapy (SLIT). Journal of Allergy and Clinical Immunology 123(2): S215–S215.

Worm, M., Rak, S., de Blay, F., Malling, H. J., Melac, M., Cadic, V., and Zeldin, R. K. (2014). Sustained efficacy and safety of a 300 IR daily dose of a sublingual solution of birch pollen allergen extract in adults with allergic rhinoconjunctivitis: results of a double-blind, placebo-controlled study. Clinical and Translational Allergy 4(1): 7.

Yang, Y. H., and Chiang, B. L. (2014). Novel Approaches to Food Allergy. Clinical Reviews in Allergy and Immunology 46(3): 250–257.

Zhu, F. G., Kandimalla, E. R., Yu, D., Tang, J. X., and Agrawal, S. (2004). Modulation of ovalbumin-induced Th2 responses by second-generation immunomodulatory oligonucleotides in mice. International Immunopharmacology 4(7): 851–862.

Zuidmeer-Jongejan, L., Fernandez-Rivas, M., Poulsen, L. K., Neubauer, A., Asturias, J., Blom, L., Boye, J., Bindslev-Jensen, C., Clausen, M., Ferrara, R., Garosi, P., Huber, H., Jensen, B. M., Koppelman, S., Kowalski, M. L., Lewandowska-Polak, A., Linhart, B., Maillere, B., Mari, A., Martinez, A., Mills, C. E., Nicoletti, C., Opstelten, D. J., Papadopoulos, N. G., Portoles, A., Rigby, N., Scala, E., Schnoor, H. J., Sigurdardottir, S. T., Stavroulakis, G., Stolz, F., Swoboda, I., Valenta, R., van den Hout, R., Versteeg, S. A., Witten, M., and van Ree, R. (2012). FAST: towards safe and effective subcutaneous immunotherapy of persistent life-threatening food allergies. Clinical and Translational Allergy 2(1): 5.

CHAPTER 5

Advances in Seafood Allergy Research

Allergen Detection and Allergen-Specific Immunotherapy

Nicki Y.H. Leung,[1] *Christine Y.Y. Wai,*[1] *Ka Hou Chu*[1] *and Patrick S.C. Leung*[2,*]

Introduction

Seafood is considered one of the most popular food choice because of its low-fat content and high-quality proteins (Bourre and Paquotte, 2008). A number of studies have reported the potential benefits of high seafood consumption, such as providing valuable sources of omega-3 fatty acids, taurine and selenium as well as its association with reduced risk of chronic diseases such as coronary heart disease, rheumatoid arthritis, cancers, etc. (Aadland *et al.*, 2015; Lund, 2013). As of 2011, the global production of seafood nearly doubled from two decades ago, reaching 129.6 million tons. The per capita consumption of seafood in 2014 also increased to an all-time high of 20.1 kg/capita/year (F.A.O., 2016). As seafood consumption continues to increase, the adverse allergic reactions to seafood intake have become an eminent global health issue, particularly in countries where consumption of seafood happens early in life (Lopata and Lehrer, 2009) or seafood consumption is frequent due to tradition or habits (Jacobs *et al.*, 2015).

[1] School of Life Sciences, The Chinese University of Hong Kong, HKSAR.
  Emails: nyhleung@cuhk.edu.hk; christineyywai@cuhk.edu.hk; kahouchu@cuhk.edu.hk
[2] Division of Rheumatology/Allergy, School of Medicine, University of California, Davis, CA 95616, USA.
* Corresponding author: psleung@ucdavis.edu

The prevalence of self-reported fish and shellfish allergies were 0.6 and 1.1%, respectively while the rates of symptoms with sensitization were slightly lower at 0.2 and 0.6%, respectively, according to a meta-analysis (Rona *et al.*, 2007). However, in some coastal countries where seafood is a major part of the daily diet, the prevalence of seafood allergies could be significantly higher. For instance, the prevalence of fish allergy in Norway and Australia was reported to be 3.0 and 5.6%, respectively (Sharp and Lopata, 2014). Shellfish is the top causative food for food-induced anaphylactic events in the USA (Ross *et al.*, 2008) and also the dominant sensitizing and anaphylaxis-inducing allergens in many Asian countries (Hajeb and Selamat, 2012; Lopata and Lehrer, 2009). More importantly, unlike cow's milk or egg allergy, fish and shellfish allergy tends to persist throughout life, thus imposing a severe healthcare economic burden and affecting the quality of life of allergic patients.

Similar to other types of food allergies, the current management of seafood allergies mainly relies on strict avoidance of intake. Parvalbumin and tropomyosin have long been identified as the major fish and shellfish allergens, respectively, and extensive efforts have been directed to characterize the allergenic properties of these two allergens in different species (Leung *et al.*, 2014). However, no preventive or curative treatment is currently available for seafood allergies, as immunotherapy for food allergies is often met with a high frequency of anaphylactic side effects (Nelson *et al.*, 1997). Recent advances in molecular cloning techniques have enabled the design of hypoallergenic derivatives of allergens, which may serve as a safe alternative to use in immunotherapies in the near future. In this chapter, we discuss the current understanding of the molecular characteristics of seafood allergens, such as the molecular identity, cross-reactivity, effects of food processing and the methods of detection of seafood allergens. We also discuss established animal models of seafood hypersensitivity and cutting edge strategies towards designing safe and effective therapeutic treatments for seafood allergies, including potential disease-modifying allergen-specific immunotherapies.

Molecular Basis of Seafood Allergy

Fish allergens

Parvalbumin was identified as the first fish allergen in the Baltic cod (Aas, 1969; Elsayed and Aas, 1970). This skeletal muscle protein regulating calcium switching was subsequently regarded as a major fish pan-allergen where it was reported as allergenic in a vast range of commonly consumed fish species and recognized by a majority of fish allergic patients (Sharp and Lopata, 2014). Parvalbumins have low molecular weights of 10–13 kDa, and they are generally heat stable and resistant to proteolytic digestion. Both linear and conformational epitopes have been reported for parvalbumin in four independent studies (Elsayed and Apold, 1983; Perez-Gordo *et al.*, 2012; Untersmayr *et al.*, 2006;

Yoshida *et al.*, 2008), and interestingly only modest sequence identity was shown between the identified epitopes. Although these results could be due to the different methods or fish species used for elucidating the IgE binding epitopes, the heterogeneity of IgE binding epitopes in parvalbumin has inevitably made the detection and treatment of fish allergy challenging.

In addition to parvalbumin, several other fish allergens have been identified over the last two decades. Enolase, an essential glycolytic enzyme found in fish muscle, was recently identified as an IgE-binding protein in the blunt snout bream (Liu *et al.*, 2011b), cod, salmon and tuna (Kuehn *et al.*, 2013), and designated as group II fish allergens. Aldolase, another group of glycolytic enzyme, have been identified as group III fish allergens (Kuehn *et al.*, 2013). Group IV fish allergens constitute of the invertebrate pan-allergen tropomyosin, where Liu *et al.* (Liu *et al.*, 2013) reported the binding of serum IgE to tropomyosin in tilapia allergic patients. Yet the authors suggested that fish tropomyosin is more likely reactive towards the human tropomyosin-specific auto-antibodies, suggesting that immune responses against fish tropomyosin run close to autoimmune responses rather than allergic reactions. In addition to the above four muscle proteins, the egg yolk precursor protein vitellogenin was also reported as an allergen in caviar (Perez-Gordo *et al.*, 2008) and salmon roe (Shimizu *et al.*, 2014), and designated as group V allergens. IgE reactivity has also been reported for other fish proteins such as collagen (Hamada *et al.*, 2001; Sakaguchi *et al.*, 2000), aldehyde phosphate dehydrogenase (Das Dores *et al.*, 2002), triosephosphate isomerase (Wang *et al.*, 2011) and muscle creatine kinase (Liu *et al.*, 2011b). However, these proteins have not been formally included as allergens by the WHO/IUIS allergen nomenclature sub-committee. A list of fish allergens is summarized in Table 5.1.

Shellfish allergens

Shellfish is a generic term to describe marine animals with an exoskeleton or shell. Crustaceans such as shrimps, lobsters and crabs, together with mollusks such as squids, clams and oysters, are the commonly consumed shellfish. Early in the 1990s, the muscle protein tropomyosin was identified as the major allergen in shrimp (Daul *et al.*, 1994; Leung *et al.*, 1994; Shanti *et al.*, 1993) and subsequently implicated as a major pan-allergen across invertebrates, including the house dust mite (Witteman *et al.*, 1994). The allergenicity of tropomyosin has been reported in numerous shellfish species, including shrimp, lobster, crab, krill, barnacle, abalone, whelk, scallop, mussel, clam, squid, etc. (reviewed by Leung *et al.*, 2014). Tropomyosin belongs to the highly conserved family of actin filament binding proteins with a simple coiled-coiled secondary structure formed by two identical alpha helical peptide chains, each around 300 amino acids in length. Similar to parvalbumin, it is extremely heat stable and resistant to proteolytic digestion. With a relatively simple secondary structure, only linear IgE-binding epitopes have been reported thus far (Ayuso *et al.*, 2002; Subba Rao *et al.*, 1998; Wai *et al.*, 2014). The immunodominant T

Table 5.1: List of fish and shellfish allergens.

Species	Allergens	Molecular identity	Remarks	References
Fish	Group I allergens (Gad c 1, Sal s 1, Sco j 1, etc.)	Parvalbumin		Aas and Elsayed, 1969; Elsayed and Aas, 1970
	Group II allergens (Gad m 2, Sal s 2)	Enolase		Liu et al., 2011b; Kuehn et al., 2013
	Group III allergens (Gad m 3, Sal s 3)	Aldolase		Kuehn et al., 2013
	Group IV allergens (Ore m 4)	Tropomyosin	First tropomyosin allergen identified in vertebrates	Liu et al., 2013
	Group V allergens (Onc k 5)	Vitellogen	Found in caviar	Perez-Gordo et al., 2008
	Ungrouped	Collagen		Sakaguchi et al., 2000; Hamada et al., 2001
	Ungrouped	Aldehyde phosphate dehydrogenase		Das Dores et al., 2002
	Ungrouped	Triosephosphate isomerase		Wang et al., 2011
	Ungrouped	Muscle creatine kinase		Liu et al., 2011b
Shellfish	Group I allergens (Met e 1, Pen a 1, etc.)	Tropomyosin	Major cross-reactive allergen among arthropods	Shanti et al., 1993; Daul et al., 1994; Leung et al., 1994
	Group II allergens (Pen m 2, Cra c 2, etc.)	Arginine kinase	Cross-reactivity reported among arthropods	Yu et al., 2003; Garcia-Orozco et al., 2007; Bauermeister et al., 2011; Abdel Rahman et al., 2011; Abdel Rahman et al., 2013
	Group III/V allergens (Lit v 3, Cra c 5)	Myosin light chain	Group III & V are different isoforms of myosin light chain	Ayuso et al., 2008; Bauermeister et al., 2011

Table 3.1 contd. …

Table 3.1 contd.

Species	Allergens	Molecular identity	Remarks	References
	Group IV allergens (Lit v 4, Cra c 4, etc.)	Sarcoplasmic calcium-binding proteins		Ayuso et al., 2009; Shiomi et al., 2008; Bauermeister et al., 2011; Abdel Rahman et al., 2013
	Group VI allergens (Cra c 6, Pen m 6)	Troponin C		Bauermeister et al., 2011; Abdel Rahman et al., 2013; Kalyanasundaram and Santiago, 2015
	Group VII allergens (Pon l 7)	Troponin I	Non-published data	WHO/IUIS
	Group VIII allergens (Cra c 8)	Triosephosphate isomerase		Bauermeister et al., 2011
Shellfish	Ungrouped	α-actin		Abdel Rahman et al., 2011
	Ungrouped	Smooth endoplasmic reticulum Ca²⁺ ATPase		Abdel Rahman et al., 2011
	Ungrouped	Glyceraldehyde-3-phosphate dehydrogenase		Abdel Rahman et al., 2013
	Ungrouped	Myosin heavy chain		Abdel Rahman et al., 2013
	Ungrouped	Hemocyanin	Identified in freshwater shrimp	Piboonpocanun et al., 2011
	Ungrouped	Paramyosin	Cross-reactive to molluscan tropomyosin; no report on cross-reactivity with crustaceans	Suzuki et al., 2011

cell epitopes were also extensively characterized (Ravkov *et al.*, 2013; Subba Rao *et al.*, 1998; Wai *et al.*, 2014).

In addition to tropomyosin, several other shellfish allergens have been identified, where most of them were isolated from shrimp species with high commercial value. Arginine kinase from both shrimps (Abdel Rahman *et al.*, 2013; Garcia-Orozco *et al.*, 2007; Yadzir *et al.*, 2012; Yu *et al.*, 2003) and crabs (Abdel Rahman *et al.*, 2011; Rosmilah *et al.*, 2012; Shen *et al.*, 2011; Yu *et al.*, 2013) was identified as an allergen and designated as group II allergens, even though only a minority of shellfish allergic patients are sensitized by this enzyme abundant in the muscle. Group III and group V allergens are different isoforms of the same muscle protein myosin light chain, they were identified as an allergen in three different shrimp species, *Litopenaeus vannamei* (Ayuso *et al.*, 2008), *Crangon crangon* (Bauermeister *et al.*, 2011) and *Pandalus borealis* (Abdel Rahman *et al.*, 2013). Sarcoplasmic calcium-binding protein from a number of shrimp species was also reported to be IgE-binding and designated as group IV allergens (Abdel Rahman *et al.*, 2013; Ayuso *et al.*, 2009; Bauermeister *et al.*, 2011; Shiomi *et al.*, 2008). Two proteins of the troponin complex, troponin C and troponin I were identified as group VI and group VII allergens, respectively and recognized by a minority of shrimp allergic patients (Abdel Rahman *et al.*, 2013; Bauermeister *et al.*, 2011; Kalyanasundaram and Santiago, 2015). IgE from patients with shellfish allergy also recognize triosephosphate isomerase (Cra c 8) from the North Sea shrimp *Crangon crangon* but the allergenicity and prevalence of its sensitization remain largely unknown in other shrimp species (Bauermeister *et al.*, 2011). Using an allergenomic approach, Abdel Rahman *et al.* (Abdel Rahman *et al.*, 2011) identified a number of novel IgE binding proteins, such as α-actin and smooth endoplasmic reticulum Ca^{2+} ATPase in the snow crab *Chionoecetes opilio*, as well as actin, Glyceraldehyde-3-phosphate dehydrogenase and myosin heavy chain in the Northern shrimp *Pandalus borealis*. In addition to the allergens identified in marine crustaceans, the oxygen-carrying protein hemocyanin was also identified as an allergen in the giant river shrimp *Macrobrachium rosenbergii* (Piboonpocanun *et al.*, 2011). Notably, except for tropomyosin and arginine kinase, the crustacean allergens stated above are not reported to be allergenic in mollusks. One allergen exclusively identified in the mollusks is the paramyosin identified in abalone (Suzuki *et al.*, 2011), where it demonstrated certain cross-reactivity with molluscan tropomyosin. A list of shellfish allergens is summarized in Table 5.1.

Cross-Reactivity of Seafood Allergens

Parvalbumin

Parvalbumins are highly conserved proteins belonging to the EF-hand calcium-binding protein family. They are abundant in the muscle and expressed as different isoforms in the fish. While the primary structure of different isoforms might differ (Saptarshi *et al.*, 2014; Sharp *et al.*, 2014), they have highly conserved tertiary structure (Arif, 2009) which could account for the substantial cross-reactivity of parvalbumins among different fish species. Earlier studies demonstrated that cod allergic patients were also sensitive to other commonly consumed fish species such as mackerel, salmon, tuna, flounder, etc. (reviewed by Leung *et al.* (2014) and Sharp and Lopata (2014)). Saptarshi *et al.* (Saptarshi *et al.*, 2014) demonstrated that parvalbumins from 18 out of 19 commonly consumed bony or cartilaginous fish species could be detected with an anti-frog parvalbumin monoclonal antibody, suggesting a high degree of cross-reactivity among fish parvalbumins, even in phylogenetically distant cartilaginous fishes. In a similar study, Sharp *et al.* (Sharp *et al.*, 2015) generated highly cross-reactive anti-parvalbumin antibodies in four distantly related fishes. All these evidence suggest that it is likely the IgE-binding epitopes are conserved between fishes due to the high degree of structural similarity.

Tropomyosin

Cross-reactivity of the major allergen tropomyosin among the crustaceans, mollusks or between the two has long been reported and demonstrated in numerous studies (reviewed by Leung *et al.*, 2014). Sequence homology of tropomyosins from crustaceans and mollusks is 93.8 and 77.2%, respectively while the sequence homology between the two groups is 61.4% (Leung *et al.*, 2014). In addition, we have also revealed a highly conserved epitope region at positions 92–101 between the crustaceans and mollusks. The extensive cross-reactivity across shellfish groups is thus essentially due to the highly conserved epitopes and structural features of tropomyosins. The conserved epitope at positions 92–101 is also present in tropomyosins of mites and insects, indicating a molecular basis for the tropomyosin as a pan-allergen across invertebrates (Leung *et al.*, 2014).

Arginine kinase

Apart from tropomyosins, arginine kinase was also reported as an allergen shared among shellfish such as shrimps, crabs and octopus, as well as in insects such as cricket (Srinroch *et al.*, 2015), cockroach (Brown *et al.*, 2004) and silkworm (Liu *et al.*, 2009). It is very likely that arginine kinase is also an invertebrate pan-allergen like the tropomyosins, although concrete molecular evidence is yet to be revealed.

Effects of Food Processing on Seafood Allergenicity

Fish allergenicity

Methods in food preparation can have highly distinct and profound effects on the allergenicity of food allergens. In western countries, most fish are deep-fried while in Asian countries the fish are often steamed or even eaten in an unprocessed style (e.g., sashimi in Japan). It is important to elucidate the changes in allergenicity with the differences in ways of food processing. The major fish allergen parvalbumin is known to be a heat-stable protein and the allergenicity remains upon cooking or even when combined with high pressure (Arif and Hasnain, 2010; Somkuti *et al.*, 2012). Chatterjee *et al.* (Chatterjee *et al.*, 2006) examined the effect of different heat processing methods (raw, boiled, fried) on the allergenicity of extracts from four fishes, pomfret, hilsa, bhetki and mackerel, and reported that the results were largely species-specific. While raw extracts from all four fishes were allergenic, the allergenicity could be altered differently in each fish upon boiling or frying. Interestingly in some species like the yellow fin tuna, the antibody reactivity to parvalbumin could only be detected in the heated extract but not the raw extract (Sharp *et al.*, 2015). Moreover, Greismeier *et al.* (Griesmeier *et al.*, 2010) reported that the whiff parvalbumin dimerized upon heating and became more resistant to proteolytic digestion, whereas untreated parvalbumins are usually susceptible to gastric or enzymatic digestion (Aas and Elsayed, 1969; Leung *et al.*, 2014; Untersmayr *et al.*, 2005). De Jongh *et al.* (de Jongh *et al.*, 2013) also reported that glycosylated parvalbumin tends to form multimers and exhibits stronger IgE-binding capacity. Hence, the differential effect of food processing on the allergenicity of parvalbumins must be taken into account in designing future therapeutics or diagnostics for parvalbumins.

Shellfish allergenicity

The effect of heating or boiling on the allergenicity of shellfish extracts has been controversial. Samson *et al.* (Samson *et al.*, 2004) reported a higher percentage of shellfish allergic patients possess IgE reactivity to tropomyosin in raw shrimp extracts than to boiled shrimp extracts. In contrast, Carnes *et al.* (Carnes *et al.*, 2007) reported that boiled shrimp extract could induce a larger wheal size in an *in vivo* skin prick test compared to raw shrimp extract. Notably, Liu *et al.* (Liu *et al.*, 2010b) highlighted the difference between allergenic properties of protein extracts or purified tropomyosin in the raw or boiled state. It was found that boiled shrimp extract contained less low and high molecular weight proteins and bound weaker to IgE than the raw extract. However, purified tropomyosin from boiled extract exhibited a higher IgE binding capacity compared to tropomyosin purified from raw extracts. This could be explained by the masking of IgE epitopes on tropomyosin by degraded proteins in boiled extracts. However, the effect of heating or boiling on the allergenicity of purified tropomyosin remains elusive as subsequent studies showed that boiling could either enhance (Kamath *et al.*, 2013), reduce (Long *et al.*, 2015) or have no effect (Usui *et al.*, 2015) on the IgE binding reactivity. These controversial results could be due to the different heating protocol or the antibodies used for reactivity determination. It was also reported that tropomyosin has a high structural versatility that allows refolding of the protein after cooling down from boiling (Usui *et al.*, 2013). Future studies on elucidating the pressure-temperature phase diagram of tropomyosin might help resolve the controversy of the effect of heating on the allergenicity of this major allergen.

Gamez *et al.* (Gamez *et al.*, 2015) reported that pepsin or simulated gastric fluid could readily digest the majority of shrimp proteins, except for the major allergen tropomyosin. Shrimp tropomyosin was reported to be resistant to pepsin and pancreatic digestion despite showing decreased allergenicity with increased digestion time (Gamez *et al.*, 2015; Toomer *et al.*, 2015). It was also shown that tropomyosins from shrimp and crab were not degraded by Simulated Gastric Fluid (SGF) or Simulated Intestinal Fluid (SIF), although a longer digestion time could reduce their allergenicity (Huang *et al.*, 2010; Liu *et al.*, 2010a; Liu *et al.*, 2011a). The digestibility of tropomyosins could also be enhanced by prior treatment with heat, ultrasound and high-pressure steam (Jin *et al.*, 2015; Yu *et al.*, 2011). These studies could inspire a comprehensive method to alleviate the allergenicity of tropomyosin or other shellfish allergens.

Methods for Detection of Seafood Allergens

Fish allergens

Since fish is one of the "big eight" allergenic food, labeling of fish ingredients on the package is mandatory in many developed countries. In order to abide with enforced food labeling, it is important to develop fast and effective assays to detect the presence of potential allergens in food. Currently, DNA and protein detection assays are commonly used in detecting food allergens. DNA detection assays, mostly PCR-based, can detect the presence of genetic materials of the allergenic food and serve as the surrogate of the allergenic protein. Several PCR-based methods have been proposed for the detection of fish major allergen parvalbumin (Hildebrandt, 2010; Sun *et al.*, 2009; Unterberger *et al.*, 2014). The advantage of PCR-based methods is that the DNA probes can be specifically designed for each species. Protein-based assays are mostly immunoassays that make use of anti-parvalbumin monoclonal antibodies (Chen *et al.*, 2006; Faeste and Plassen, 2008; Lopata *et al.*, 2005; Taylor *et al.*, 2000). In addition to conventional methods like the sandwich ELISA, immobilized anti-parvalbumin antibodies have also been used together with superparamagnetic nanoparticle (Zheng *et al.*, 2012) and surface plasmon resonance biosensor (Lu *et al.*, 2004) for the detection of fish parvalbumins. Carrera *et al.* (Carrera *et al.*, 2012) developed a method based on ion monitoring mass spectrometry that detects a number of peptide markers derived from trypsin digestion of parvalbumin. Both DNA- and protein-based approaches can detect effectively the presence of fish parvalbumins and show little cross-reactivity to irrelevant species.

Shellfish allergens

The labeling of shellfish ingredients is compulsory in food labeling in the United States and European Union member states. Unfortunately, the detection of shellfish allergens in food seems to lag behind the fish allergen tests. PCR-based methods have been developed for detecting the presence of shellfish in processed food (Eischeid, 2016; Eischeid *et al.*, 2013; Herrero *et al.*, 2012; Taguchi *et al.*, 2011; Unterberger *et al.*, 2014). Unlike the fish detection tests where the DNA probes are parvalbumin-specific, the probes for shellfish mainly target mitochondrial DNA with no relevance to the shellfish allergens. There are also protein-based assays that mostly make use of the sandwich ELISA method (Jeoung *et al.*, 1997; Kamath *et al.*, 2014; Seiki *et al.*, 2007; Zhang *et al.*, 2014) and mass spectrometry (Abdel Rahman *et al.*, 2012; Abdel Rahman *et al.*, 2013). Koizumi *et al.* (Koizumi *et al.*, 2014) recently developed a lateral flow assay for the detection of crustacean tropomyosin, which can be done in 20 minutes without the need of sophisticated equipment. By detecting the allergenic protein itself, protein-based methods could better predict the potential allergenicity of the food. However, as previously discussed, tropomyosins are highly conserved across crustaceans and mollusks and the monoclonal antibodies applied in the protein-based assays might not be able to distinguish different groups of shellfish. This could impose certain limitations as food labels often require the type of crustaceans specified. It might be interesting to use both approaches as a complementary strategy to obtain the best results. The current methods for detection of seafood allergens are summarized in Table 5.2.

Animal Models of Seafood Allergy

Fish allergy

Animal models are valuable tools to improve clinical management of seafood allergy disorders, by dissecting the immunopathological mechanisms of food allergies, as well as identifying and validating novel preventive and therapeutic strategies that cannot be performed on human subjects. However, we should note that the mechanisms underlying the breach of oral tolerance in food allergic subjects are still unclear. In most animal models of food allergy, Th2-promoting adjuvants are needed to establish these isomorphic food allergy models.

Despite the extensive characterization of fish allergens, a "true" murine model of fish allergy is not yet available. Only a murine model for investigating the role of antacids in the pathophysiology of fish allergy was reported (Untersmayr *et al.*, 2003). Briefly, BALB/c mice were intragastrically

Table 5.2: Methods for detection of seafood allergens.

	Method	Species	Probe/Target	Sensitivity	Specificity/Cross-reactivity	References
DNA-based	Real-time PCR	Fish	Universal fish parvalbumin	5 pg of DNA extracts	No reported cross-reactivity	Sun et al., 2009
	xMAP technology	Fish	Species-specific parvalbumin	0.01–0.04% of weight in processed food		Hildebrandt, 2010
	Ligation-dependent probe amplification	Crustacean, mollusk, fish	Species-specific genes (H3, tropomyosin, parvalbumin)	20–100 mg kg^{-1} processed food	Cross-reactivity with plant family Apiacea	Unterberger et al., 2014
	PCR + post-amplification digestion	Shrimp and crab	Species-specific 16S rRNA	5 pg of DNA extracts; 10 ppm of processed food	Cross-reactivity with other non-target crustaceans	Taguchi et al., 2011
	Real-time PCR	Crustacean	Crustacean-specific 16S rRNA	12.5 pg DNA extracts	No reported cross-reactivity	Herrero et al., 2012
	Real-time PCR	Shrimp and crab	Shrimp 12S and 16S rRNA; Crab COI and cyt-b	0.1–1 ppm in processed food	Low cross-reactivity with other crustaceans; Shrimp 12S rRNA cross-react with blue crab	Eischeid et al., 2013
	Real-time PCR	Lobster	Lobster-specific 12S rRNA	0.1–1 ppm in processed food	No reported cross-reactivity	Eischeid et al., 2016
Protein-based	Inhibition radioimmunoassay	Fish (aerosolized allergens)	IgE from fish-sensitive patients	2 ng	No reported cross-reactivity	Taylor et al., 2000
	Inhibition ELISA	Fish (aerosolized allergens)	Polyclonal rabbit anti-fish extract IgG	0.5 µg/ml		Lopata et al., 2005
	Sandwich ELISA	Fish	Polyclonal rabbit anti-cod parvalbumin IgG	0.01 mg parvalbumin /kg food; 5 mg fish/kg food		Faeste and Plassen, 2008
	Quantitative lateral flow immunoassay	Fish	Monoclonal mouse anti-tuna parvalbumin IgG	5 µg/mL	Other vertebrate parvalbumins	Zheng et al., 2012

Method	Sample	Antibody/Peptide	Detection limit	Cross-reactivity	Reference
Surface plasmon resonance biosensor	Fish	Monoclonal mouse anti-tuna parvalbumin IgG	3.55 µg/L	Other vertebrate parvalbumins	Lu et al., 2004
MS/MS ion monitoring mass spectrometry	Fish (Peptide fragments of digested parvalbumin)	Linear ion trap mass spectrometer	/	No reported cross-reactivity	Carrera et al., 2012
Sandwich ELISA	Shrimp, crab and lobster	Monoclonal mouse anti-shrimp tropomyosin IgG	4 ng/ml	No reported cross-reactivity	Jeoung et al., 1997
Sandwich ELISA	Crustacean	Monoclonal mouse anti-shrimp tropomyosin IgG + Polyclonal rabbit anti-shrimp tropomyosin IgG	1.56 ng/ml	Specific to Decapoda tropomyosins; minor cross-reactivity to other crustaceans and mollusks	Seiki et al., 2007
Sandwich ELISA	Invertebrates	Monoclonal mouse anti-shellfish tropomyosin IgG (raised against C-terminal dominant IgE-binding epitopes of shellfish tropomyosins)	0.09–0.64 ng/ml	No reported cross-reactivity	Zhang et al., 2014
Sandwich ELISA	Crab (aerosolized allergens)	Polyclonal rabbit-anti shrimp tropomyosin IgG	60 pg/mL	Cross-reactivity with other invertebrates	Kamath et al., 2014
Tandem mass spectrometry	Crab (aerosolized allergens)	Signature peptides of snow crab tropomyosin and arginine kinase	1 nM	Specific to snow crab tropomyosin and arginine kinase	Abdel Rahman et al., 2010; Abdel Rahman et al., 2012
Tandem mass spectrometry	Shrimp (aerosolized allergens)	Signature peptides for Northern shrimp tropomyosin and arginine kinase	1 nM	Specific to Northern shrimp tropomyosin and arginine kian	Abdel Rahman et al., 2013
Lateral flow assay	Crustacean	Monoclonal mouse anti-shrimp tropomyosin IgG + Polyclonal rabbit anti-shrimp tropomyosin IgG	25 µg/L	Specific to Decapoda tropomyosins; minor cross-reactivity to other crustaceans and mollusks	Koizumi et al., 2014

immunized with caviar extract or the major fish allergen parvalbumin on days 0 and 28 with/without ranitidine hydrochloride, sucralfate or omeprazole. These mice then received oral provocation on day 92 and thereafter evaluated for inflammatory responses. The authors detected a significant increase of caviar- and parvalbumin-specific IgE antibodies only after the first oral immunization on day 28 and elevated counts of mast cells and eosinophils in the gastrointestinal tract after oral protein challenge. This experiment therefore strongly suggests that medication with the above antacids that directly interfere with acid production and peptic digestion could allow the preservation of the native structure of the proteins and therefore increase the risk of IgE-mediated food allergy.

Shellfish allergy

Mouse models of shellfish allergy are, on the other hand, better established. Our laboratory has developed a mouse model of shrimp tropomyosin-induced hypersensitivity (Leung *et al.*, 2008). BALB/c mice were intragastrically sensitized with 0.1 mg recombinant tropomyosin from *Metapenaeus ensis* (rMet e 1) together with 10 µg of cholera toxin as an adjuvant on days 0, 12, 19 and 26, followed by a high dose rMet e 1 challenge (0.5–1 mg) on day 33. In addition to having systemic allergic reactions, elevated levels of serological specific IgE, and increased IL-4, IL-5 and IL-13 in the splenocyte culture supernatants, these mice also displayed a local up-regulated expression of IL-4 and IL-6 in the jejunum 24 hours after tropomyosin challenge. We also reported the regional and temporal differences in the gut upon shrimp tropomyosin sensitization (Lam *et al.*, 2015). Specifically, significant accumulation of mast cells, eosinophils and goblet cells was most obvious in the duodenum, but gradually decreased from the duodenum, jejunum and to the ileum. The number of mast cells and goblet cells, as well as over-expression of mMCP-1 clearly increased 72 hours after challenge compared to 24 hours after challenge, whereas a lower count of eosinophils could be found at 72 hours after challenge. Similar mouse models of tropomyosin induced hypersensitivity have been reported (Capobianco *et al.*, 2008; Guo *et al.*, 2008).

Liu *et al.* (Liu *et al.*, 2012) reported the purification of tropomyosin and arginine kinase from the mud crab *Scylla paramamosain* and the establishment of mouse models for these two allergens. BALB/c mice were intraperitoneally sensitized with 0.1 mg tropomyosin or arginine kinase using Freund's complete adjuvant on days 0, 14 and 21, followed by an intragastric challenge with either of the allergen at 600 µg on day 33. These challenged mice showed allergic symptoms and had elevated levels of histamine, allergen-specific IgE, as well as IL-4, IL-13 and IFN-γ in their splenocyte cultures. The availability of these mouse models of shrimp allergy can greatly facilitate the design and testing of different therapeutic interventions that cannot be performed on human subjects.

Allergen-Specific Immunotherapy (AIT) (See Chapter 7 Aziz Sheikh and Bright Nwaru)

Fish allergy

Hypoallergens are modified allergens with reduced allergenicity that can be used for promoting T cell tolerance and generating blocking antibodies in AIT. A hypoallergen of the major fish allergen parvalbumin was described by Swoboda *et al.* (Swoboda *et al.*, 2007). A previous observation suggested that calcium depletion significantly reduced the IgE-binding capacity of the carp parvalbumin Cyp c 1. The authors, therefore, replaced the acidic amino acids by non-polar alanine residues in the two functional calcium-binding sites of Cyp c 1 (CD and EF domains). Three mutants of Cyp c 1 were constructed, including two single mutants Mut-CD and Mut-EF, as well as one double mutant Mut-CD/EF. A significant conformational change in the purified protein could only be found in the double mutant Mut-CD/EF. This mutant displayed the most significant reduction in IgE reactivity (< 5% reactivity remained) and allergenicity (~ 100-fold reduction) as confirmed by dot immunoblotting, histamine release assay and skin prick test. Mut-CD/EF also retained a strong immunogenicity in inducing Cyp c 1-specific IgG and these IgG antibodies could block 67–76% patient IgE from binding to Cyp c 1.

An important step forward in the management of fish allergy is the initiation of the EU-funded Food Allergy Specific Immunotherapy (FAST) collaborative project in 2008 (Zuidmeer-Jongejan *et al.*, 2012). This project aims at developing safe and effective subcutaneous AIT towards fish allergy using hypoallergenic proteins. Apart from Mut-CD/EF described above, another chemically-modified hypoallergen constructed by glutaraldehyde treatment is also included in this project. The FAST project is divided into three main stages. The first stage involves the production of hypoallergens under good manufacturing practice for clinical use. In this context, the pre-clinical development of Mut-CD/EF was recently reported, in which the mutant exhibited no toxic effects when adsorbed to aluminum hydroxide (Zuidmeer-Jongejan *et al.*, 2015). The second stage of the project will proceed to test the efficacies of the hypoallergen-based subcutaneous therapy in mouse models. The evaluation will be based on *in vivo* parameters such as symptom scores, vascular leakage and immediate skin tests, as well as *in vitro* parameters such as serological antibody levels, cellular responses in spleen and lymph node, histamine level and histological tests in the lung and intestine. The final stage of the project will be Phase I/IIa and Phase IIb clinical trials to determine the safety dosages, tolerability and clinical outcome of the therapy in fish allergic subjects through double-blinded, placebo-controlled food challenge after AIT. It is anticipated that the FAST project will help in developing strategies to replace avoidance and rescue medication in the clinical management of food allergy in general.

Another AIT candidate for fish allergy is parvalbumin-specific mimotopes (Untersmayr *et al.*, 2006). Mimotopes are peptides mimicking the IgE-binding epitopes of an allergen and possess the capacity to treat allergic disease by inducing blocking antibodies against the native allergens. Through biopanning of phase-display library with purified parvalbumin-specific IgE from fish allergic subjects and further validation by capture ELISA, five most reactive mimotopes were identified (clone 1–YRGVTLAGHR; clone 2–FKGVRLDGTP; clone 3–FRGLDVAGNV; clone 4–AREYGTNRWV and clone 5–YRGARVDGLM). These mimotopes share a high degree of amino acid similarity and correspond to three major epitope areas on parvalbumin at AA23–37, 77–79 and 97–94. Most importantly, comparison of these sites to previously located epitopes on cod parvalbumin reveals overlapping areas or a close proximity of the epitopes. Although the current investigation of parvalbumin-specific mimotopes is still at the initial stage of screening and characterization, future reports concerning their therapeutic potential will be exciting.

Shellfish allergy

Compared to fish allergy, there is a more diverse exploration on potential therapeutic vaccines targeting at shellfish allergy. Reese *et al.* (Reese *et al.*, 2005) introduced a hypoallergen of the shrimp tropomyosin Pen a 1. First, eight IgE-reactive sequences were mapped on Pen a 1 within the five major previously identified reactive regions (Ayuso *et al.*, 2002). Combinatorial substitution analysis was then performed to determine critical IgE binding amino acid residues within these sequences. Based on the above results, a Pen a 1 mutant, VR9-1, was generated by site-directed mutagenesis at 12 amino acid positions. The allergenicity of VR9-1 was reduced by 10- to 40-fold, calculated as the increase in VR9-1 concentration needed to induce 50% of the maximal release on Pen a 1 determined in a mediator release assay using humanized RBL-30/25. However, the maximal release by VR9-1 was often similar to that of Pen a 1, suggesting the presence of other IgE-reactive epitopes, and/or that the substitutions were not sufficient to markedly abolish the allergenicity of the mutant. These, therefore, limit the subsequent use of this VR9-1 mutant as AIT candidate vaccine.

Recently, our laboratory has extensively investigated an array of potential AIT vaccines, which are highlighted below. Wai *et al.* (Wai *et al.*, 2014) have reported the design of two hypoallergens of Met e 1. The first hypoallergen was constructed by comparing the nine major IgE-binding epitopes of Met e 1 to the homologous tropomyosin sequences of four edible fish species (Atlantic salmon, orange-spotted grouper, Mandarin fish and Atlantic blue-fin tuna). Forty-nine amino acid residues within these epitopes were found to differ and then point mutations were introduced into these sites to generate the first mutant MEM49. The second mutant MED171, on the other hand, was constructed by deleting all the nine IgE-binding epitopes of Met e 1, thus generating a smaller protein with only 171 amino acid residues. Both MEM49 and MED171 had a significant reduction (> 70%) in their *in vitro* IgE reactivity and *in vivo* allergenicity in passive cutaneous anaphylaxis assay and immunization experiments. Sera of MEM49- or MED171-immunized mice also contained Met e 1-recognizing IgG antibodies, in particular, the IgG_{2a} isotype that was validated to have a blocking ability against IgE of shrimp allergic subjects and Met e 1-sensitized BALB/c mice. Such capacity in inducing blocking antibody makes MEM49 and MED171 the desired AIT modulators since the antibodies induced by these hypoallergens can act against allergic reactions in a fast-responding manner (Wai *et al.*, 2015). Presently, our work is extended to evaluate the prophylactic and therapeutic effects of these hypoallergens when they are delivered in the form of DNA vaccines.

The second candidate is T cell epitopes of the shrimp tropomyosin Met e 1 (Wai *et al.*, 2016). Six major T cell epitopes of Met e 1 (T1–T6, AA26–45, 56–75, 86–105, 146–165, 221–240 and 251–270) were mapped by both proliferation and cytokine assays using spleen cells from BALB/c mice orally sensitized to Met e 1. These respective sequences are in consensus with the reactive regions mapped on Pen a 1 using T cell lines generated from shrimp allergic subjects (Ravkov *et al.*, 2013). Oral administration of a mixture of these T cell epitope peptides remarkably suppressed Th2 allergic responses to shrimp tropomyosin, including a reduction in the severity of systemic allergic symptoms, the level of Met e 1-specific IgE, levels of IL-4 and IL-5 in the splenocyte culture and expression of IL-5 and IL-13 in the ileum. Apart from the restoration of the Th1/Th2 immune balance, the induction of Treg-like responses and synthesis of IgG_{2a} antibody that possesses both *in vitro* and *in vivo* blocking abilities were also present in the T cell peptide-treated mice. These results strongly suggest the great immunotherapeutic potential of these epitope peptides and further optimization will certainly advance their clinical use for the treatment of shellfish allergy disorders.

A third candidate vaccine is tropomyosin-specific mimotopes. We reported the use of a One-Bead-One-Compound (OBOC) combinatorial peptide library in identifying 25 mimotopes that correspond to six IgE-reactive regions of the shrimp tropomyosin Met e 1 (Leung *et al.*, 2017). Immunization of BALB/c mice with six of these mimotopes induced Met e 1-specific IgG antibody, suggesting not only the mimicry ability of these mimotopes, but also the potential of these mimotopes in inducing blocking IgG antibody when employed in AIT (Leung *et al.*, 2015). Currently, the therapeutic efficacy of a mimotope cocktail is under investigation. Illustration of novel strategies for AIT is summarized in Fig. 5.1.

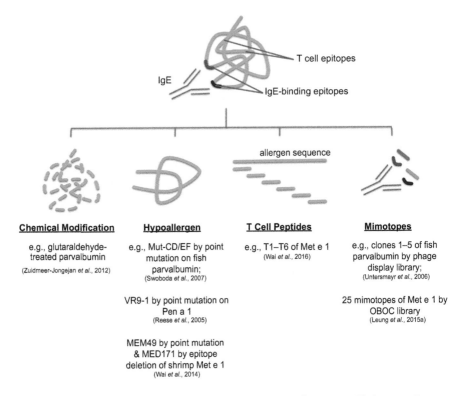

Chemical Modification

e.g., glutaraldehyde-
treated parvalbumin
(Zuidmeer-Jongejan *et al.*, 2012)

Hypoallergen

e.g., Mut-CD/EF by point
mutation on fish
parvalbumin;
(Swoboda *et al.*, 2007)

VR9-1 by point mutation on
Pen a 1
(Reese *et al.*, 2005)

MEM49 by point mutation
& MED171 by epitope
deletion of shrimp Met e 1
(Wai *et al.*, 2014)

T Cell Peptides

e.g., T1–T6 of Met e 1
(Wai *et al.*, 2016)

Mimotopes

e.g., clones 1–5 of fish
parvalbumin by phage
display library;
(Untersmayr *et al.*, 2006)

25 mimotopes of Met e 1 by
OBOC library
(Leung *et al.*, 2015a)

Fig. 5.1: Schematic illustration of four different strategies in allergen-specific immunotherapy for seafood allergy. These strategies include the direct chemical modification of the allergen, the design of hypoallergens, T cell peptides and allergen-specific mimotopes.

Alternative Treatments of Seafood Allergy

Probiotics

Other than the allergen-specific therapies discussed above, non-allergen specific treatments have also been evaluated for tackling against fish and shellfish allergies. The use of probiotic VSL#3 represents an example of these treatments (Schiavi *et al.*, 2011). This probiotic preparation contains a high concentration of eight live freeze-dried Gram-positive bacteria species, including *Lactobacillus acidophilus, L. delbrueckii* subsp. *bulgaricus, L. casei, L. plantarum, Bifadobacterium longum, B. infantis, B. breve* and *Streptococcus salvarius* subsp. *thermophilus*. Shrimp tropomyosin sensitized- and challenged-C3H/HeJ mice were orally treated with 50 µl of VSL#3 that correspond to 7.5 x 10^8 bacteria daily for three weeks. On the second shrimp tropomyosin challenge, the anaphylactic symptom scores, levels of fecal histamine and serological IgE, as well as Th2 cytokine expression in jejunum were significantly reduced. In addition, there was also a significant increase in the level of fecal IgA and serological IgG_{2a} antibodies. Such microbial-mediated therapeutic effects might be a result of the interaction between microbial products with toll-like receptors that fine-tune the expression of IL-12, thereby modulating Th2 cells-mediated inflammation.

Herbal medicine

Chinese medicine has a long history of human use and a Food Allergy Herbal Formula-2 (FAHF-2) containing nine herbal extracts was developed by Wu Mei Wan for treating parasitic infection and food allergy-like symptoms (Bensky and Barolet, 1990). Srivastava *et al.* (Srivastava *et al.*, 2012) tested the efficacy of this formula in C3H/HeJ mice concurrently sensitized to codfish, peanut and egg. The mice were sensitized to 2.5 mg protein per each homogenized food, followed by two boosts with 12.5 mg protein. Mice were then orally treated with 27 mg FAHF-2 in 0.5 ml drinking water twice a day for 7 weeks and received a separate food challenge. Unlike the untreated mice showing obvious allergic symptoms and decrease in body temperature on fish protein challenge, FAHF-2-treated mice were protected from these reactions and had persistent decrease in IgE but increase in IgG_{2a} level at 14 weeks post-therapy. Although the levels of Th2 cytokines were decreased in both the cultured splenocytes and mesenteric lymph node cells, only IFN-γ but not TGF-β level was found enhanced. These data suggest that the redirecting action by FAHF-2 is Th1-rather than Treg-mediated.

This herbal formula was put into Phase I studies to study its safety and efficacy (Patil *et al.*, 2011). Eighteen patients with multiple food allergies to peanut, tree nut, fish or shellfish were recruited and instructed to take six tablets of FAHF-2 (3.3 g) three times per day for 6 months. Throughout the treatment, no patient reported any food-induced allergic reactions, suggesting the high safety profile and tolerability of FAHF-2. Recipients also had significant reduction in their basophil activity and percentage of circulating basophils after 4 to 6 months of therapy. A Phase II study has been planned and future reports are awaited to ensure the immunological effects of this herbal formulation.

Summary

1. A number of fish and shellfish allergens have been identified in the past two decades in addition to the major allergens parvalbumin and tropomyosin. While the molecular identities of these novel allergens are well documented, their allergenic properties remain largely elusive. Further characterization of these novel allergens could help elucidate the sensitization pattern and improve the accuracy of diagnostic tests.

2. The effects of different food processing methods on the allergenicity of seafood allergens have been studied extensively, but the results from different studies using different species are often contradicting. The

contradicting results could be due to the different treatment methods, but the possibility of differential species-specific properties should not be overlooked.

3. DNA- and protein-based detection assays are commonly used in detecting food allergens and both methods have their own advantages and disadvantages. DNA detection methods are species-specific but may detect targets that are irrelevant to the allergen itself, while protein detection methods are allergen-specific but often demonstrate significant cross-reactivity with other irrelevant species. Both methods may be used in a complementary for the detection of food allergens.

4. Animal models of seafood allergies are valuable tools for evaluating different therapeutic strategies and facilitate the development of novel AIT strategies. Hypoallergens of parvalbumin and tropomyosin have been designed for use in AIT and exhibit exciting potential as a safe and effective treatment in the mouse models. It is expected that a safe and effective immunotherapy for treating seafood allergy will come to life rather sooner than later.

Acknowledgements

The work on seafood allergy of the authors was supported by grants from the Research Grants Council (CUHK 463911) and the Health and Medical Research Fund (02130206), Hong Kong Special Administrative Region, China.

Keywords: Allergen-specific immunotherapy, cross-reactivity, hypoallergen, mimotope, parvalbumin, T cell epitope, tropomyosin

References

Aadland, E. K., Lavigne, C., Graff, I. E., Eng, O., Paquette, M., Holthe, A., Mellgren, G., Jacques, H., and Liaset, B. (2015). Lean-seafood intake reduces cardiovascular lipid risk factors in healthy subjects: results from a randomized controlled trial with a crossover design. The American Journal of Clinical Nutrition 102(3): 582–592.

Aas, K. (1969). Antigens and allergens of fish. International Archives of Allergy and Applied Immunology 36(1): 152–155.

Aas, K., and Elsayed, S. M. (1969). Characterization of a major allergen (cod). Effect of enzymic hydrolysis on the allergenic activity. The Journal of Allergy 44(6): 333–343.

Abdel Rahman, A. M., Kamath, S. D., Lopata, A. L., Robinson, J. J., and Helleur, R. J. (2011). Biomolecular characterization of allergenic proteins in snow crab (*Chionoecetes opilio*) and *de novo* sequencing of the second allergen arginine kinase using tandem mass spectrometry. Journal of Proteomics 74(2): 231–241.

Abdel Rahman, A. M., Gagne, S., and Helleur, R. J. (2012). Simultaneous determination of two major snow crab aeroallergens in processing plants by use of isotopic dilution tandem mass spectrometry. Analytical and Bioanalytical Chemistry 403(3): 821–831.

Abdel Rahman, A. M., Kamath, S. D., Gagne, S., Lopata, A. L., and Helleur, R. (2013). Comprehensive proteomics approach in characterizing and quantifying allergenic proteins from northern shrimp: toward better occupational asthma prevention. Journal of Proteome Research 12(2): 647–656.

Arif, S. H. (2009). A Ca^{2+}-binding protein with numerous roles and uses: parvalbumin in molecular biology and physiology. BioEssays: News and Reviews in Molecular, Cellular and Developmental Biology 31(4): 410–421.

Arif, S. H., and Hasnain, A. (2010). A major cross-reactive fish allergen with exceptional stability: parvalbumin. African Journal of Food Science 4(3): 109–114.

Ayuso, R., Lehrer, S. B., and Reese, G. (2002). Identification of continuous, allergenic regions of the major shrimp allergen Pen a 1 (tropomyosin). International Archives of Allergy and Immunology 127(1): 27–37.

Ayuso, R., Grishina, G., Bardina, L., Carrillo, T., Blanco, C., Ibanez, M. D., Sampson, H. A., and Beyer, K. (2008). Myosin light chain is a novel shrimp allergen, Lit v 3. The Journal of Allergy and Clinical Immunology 122(4): 795–802.

Ayuso, R., Grishina, G., Ibanez, M. D., Blanco, C., Carrillo, T., Bencharitiwong, R., Sanchez, S., Nowak-Wegrzyn, A., and Sampson, H. A. (2009). Sarcoplasmic calcium-binding protein is an EF-hand-type protein identified as a new shrimp allergen. The Journal of Allergy and Clinical Immunology 124(1): 114–120.

Bauermeister, K., Wangorsch, A., Garoffo, L. P., Reuter, A., Conti, A., Taylor, S. L., Lidholm, J., Dewitt, A. M., Enrique, E., Vieths, S., Holzhauser, T., Ballmer-Weber, B., and Reese, G. (2011). Generation of a comprehensive panel of crustacean allergens from the North Sea Shrimp *Crangon crangon*. Molecular Immunology 48(15-16): 1983–1992.

Bensky, D., and Barolet, R. (1990). Chinese Herbal Medicine: Formulas and Strategies. Seattle: Eastland Press.

Bourre, J. M., and Paquotte, P. (2008). Seafood (wild and farmed) for the elderly: contribution to the dietary intakes of iodine, selenium, DHA and vitamins B12 and D. The Journal of Nutrition, Health and Aging 12(3): 186–192.

Brown, A. E., France, R. M., and Grossman, S. H. (2004). Purification and characterization of arginine kinase from the American cockroach (*Periplaneta americana*). Archives of Insect Biochemistry and Physiology 56(2): 51–60.

Capobianco, F., Butteroni, C., Barletta, B., Corinti, S., Afferni, C., Tinghino, R., Boirivant, M., and Di Felice, G. (2008). Oral sensitization with shrimp tropomyosin induces in mice allergen-specific IgE, T cell response and systemic anaphylactic reactions. International Immunology 20(8): 1077–1086.

Carnes, J., Ferrer, A., Huertas, A. J., Andreu, C., Larramendi, C. H., and Fernandez-Caldas, E. (2007). The use of raw or boiled crustacean extracts for the diagnosis of seafood allergic individuals. Annals of Allergy, Asthma and Immunology 98(4): 349–354.

Carrera, M., Canas, B., and Gallardo, J. M. (2012). Rapid direct detection of the major fish allergen, parvalbumin, by selected MS/MS ion monitoring mass spectrometry. Journal of Proteomics 75(11): 3211–3220.

Chatterjee, U., Mondal, G., Chakraborti, P., Patra, H. K., and Chatterjee, B. P. (2006). Changes in the allergenicity during different preparations of Pomfret, Hilsa, Bhetki and mackerel fish as illustrated by enzyme-linked immunosorbent assay and immunoblotting. International Archives of Allergy and Immunology 141(1): 1–10.

Chen, L., Hefle, S. L., Taylor, S. L., Swoboda, I., and Goodman, R. E. (2006). Detecting fish parvalbumin with commercial mouse monoclonal anti-frog parvalbumin IgG. Journal of Agricultural and Food Chemistry 54(15): 5577–5582.

Das Dores, S., Chopin, C., Romano, A., Galland-Irmouli, A. V., Quaratino, D., Pascual, C., Fleurence, J., and Gueant, J. L. (2002). IgE-binding and cross-reactivity of a new 41 kDa allergen of codfish. Allergy 57: 84–87.

Daul, C. B., Slattery, M., Reese, G., and Lehrer, S. B. (1994). Identification of the major brown shrimp (*Penaeus aztecus*) allergen as the muscle protein tropomyosin. International Archives of Allergy and Immunology 105(1): 49–55.

de Jongh, H. H., Robles, C. L., Timmerman, E., Nordlee, J. A., Lee, P. W., Baumert, J. L., Hamilton, R. G., Taylor, S. L., and Koppelman, S. J. (2013). Digestibility and IgE-binding of glycosylated codfish parvalbumin. BioMed Research International 2013: 756789.

Eischeid, A. C., Kim, B. H., and Kasko, S. M. (2013). Two quantitative real-time PCR assays for the detection of penaeid shrimp and blue crab, crustacean shellfish allergens. Journal of Agricultural and Food Chemistry 61(24): 5669–5674.

Eischeid, A. C. (2016). Development and evaluation of a real-time PCR assay for detection of lobster, a crustacean shellfish allergen. Food Control 59: 393–399.

Elsayed, S., and Apold, J. (1983). Immunochemical analysis of cod fish allergen M: locations of the immunoglobulin binding sites as demonstrated by the native and synthetic peptides. Allergy 38(7): 449–459.

Elsayed, S. M., and Aas, K. (1970). Characterization of a major allergen (cod.) chemical composition and immunological properties. International Archives of Allergy and Applied Immunology 38(5): 536–548.

F.A.O. (2016). The State of World Fisheries and Aquaculture 2016.

Faeste, C. K., and Plassen, C. (2008). Quantitative sandwich ELISA for the determination of fish in foods. Journal of Immunological Methods 329(1-2): 45–55.

Gamez, C., Zafra, M. P., Sanz, V., Mazzeo, C., Ibanez, M. D., Sastre, J., and del Pozo, V. (2015). Simulated gastrointestinal digestion reduces the allergic reactivity of shrimp extract proteins and tropomyosin. Food Chemistry 173: 475–481.

Garcia-Orozco, K. D., Aispuro-Hernandez, E., Yepiz-Plascencia, G., Calderon-de-la-Barca, A. M., and Sotelo-Mundo, R. R. (2007). Molecular characterization of arginine kinase, an allergen from the shrimp *Litopenaeus vannamei*. International Archives of Allergy and Immunology 144(1): 23–28.

Griesmeier, U., Bublin, M., Radauer, C., Vazquez-Cortes, S., Ma, Y., Fernandez-Rivas, M., and Breiteneder, H. (2010). Physicochemical properties and thermal stability of Lep w 1, the major allergen of whiff. Molecular Nutrition and Food Research 54(6): 861–869.

Guo, Y., Li, Z., and Lin, H. (2008). Mouse model in food allergy: dynamic determination of shrimp allergenicity. African Journal of Biotechnology 7(18): 3352–3356.

Hajeb, P., and Selamat, J. (2012). A contemporary review of seafood allergy. Clinical Reviews in Allergy and Immunology 42(3): 365–385.

Hamada, Y., Nagashima, Y., and Shiomi, K. (2001). Identification of collagen as a new fish allergen. Bioscience, Biotechnology, and Biochemistry 65(2): 285–291.

Herrero, B., Vieites, J. M., and Espineira, M. (2012). Fast real-time PCR for the detection of crustacean allergen in foods. Journal of Agricultural and Food Chemistry 60(8): 1893–1897.

Hildebrandt, S. (2010). Multiplexed identification of different fish species by detection of parvalbumin, a common fish allergen gene: a DNA application of multi-analyte profiling (xMAP) technology. Analytical and Bioanalytical Chemistry 397(5): 1787–1796.

Huang, Y. Y., Liu, G. M., Cai, Q. F., Weng, W. Y., Maleki, S. J., Su, W. J., and Cao, M. J. (2010). Stability of major allergen tropomyosin and other food proteins of mud crab (*Scylla serrata*) by *in vitro* gastrointestinal digestion. Food and Chemical Toxicology 48(5): 1196–1201.

Jacobs, S., Sioen, I., Pieniak, Z., De Henauw, S., Maulvault, A. L., Reuver, M., Fait, G., Cano-Sancho, G., and Verbeke, W. (2015). Consumers' health risk-benefit perception of seafood and attitude toward the marine environment: Insights from five European countries. Environmental Research 143: 11–19.

Jeoung, B. J., Reese, G., Hauck, P., Oliver, J. B., Daul, C. B., and Lehrer, S. B. (1997). Quantification of the major brown shrimp allergen Pen a 1 (tropomyosin) by a monoclonal antibody-based sandwich ELISA. The Journal of Allergy and Clinical Immunology 100(2): 229–234.

Jin, Y., Deng, Y., Qian, B., Zhang, Y., Liu, Z., and Zhao, Y. (2015). Allergenic response to squid (*Todarodes pacificus*) tropomyosin Tod p 1 structure modifications induced by high hydrostatic pressure. Food and Chemical Toxicology 76: 86–93.

Kalyanasundaram, A., and Santiago, T. C. (2015). Identification and characterization of new allergen troponin C (Pen m 6.0101) from Indian black tiger shrimp *Penaeus monodon*. European Food Research Technology 240(3): 509–515.

Kamath, S. D., Abdel Rahman, A. M., Komoda, T., and Lopata, A. L. (2013). Impact of heat processing on the detection of the major shellfish allergen tropomyosin in crustaceans and molluscs using specific monoclonal antibodies. Food Chemistry 141(4): 4031–4039.

Kamath, S. D., Thomassen, M. R., Saptarshi, S. R., Nguyen, H. M., Aasmoe, L., Bang, B. E., and Lopata, A. L. (2014). Molecular and immunological approaches in quantifying the air-borne food allergen tropomyosin in crab processing facilities. International Journal of Hygiene and Environmental Health 217(7): 740–750.

Koizumi, D., Shirota, K., Akita, R., Oda, H., and Akiyama, H. (2014). Development and validation of a lateral flow assay for the detection of crustacean protein in processed foods. Food Chemistry 150: 348–352.

Kuehn, A., Hilger, C., Lehners-Weber, C., Codreanu-Morel, F., Morisset, M., Metz-Favre, C., Pauli, G., de Blay, F., Revets, D., Muller, C. P., Vogel, L., Vieths, S., and Hentges, F. (2013). Identification of enolases and aldolases as important fish allergens in cod, salmon and tuna: component resolved diagnosis using parvalbumin and the new allergens. Clinical and Experimental Allergy 43(7): 811–822.

Lam, Y. F., Tong, K. K., Kwan, K. M., Tsuneyama, K., Shu, S. A., Leung, P. S., and Chu, K. H. (2015). Gastrointestinal immune response to the shrimp allergen tropomyosin: Histological and immunological analysis in an animal model of shrimp tropomyosin hypersensitivity. International Archives of Allergy and Immunology 167(1): 29–40.

Leung, N. Y., Wai, C. Y., Shu, S., Wang, J., Kenny, T. P., Chu, K. H., and Leung, P. S. (2014). Current immunological and molecular biological perspectives on seafood allergy: a comprehensive review. Clinical Reviews in Allergy and Immunology 46(3): 180–197.

Leung, N. Y., Wai, C. Y., Ho, M. H., Liu, R., Lam, K. S., Wang, J. J., Shu, S. A., Chu, K. H., and Leung, P. S. (2017). Screening and identification of mimotopes of the major shrimp allergen tropomyosin using one-bead-one-compound peptide libraries. Cellular and Molecular Immunology 17: 308–318.

Leung, N. Y., Wai, C. Y., Leung, P. S., and Chu, K. H. (2015). Mimotopes of the major shellfish allergen tropomyosin suppress splenocyte proliferation and local cytokine expression in a mouse model of shellfish allergy. Paper Presented at the World Allergy Congress, Seoul, Korea.

Leung, P. S., Chu, K. H., Chow, W. K., Ansari, A., Bandea, C. I., Kwan, H. S., Nagy, S. M., and Gershwin, M. E. (1994). Cloning, expression, and primary structure of *Metapenaeus ensis* tropomyosin, the major heat-stable shrimp allergen. The Journal of Allergy and Clinical Immunology 94(5): 882–890.

Leung, P. S., Lee, Y. S., Tang, C. Y., Kung, W. Y., Chuang, Y. H., Chiang, B. L., Fung, M. C., and Chu, K. H. (2008). Induction of shrimp tropomyosin-specific hypersensitivity in mice. International Archives of Allergy and Immunology 147(4): 305–314.

Liu, Z., Xia, L., Wu, Y., Xia, Q., Chen, J., and Roux, K. H. (2009). Identification and characterization of an arginine kinase as a major allergen from silkworm (*Bombyx mori*) larvae. International Archives of Allergy and Immunology 150(1): 8–14.

Liu, G. M., Cao, M. J., Huang, Y. Y., Cai, Q. F., Weng, W. Y., and Su, W. J. (2010a). Comparative study of *in vitro* digestibility of major allergen tropomyosin and other food proteins of Chinese mitten crab (*Eriocheir sinensis*). Journal of the Science of Food and Agriculture 90(10): 1614–1620.

Liu, G. M., Cheng, H., Nesbit, J. B., Su, W. J., Cao, M. J., and Maleki, S. J. (2010b). Effects of boiling on the IgE-binding properties of tropomyosin of shrimp (*Litopenaeus vannamei*). Journal of Food Science 75(1): T1–5.

Liu, G. M., Huang, Y. Y., Cai, Q. F., Weng, W. Y., Su, W. J., and Cao, M. J. (2011a). Comparative study of *in vitro* digestibility of major allergen, tropomyosin and other proteins between Grass prawn (*Penaeus monodon*) and Pacific white shrimp (*Litopenaeus vannamei*). Journal of the Science of Food and Agriculture 91(1): 163–170.

Liu, R., Krishnan, H. B., Xue, W., and Liu, C. (2011b). Characterization of allergens isolated from the freshwater fish blunt snout bream (*Megalobrama amblycephala*). Journal of Agricultural and Food Chemistry 59(1): 458–463.

Liu, G. M., Li, B., Yu, H. L., Cao, M. J., Cai, Q. F., Lin, J. W., and Su, W. J. (2012). Induction of mud crab (*Scylla paramamosain*) tropomyosin and arginine kinase specific hypersensitivity in BALB/c mice. Journal of the Science of Food and Agriculture 92(2): 232–238.

Liu, R., Holck, A. L., Yang, E., Liu, C., and Xue, W. (2013). Tropomyosin from tilapia (*Oreochromis mossambicus*) as an allergen. Clinical and Experimental Allergy 43(3): 365–377.

Long, F., Yang, X., Wang, R., Hu, X., and Chen, F. (2015). Effects of combined high pressure and thermal treatments on the allergenic potential of shrimp (*Litopenaeus vannamei*) tropomyosin in a mouse model of allergy. Innovative Food Science and emerging Technologies 29: 119–124.

Lopata, A. L., Jeebhay, M. F., Reese, G., Fernandes, J., Swoboda, I., Robins, T. G., and Lehrer, S. B. (2005). Detection of fish antigens aerosolized during fish processing using newly developed immunoassays. International Archives of Allergy and Immunology 138(1): 21–28.

Lopata, A. L., and Lehrer, S. B. (2009). New insights into seafood allergy. Current Opinion in Allergy and Clinical Immunology 9(3): 270–277.

Lu, Y., Ohshima, T., and Ushio, H. (2004). Rapid detection of fish major allergen parvalbumin by surface plasmon resonance biosensor. Journal of Food Science 69(8): 652–658.

Lund, E. K. (2013). Health benefits of seafood; is it just the fatty acids? Food Chemistry 140(3): 413–420.

Nelson, H. S., Lahr, J., Rule, R., Bock, A., and Leung, D. (1997). Treatment of anaphylactic sensitivity to peanuts by immunotherapy with injections of aqueous peanut extract. The Journal of Allergy and Clinical Immunology 99: 744–751.

Patil, S. P., Wang, J., Song, Y., Noone, S., Yang, N., Wallenstein, S., Sampson, H. A., and Li, X. M. (2011). Clinical safety of Food Allergy Herbal Formula-2 (FAHF-2) and inhibitory effect on basophils from patients with food allergy: Extended phase I study. The Journal of Allergy and Clinical Immunology 128(6): 1259–1265.

Perez-Gordo, M., Sanchez-Garcia, S., Cases, B., Pastor, C., Vivanco, F., and Cuesta-Herranz, J. (2008). Identification of vitellogenin as an allergen in Beluga caviar allergy. Allergy 63(4): 479–480.

Perez-Gordo, M., Lin, J., Bardina, L., Pastor-Vargas, C., Cases, B., Vivanco, F., Cuesta-Herranz, J., and Sampson, H. A. (2012). Epitope mapping of Atlantic salmon major allergen by peptide microarray immunoassay. International Archives of Allergy and Immunology 157(1): 31–40.

Piboonpocanun, S., Jirapongsananuruk, O., Tipayanon, T., Boonchoo, S., and Goodman, R. E. (2011). Identification of hemocyanin as a novel non-cross-reactive allergen from the giant freshwater shrimp *Macrobrachium rosenbergii*. Molecular Nutrition and Food Research 55(10): 1492–1498.

Ravkov, E. V., Pavlov, I. Y., Martins, T. B., Gleich, G. J., Wagner, L. A., Hill, H. R., and Delgado, J. C. (2013). Identification and validation of shrimp-tropomyosin specific CD4 T cell epitopes. Human Immunology 74(12): 1542–1549.

Reese, G., Viebranz, J., Leong-Kee, S. M., Plante, M., Lauer, I., Randow, S., Moncin, M. S., Ayuso, R., Lehrer, S. B., and Vieths, S. (2005). Reduced allergenic potency of VR9-1, a mutant of the major shrimp allergen Pen a 1 (tropomyosin). Journal of Immunology 175(12): 8354–8364.

Rona, R. J., Keil, T., Summers, C., Gislason, D., Zuidmeer, L., Sodergren, E., Sigurdardottir, S. T., Lindner, T., Goldhahn, K., Dahlstrom, J., McBride, D., and Madsen, C. (2007). The prevalence of food allergy: a meta-analysis. The Journal of Allergy and Clinical Immunology 120(3): 638–646.

Rosmilah, M., Shahnaz, M., Zailatul, H. M., Noormalin, A., and Normilah, I. (2012). Identification of tropomyosin and arginine kinase as major allergens of *Portunus pelagicus* (blue swimming crab). Tropical Biomedicine 29(3): 467–478.

Ross, M. P., Ferguson, M., Street, D., Klontz, K., Schroeder, T., and Luccioli, S. (2008). Analysis of food-allergic and anaphylactic events in the National Electronic Injury Surveillance System. The Journal of Allergy and Clinical Immunology 121(1): 166–171.

Sakaguchi, M., Toda, M., Ebihara, T., Irie, S., Hori, H., Imai, A., Yanagida, M., Miyazawa, H., Ohsuna, H., Ikezawa, Z., and Inouye, S. (2000). IgE antibody to fish gelatin (type I collagen) in patients with fish allergy. The Journal of Allergy and Clinical Immunology 106(3): 579–584.

Samson, K. T., Chen, F. H., Miura, K., Odajima, Y., Iikura, Y., Naval Rivas, M., Minoguchi, K., and Adachi, M. (2004). IgE binding to raw and boiled shrimp proteins in atopic and nonatopic patients with adverse reactions to shrimp. International Archives of Allergy and Immunology 133(3): 225–232.

Saptarshi, S. R., Sharp, M. F., Kamath, S. D., and Lopata, A. L. (2014). Antibody reactivity to the major fish allergen parvalbumin is determined by isoforms and impact of thermal processing. Food Chemistry 148: 321–328.

Schiavi, E., Barletta, B., Butteroni, C., Corinti, S., Boirivant, M., and Di Felice, G. (2011). Oral therapeutic administration of a probiotic mixture suppresses established Th2 responses and systemic anaphylaxis in a murine model of food allergy. Allergy 66(4): 499–508.

Seiki, K., Oda, H., Yoshioka, H., Sakai, S., Urisu, A., Akiyama, H., and Ohno, Y. (2007). A reliable and sensitive immunoassay for the determination of crustacean protein in processed foods. Journal of Agricultural and Food Chemistry 55(23): 9345–9350.

Shanti, K. N., Martin, B. M., Nagpal, S., Metcalfe, D. D., and Rao, P. V. (1993). Identification of tropomyosin as the major shrimp allergen and characterization of its IgE-binding epitopes. Journal of Immunology 151(10): 5354–5363.

Sharp, M. F., Kamath, S. D., Koeberl, M., Jerry, D. R., O'Hehir, R. E., Campbell, D. E., and Lopata, A. L. (2014). Differential IgE binding to isoallergens from Asian seabass (*Lates calcarifer*) in children and adults. Molecular Immunology 62(1): 77–85.

Sharp, M. F., and Lopata, A. L. (2014). Fish allergy: in review. Clinical Reviews in Allergy and Immunology 46(3): 258–271.

Sharp, M. F., Stephen, J. N., Kraft, L., Weiss, T., Kamath, S. D., and Lopata, A. L. (2015). Immunological cross-reactivity between four distant parvalbumins-Impact on allergen detection and diagnostics. Molecular Immunology 63(2): 437–448.

Shen, Y., Cao, M. J., Cai, Q. F., Su, W. J., Yu, H. L., Ruan, W. W., and Liu, G. M. (2011). Purification, cloning, expression and immunological analysis of *Scylla serrata* arginine kinase, the crab allergen. Journal of the Science of Food and Agriculture 91(7): 1326–1335.

Shimizu, Y., Kishimura, H., Kanno, G., Nakamura, A., Adachi, R., Akiyama, H., Watanabe, K., Hara, A., Ebisawa, M., and Saeki, H. (2014). Molecular and immunological characterization of β'-component (Onc k 5), a major IgE-binding protein in chum salmon roe. International Immunology 26(3): 139–147.

Shiomi, K., Sato, Y., Hamamoto, S., Mita, H., and Shimakura, K. (2008). Sarcoplasmic calcium-binding protein: identification as a new allergen of the black tiger shrimp *Penaeus monodon*. International Archives of Allergy and Immunology 146(2): 91–98.

Somkuti, J., Bublin, M., Breiteneder, H., and Smeller, L. (2012). Pressure-temperature stability, Ca^{2+} binding, and pressure-temperature phase diagram of cod parvalbumin: Gad m 1. Biochemistry 51(30): 5903–5911.

Srinroch, C., Srisomsap, C., Chokchaichamnankit, D., Punyarit, P., and Phiriyangkul, P. (2015). Identification of novel allergen in edible insect, *Gryllus bimaculatus* and its cross-reactivity with *Macrobrachium* spp. allergens. Food Chemistry 184: 160–166.

Srivastava, K. D., Bardina, L., Sampson, H. A., and Li, X. M. (2012). Efficacy and immunological actions of FAHF-2 in a murine model of multiple food allergies. Annals of Allergy, Asthma and Immunology 108(5): 351–358.

Subba Rao, P. V., Rajagopal, D., and Ganesh, K. A. (1998). B- and T-cell epitopes of tropomyosin, the major shrimp allergen. Allergy 53(46 Suppl): 44–47.

Sun, M., Liang, C., Gao, H., Lin, C., and Deng, M. (2009). Detection of parvalbumin, a common fish allergen gene in food, by real-time polymerase chain reaction. Journal of AOAC International 92(1): 234–240.

Suzuki, M., Kobayashi, Y., Hiraki, Y., Nakata, H., and Shiomi, K. (2011). Paramyosin of the disc abalone *Haliotis discus discus*: identification as a new allergen and cross-reactivity with tropomyosin. Food Chemistry 124: 921–926.

Swoboda, I., Bugajska-Schretter, A., Linhart, B., Verdino, P., Keller, W., Schulmeister, U., Sperr, W. R., Valent, P., Peltre, G., Quirce, S., Douladiris, N., Papadopoulos, N. G., Valenta, R., and Spitzauer, S. (2007). A recombinant hypoallergenic parvalbumin mutant for immunotherapy of IgE-mediated fish allergy. Journal of Immunology 178(10): 6290–6296.

Taguchi, H., Watanabe, S., Temmei, Y., Hirao, T., Akiyama, H., Sakai, S., Adachi, R., Sakata, K., Urisu, A., and Teshima, R. (2011). Differential detection of shrimp and crab for food labeling using polymerase chain reaction. Journal of Agricultural and Food Chemistry 59(8): 3510–3519.

Taylor, A. V., Swanson, M. C., Jones, R. T., Vives, R., Rodriguez, J., Yunginger, J. W., and Crespo, J. F. (2000). Detection and quantitation of raw fish aeroallergens from an open-air fish market. The Journal of Allergy and Clinical Immunology 105(1 Pt 1): 166–169.

Toomer, O. T., Do, A. B., Fu, T. J., and Williams, K. M. (2015). Digestibility and immunoreactivity of shrimp extracts using an *in vitro* digestibility model with pepsin and pancreatin. Journal of Food Science 80(7): T1633–1639.

Unterberger, C., Luber, F., Denmel, A., Grunwald, K., Huber, I., Engel, K., and Busch, U. (2014). Simultaneous detection of allergenic fish, cephalopods and shellfish in food by multiplex ligation-dependent probe amplification. European Food Research Technology 239(4): 559–566.

Untersmayr, E., Scholl, I., Swoboda, I., Beil, W. J., Forster-Waldl, E., Walter, F., Riemer, A., Kraml, G., Kinaciyan, T., Spitzauer, S., Boltz-Nitulescu, G., Scheiner, O., and Jensen-Jarolim, E. (2003). Antacid medication inhibits digestion of dietary proteins and causes food allergy: a fish allergy model in BALB/c mice. The Journal of Allergy and Clinical Immunology 112(3): 616–623.

Untersmayr, E., Poulsen, L. K., Platzer, M. H., Pedersen, M. H., Boltz-Nitulescu, G., Skov, P. S., and Jensen-Jarolim, E. (2005). The effects of gastric digestion on codfish allergenicity. The Journal of Allergy and Clinical Immunology 115(2): 377–382.

Untersmayr, E., Szalai, K., Riemer, A. B., Hemmer, W., Swoboda, I., Hantusch, B., Scholl, I., Spitzauer, S., Scheiner, O., Jarisch, R., Boltz-Nitulescu, G., and Jensen-Jarolim, E. (2006). Mimotopes identify conformational epitopes on parvalbumin, the major fish allergen. Molecular Immunology 43(9): 1454–1461.

Usui, M., Harada, A., Ishimaru, T., Sakumichi, E., Saratani, F., Sato-Minami, C., Azakami, H., Miyasaki, T., and Hanaoka, K. (2013). Contribution of structural reversibility to the heat stability of the tropomyosin shrimp allergen. Bioscience, Biotechnology, and Biochemistry 77(5): 948–953.

Usui, M., Harada, A., Yasumoto, S., Sugiura, Y., Nishidai, A., Ikarashi, M., Takaba, H., Miyasaki, T., Azakami, H., and Kondo, M. (2015). Relationship between the risk for a shrimp allergy and freshness or cooking. Bioscience, Biotechnology, and Biochemistry 79(10): 1698–1701.

Wai, C. Y., Leung, N. Y., Ho, M. H., Gershwin, L. J., Shu, S. A., Leung, P. S., and Chu, K. H. (2014). Immunization with hypoallergens of shrimp allergen tropomyosin inhibits shrimp tropomyosin specific IgE reactivity. PloS One 9(11): e111649.

Wai, C. Y., Leung, N. Y., Leung, P. S., and Chu, K. H. (2015). Hypoallergen-encoding DNA plasmids as immunoprophylactic vaccines of shrimp tropomyosin hypersensitivity. Paper Presented at the World Allergy Congress, Seoul, Korea.

Wai, C. Y., Leung, N. Y., Leung, P. S., and Chu, K. H. (2016). T cell epitope immunotherapy ameliorates allergic responses in a murine model of shrimp allergy. Clinical and Experimental Allergy 46(3): 491–503.

Wang, B., Li, Z., Zheng, L., Liu, Y., and Lin, H. (2011). Identification and characterization of a IgE-binding protein in mackerel (*Scromber japonicus*) by MALDI-TOF-MS. Journal of Ocean University of China 10(1): 93–98.

Witteman, A. M., Akkerdaas, J. H., van Leeuwen, J., van der Zee, J. S., and Aalberse, R. C. (1994). Identification of a cross-reactive allergen (presumably tropomyosin) in shrimp, mite and insects. International Archives of Allergy and Immunology 105(1): 56–61.

Yadzir, Z. H., Misnan, R., Abdullah, N., Bakhtiar, F., Arip, M., and Murad, S. (2012). Identification of the major allergen of *Macrobrachium rosenbergii* (giant freshwater prawn). Asian Pacific Journal of Tropical Biomedicine 2(1): 50–54.

Yoshida, S., Ichimura, A., and Shiomi, K. (2008). Elucidation of a major IgE epitope of Pacific mackerel parvalbumin. Food Chemistry 111(4): 857–861.

Yu, C. J., Lin, Y. F., Chiang, B. L., and Chow, L. P. (2003). Proteomics and immunological analysis of a novel shrimp allergen, Pen m 2. Journal of Immunology 170(1): 445–453.

Yu, H. L., Cao, M. J., Cai, Q. F., Weng, W. Y., Su, W. J., and Liu, G. M. (2011). Effects of different processing methods on digestibility of *Scylla paramamosain* allergen (tropomyosin). Food and Chemical Toxicology 49(4): 791–798.

Yu, H. L., Ruan, W. W., Cao, M. J., Cai, Q. F., Shen, H. W., and Liu, G. M. (2013). Identification of physicochemical properties of *Scylla paramamosain* allergen, arginin kinase. Journal of the Science of Food and Agriculture 93(2): 245–253.

Zhang, H., Lu, Y., Ushio, H., and Shiomi, K. (2014). Development of sandwich ELISA for detection and quantification of invertebrate major allergen tropomyosin by a monoclonal antibody. Food Chemistry 150: 151–157.

Zheng, C., Wang, X., Lu, Y., and Liu, Y. (2012). Rapid detection of fish major allergen parvalbumin using superparamagnetic nanoparticle-based lateral flow immunoassay. Food Control 26(2): 446–452.

Zuidmeer-Jongejan, L., Fernandez-Rivas, M., Poulsen, L. K., Neubauer, A., Asturias, J., Blom, L., Boye, J., Bindslev-Jensen, C., Clausen, M., Ferrara, R., Garosi, P., Huber, H., Jensen, B. M., Koppelman, S., Kowalski, M. L., Lewandowska-Polak, A., Linhart, B., Maillere, B., Mari, A., Martinez, A., Mills, C. E., Nicoletti, C., Opstelten, D. J., Papadopoulos, N. G., Portoles, A., Rigby, N., Scala, E., Schnoor, H. J., Sigurdardottir, S. T., Stavroulakis, G., Stolz, F., Swoboda, I., Valenta, R., van den Hout, R., Versteeg, S. A., Witten, M., and van Ree, R. (2012). FAST: towards safe and effective subcutaneous immunotherapy of persistent life-threatening food allergies. Clinical and Translational Allergy 2(1): 5.

Zuidmeer-Jongejan, L., Huber, H., Swoboda, I., Rigby, N., Versteeg, S. A., Jensen, B. M., Quaak, S., Akkerdaas, J. H., Blom, L., Asturias, J., Bindslev-Jensen, C., Bernardi, M. L., Clausen, M., Ferrara, R., Hauer, M., Heyse, J., Kopp, S., Kowalski, M. L., Lewandowska-Polak, A., Linhart, B., Maderegger, B., Maillere, B., Mari, A., Martinez, A., Mills, E. N., Neubauer, A., Nicoletti, C., Papadopoulos, N. G., Portoles, A., Ranta-Panula, V., Santos-Magadan, S., Schnoor, H. J., Sigurdardottir, S. T., Stahl-Skov, P., Stavroulakis, G., Stegfellner, G., Vazquez-Cortes, S., Witten, M., Stolz, F., Poulsen, L. K., Fernandez-Rivas, M., Valenta, R., and van Ree, R. (2015). Development of a hypoallergenic recombinant parvalbumin for first-in-man subcutaneous immunotherapy of fish allergy. International Archives of Allergy and Immunology 166(1): 41–51.

CHAPTER 6

Skin Prick/Puncture Testing in Food Allergy

Sten Dreborg

Introduction

The skin prick/puncture test (SPT) is the most common method within allergology used for screening of sensitization to food allergens and primary diagnostic tool of food allergen sensitization. There are many practice parameters and position papers on the subject, e.g., the AAAAI/ACAAI practice parameter (Bernstein *et al.*, 2008), and the EAACI position paper on Allergen standardization and skin tests (Dreborg *et al.*, 1993) and others (Genser and Schmid-Grendelmeier, 2014; Heinzerling *et al.*, 2013). However, most publications using SPT for diagnosis and/or evaluation of changes in skin sensitization do not contain relevant information on the test procedure and evaluation of results. Therefore, there is a need for discussing factors influencing SPT as well as evaluation and expression of SPT results. Furthermore, minimal criteria for performance and evaluation of SPT in clinical practice and research have recently been set up (Dreborg, 2017a, 2017b).

A positive SPT with food indicates IgE sensitization, i.e., atopy, and possible IgE-mediated allergy (Johansson *et al.*, 2004). However, the presence of IgE antibodies on mast cells in the skin or elsewhere does not prove IgE-mediated clinical allergy. A negative SPT result can be due to inadequate test material, low precision in the hands of testing personnel, many stronger sensitizations, etc. Furthermore, with increasing concentrations of allergen extract, the risk of false positive reactions increases. False positives in relation

Department of Women's and Children's Health, Department of Pediatric Allergology, University Hospital SE-751 85 Uppsala, Sweden.
Email: sten.dreborg@kbh.uu.se

to clinical allergy, while not in relation to sensitization. The results of SPT also depend on the reactivity of the skin that can be estimated by, e.g., histamine reactivity (Dreborg, 2001; Dreborg, 2015; Malling, 1984; Stuckey *et al.*, 1985).

In vitro allergen-specific serum IgE (s-IgE) tests detect circulating allergen-specific IgE antibodies with a technical lower limit, cutoff, nowadays 0.1 kU_A/L. The background guarantees all values higher than the cutoff limit really measures allergen-specific IgE, s-IgE. Patients with an IgE value higher than the cutoff are sensitized but not all individuals are clinically allergic (Johansson *et al.*, 2001; Johansson *et al.*, 2004). All patients with a positive SPT, i.e., a wheal larger than the cutoff limit, are sensitized but not all are clinically allergic.

It should be mentioned, the scratch test, formerly used by many allergists, has no place in allergy diagnosis since it introduces a trauma to the skin that is difficult to standardize. The intradermal test can be used with food extracts, since food extracts are mostly weak, and intradermal testing is about 1,000 more sensitive than the SPT. However, intradermal skin testing inherits an increased risk of general reactions, it is not recommended for routine use (Epstein *et al.*, 2016; Lockey *et al.*, 1987).

The indication for SPT or conventional *in vitro* IgE testing has been diagnosis of species specific sensitization or allergy. However, during recent years, component-resolved diagnosis using an allergen chip based technology, ISAC, has made it possible to reveal sensitization to a relatively low number of allergen protein families with cross–reacting molecules within related but even unrelated allergen source materials. This will make SPT important as a screening method for later molecular diagnosis.

This chapter is based on my recent review of the prick-prick test method and recent data on the concept of the histamine equivalent allergen concentration (Dreborg, 2017a, 2017b) aims at discussing factors influencing SPT as a diagnostic tool in food allergy, the registration, evaluation and interpretation of skin prick/puncture tests in clinical trials as well as in daily practice.

Tests Solutions and Materials—Allergens

The potency and composition of allergen extracts used in daily practice as well as in clinical studies are of great importance when discussing the SPT method and its evaluation, it is a question of using foot, yard or meter, when estimating the sensitivity of patients. The results of SPT in food allergy diagnosis depends to a great extent on the choice of allergen source material.

In this chapter, allergen means allergen extract or allergen source material whereas single purified or recombinant allergenic molecules are not discussed since they are not commercially available for skin testing. Conventional allergen extracts are aiming at containing components in naturally occurring proportions (Dreborg *et al.*, 1993; Einarsson and Dreborg, 1987; Larsen and Dreborg, 2008). Mostly, the dominating (major) allergens

(Allergen nomenclature. IUIS/WHO Allergen Nomenclature Subcommittee, 1994; Radauer *et al.*, 2014) are present in larger amounts both in nature and in extracts. In some cases allergens are rapidly degraded by enzymes in the extract, especially mold extracts.

In general, allergens used for skin testing should be standardized, i.e., with given composition and total allergenic potency and used in a form that assures stability, i.e., glycerinated, or best, freeze-dried. Tests with non-standardized allergen extracts should, therefore, be avoided, since the skin test results can never be reproduced (Bernstein *et al.*, 2008; Larsen and Dreborg, 2008).

Food allergen extracts are not only non-standardized but mostly diluted (1/10–100 w/v). The potency is lower than that of fresh or frozen foods (Ortolani *et al.*, 1989). Thus, very few patients with Oral Allergy Syndrome (OAS) are diagnosed by SPT with fruit extracts. It has been shown that phenols, naturally present in apples, degrade apple allergens rapidly (Bjorksten *et al.*, 1980), which is why crushed apple is tolerated by patients with OAS. The influence of phenols and dilution may explain the low potency and therefore low sensitivity of food allergen extracts (Varjonen *et al.*, 1996). Until better, probably concentrated and standardized, materials are available, fresh, frozen or boiled material, preferably the same locally available fruit and nut species is recommended in combination with prick-prick testing (Dreborg and Foucard, 1983). Skimmed cow's milk, hen's egg white, and other liquid foods can be frozen in small aliquots at –20°C in NUNC vials in paper-boxes for 100 vials (Fig. 6.1), and one sample thawed once a week, and then kept in a refrigerator. The same material can be kept at least for one year (Dreborg, 1991, Dreborg, 2017b) however stability studies are difficult to perform and have not been

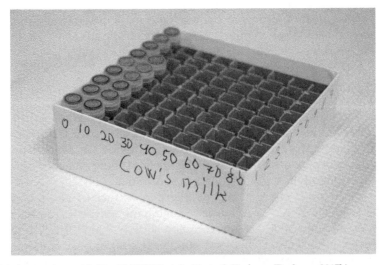

Fig. 6.1: A paper box with 10 x 10 NUNC vials. Photo S. Dreborg (Dreborg, 2017b).

reported. The same method can be applied to, e.g., wheat or rice flour. One gram is mixed with one milliliter water and dispensed in small aliquots. Nuts and fruits are preferably used fresh, stored in the fridge. Apples can be kept in the refrigerator for long periods. In trials, all patients should be tested with the same food, e.g., apple cultivar at each follow-up time. Some proposed raw materials and storage of materials are given in Table 6.1.

As shown by Begin (Begin *et al.*, 2011), as compared to fresh fruits the total allergenic potency of frozen fruits is maintained. However, after thawing, some fruits are rapidly destroyed. As mentioned both fresh and frozen fruits have a higher potency than food extracts (Rance *et al.*, 1997).

The potency and composition of allergens (allergen extracts) and raw materials is crucial. Doses of food allergen that food allergic patients are exposed to during oral challenges are at the milligram to gram level of protein, i.e., for hen's egg, hazelnut and peanut between 42 and 190 mg of fresh, or frozen food, for cow's milk 1.5–5.4 ml corresponding to 60–200 mg protein. The amount of inhalant allergen eliciting a reaction in the skin, conjunctiva or bronchi ranges from 0.01 μg to 1 mg of major allergen (Dreborg, 1987, 1990; Dreborg *et al.*, 1987; Dreborg and Einarsson, 1992). Thus, a 1/100 w/v cow's milk extract contains only 0.5–2 mg of milk protein/ml (Dreborg, 2017b).

The potency of raw materials of commercial non-standardized extracts was investigated by (Rance *et al.*, 1997). They found the wheal sizes of fresh foods being significantly larger than using commercial extracts. SPT with commercial extracts were positive in only 40% of children with positive

Table 6.1: Some examples on fresh and frozen food that can be used for prick-prick testing (Dreborg and Foucard, 1983). Stored frozen in 0.5–1 ml aliquots according to Fig. 6.1. A new vial thawed at least once a week. Some examples. From (Dreborg, 2017a).

Allergen, species	Allergen, source	Remark
Cow's milk	Skimmed milk	Frozen in aliquots, 0.5–1 ml
Hen's egg	Hen's egg white	Frozen in aliquots, 0.5–1 ml
Wheat	Wheat four	Dissolved in water, 1 g in 1–5 ml, frozen
Soy	Soy four	Dissolved in water, 1 g in 1–5 ml
Tree nuts	Fresh nut	One and the same nut per season stored in fridge
Peanut	Peanut, roasted	
	Peanut, fresh	
	Peanut butter	Stored in fridge per season
Fruits	e.g., apple, peach	
Fish	Salmon	Fresh, local products. Can be frozen in small aliquots and thawed with 2–3 days interval
	Cod	
Shellfish	Shrimp, local	
Mollusks	Mollusks, local	

Double Blind, Placebo Controlled, Food Challenges, DBPCFC, but positive in 81.3% using fresh foods for prick-prick testing. The concordance between a positive SPT and the positive challenge was 58.8% with commercial extracts and 91.7% with fresh foods and prick-prick testing. Thus, using fresh foods have a higher sensitivity then commercial extracts detecting sensitization to clinically relevant food allergens.

Conventional allergen extracts used for skin testing must be standardized with given composition and total allergenic potency and used in a form that assures stability, i.e., glycerinated or best freeze-dried and have documented diagnostic properties. Waiting for better food allergen extracts, raw or fresh frozen food using prick-prick testing is recommended.

Negative test solution

The only reasons for using a negative test is to exclude dermographism and for estimation of the background and cutoff of devices and diluents.

Patients with dermographism mostly react with wheals with surrounding erythema, all of the same size, most often 1–2 mm in diameter.

More important is documenting the background (cutoff) that should be documented per device and diluent/negative control solution (Nelson *et al.*, 1998; Oppenheimer and Nelson, 2006; Dreborg, 2017a).

Since the composition of the buffers/solutions used for extraction/ preparation of the allergen extracts have different irritant properties (Nelson *et al.*, 1996), the negative test should be done with the solution used for extraction/preparation.

When using the prick-prick method, the dry lancet, needle or multitest used should be used when documenting the background.

Positive test solutions

The most commonly used positive reference is histamine, histamine dihydrochloride or histamine phosphate, the concentration varying between manufacturers and regions. Using different concentrations does not allow comparison between studies. Therefore, I recommend histamine dihydrochloride 10 mg/ml, i.e., 53.4 mmol/L, until a WAO international agreement has been reached (Dreborg, 2017a, 2017b).

The aims of using a positive test solution are (Dreborg, 2017a):

- To test the reactivity of the skin. The histamine reactivity varies with total IgE, the number of positive allergy tests (Stuckey *et al.*, 1985; Witt *et al.*, 1987) and the degree of sensitivity to the allergen used (Dreborg *et al.*, 2016b; Dreborg *et al.*, 2012; Kuhn *et al.*, 1985). The histamine reactivity of the skin is reduced by, e.g., immunotherapy (Dreborg *et al.*, 2016b; Dreborg *et al.*, 2012; Kuhn *et al.*, 1985).

- To document the test technique of the assistant by establishing the mean histamine wheal size, in trials per test occasion and in the office at intervals, documenting changes in test technique or general sensitivity of the skin of tested individuals.

- To relate the allergen reactivity to that of histamine by establishing the histamine equivalent allergen concentration, C_{ah}. The concentration of allergen, eliciting a wheal response of the same size as that of the histamine reference, C_{ah}, can be calculated and followed (Dreborg *et al.*, 2016b; Dreborg and Holgersson, 2015). It is important that the allergen, the reference, and their strengths are the same at all follow up times.

Devices

There are many types of devices used to insert allergen into the epidermis. The physical shape of devices has varied over time and between regions. In the US, many types of devices are used, in Europe just a few. Test results depend on many other factors than the shape of the device. Every assistant has his or her SPT technique. All devices have different cutoffs depending on number of points, their shape and length and the technique used by the assistant. Basic documentation of background/cutoff and precision, the coefficient of variation, (CV) is essential.

The optimal length of the tip of devices used for prick/puncture testing is 1 mm (Osterballe and Weeke, 1979).

The type of device is not of importance, provided the precision, the background, and the cutoff of the device in the hands of the testing personnel is properly established (Dreborg, 2017a).

Test Sites

Any part of the skin can be used for SPT. However, the volar aspect of the forearms is recommended for routine use. To be able to test many allergens or concentrations of allergen at the same time, it is sometimes necessary to use the back.

It has been reported that tests on the back are larger than on the forearm. In healthy infants and small children, the difference is significant but not impressive, i.e., mean wheal diameter ± standard deviation (SD) were 4.74 ± 1.37 mm on the upper back and 3.86 ± 1.82 mm on the forearms ($p < 0.0001$) (Yuenyongviwat *et al.*, 2012).

Test Application

Tests should be performed 2–2.5 cm apart and not closer from the wrist than 50 mm in the US and 20 mm in Europe to the wrist and more than 30 mm from the antecubital fossae (Bernstein *et al.*, 2008; Heinzerling *et al.*, 2009).

This allows two rows with five tests, i.e., 10 tests on the volar aspect of each forearm. To reduce the possible influence of location on test results, duplicate tests should be applied in a mirrored, upside down fashion. When using the back it is also recommended using mirrored, upside down allocation (Dreborg *et al.*, 1987; Dreborg *et al.*, 1993) rather than randomized allocation. This is especially true for small samples of tested individuals. Sun exposed skin areas have a lower reactivity than those not exposed to the sun (King *et al.*, 2014) and sun-exposed areas should therefore be avoided, especially in diagnosis (false negatives), and when possible, in prospective trials.

It is essential to use the same area, e.g., when comparing sensitization patterns in different regions, and development of sensitization over time (Dreborg, 2017).

Prick-Puncture Testing

Methods for skin prick-puncture testing

Using food allergen extracts

The normal procedure is to apply a drop of test solution on the skin, penetrate the drop with a device, then puncturing the skin, letting a minute amount of test solution enter the superficial layer of the skin without bleeding. There are many techniques. The technique used by the technician should show a high reproducibility, i.e., C.V. < 20% (mean diameter), if possible < 10% (area 40 and 20% respectively), and use a cutoff using the same device and diluent. Any technique and device with documented c.v., background and thereby documented cutoff can be used. All wheal diameters recorded less than the cutoff limit are negative and should therefore not be discussed in trials or used in practice.

After finalizing the test, the drop can be removed by pressing a soft tissue against the skin, avoiding any spread of test material to other sites (Dreborg *et al.*, 1993).

The Prick-Prick Method with Fresh or Frozen Food

When performing the prick-prick test (Dreborg and Foucard, 1983), the fruit/food is first pricked, alternatively the device is dipped into the fresh or thawed fluid allergen source and then the skin is pricked (Dreborg, 1991). One device should be used per prick to avoid transferal of microbes from patient to the fruit or other food.

At present, due to lack of reliable standardized food allergen extracts, the prick-prick method should be preferred.

Registration of skin response

The wheals should be read after 15 minutes. The wheal should be surrounded by a flare.
Methods for registration are:

- Just looking at the wheal-and-flare reaction subjectively noting positive or negative.
- Measure the wheal diameters directly on the skin.

Or better

- Encircling the wheal by drawing a line (blue or black) on the erythema close to the wheal border (and along the border of the surrounding erythema on intact skin (red)) (Bernstein *et al.*, 2008; Dreborg *et al.*, 1993).
- Transfer the drawing by means of a translucent tape, first pressed against the drawing, then placed on a record sheet.

Either

- Measure the longest diameter (d_1) and the midpoint orthogonal diameter (d_2). Then calculating the mean diameter

(1) $(\dfrac{d_1 + d_2}{2} = D)$.

Or

- Calculate the area by planimetry or digitizer (Konstantinou *et al.*, 2010; Pijnenborg *et al.*, 1996; Poulsen *et al.*, 1993).

  Register the result on the record sheet (and in the computer's registration program).

A number of more or less sophisticated techniques have been used for estimating the skin reactivity to allergens, e.g., laser doppler imaging (Bisgaard and Kristensen, 1984; Olsson *et al.*, 1988), skin impedance (Nyren *et al.*, 1996), thermography (Phipatanakul and Slavin, 1972; Rokita *et al.*, 2011; Uematsu *et al.*, 1987), photography (dos Santos *et al.*, 2007) and 3D scanning (dos Santos *et al.*, 2008; Siebenhaar *et al.*, 2009). These techniques are of scientific interest. However, these techniques are not suitable for routine use.

All parts of the SPT procedure and evaluation are contributing to the often high C.V. Therefore, it is important to reduce the variation of SPT results by performing the tests, the registration of results and the evaluation as precise as possible. See proficiency testing. The total resulting C.V. should be less than 20% (10%) based on the mean diameter.

Drawings and measures should be preserved for possible follow-up and control.

Evaluation of skin responses

In principle, there are six possibilities (Dreborg, 2017a):

1. To use the mean of the longest and the midpoint orthogonal wheal diameters. Register the mean diameter.
2. To use the area. In the 1990-ties, Poulsen *et al.* developed a simple scanning program for estimating the wheal area (Pijnenborg *et al.*, 1996; Poulsen *et al.*, 1993). This program is no longer used, but there are modern programs for estimation of the cell areas, e.g., cellSens software (cellSens, 2015) that can be used in scientific studies.
3. To estimate the allergen concentration inducing a certain wheal size, e.g., 3 or 6 mm (Durham and Church, 2001), not correcting for changes in skin reactivity or assistant technique by using the histamine equivalent allergen concentration, C_{ah}.
4. To estimate the allergen response (wheal area) in relation to that of histamine, a non-precise, semi-quantitative method (Aas and Belin, 1973; Aas and Belin, 1974).
5. To use the size of the allergen wheal in percent of the histamine wheal.
6. To calculate the histamine equivalent allergen threshold concentration, C_{ah}.

The first three are well known. The fifth that has been described recently (Dreborg and Holgersson, 2015) and has the advantage of expressing the result as a threshold concentration (Dreborg and Holgersson, 2015).

Ad. 1. The mean wheal diameter or area is used in routine and in most published trials. This is simple and has been the common measure of skin response, but does not give any information about the sensitivity of the patient comparable to other *in vivo* threshold concentrations, e.g., PC_{20}, PD_{20}, CPT, NPT or DBPCFC threshold concentrations, and *in vitro* tests with documented cutoff.

One report suggests the longest diameter correlates better than the mean diameter with the area of the wheal (Konstantinou *et al.*, 2010). However, this correlation does not prove the longest diameter is better than the mean diameter as a measure of skin sensitivity. The better correlation may be due to some outliers with pseudopods that increases the correlation using the same basic data. The question is if there is a better correlation with the patient's sensitivity as measured by a gold standard. The s-IgE level does not measure the same parameter as the SPT and can therefore not be used as a gold standard. The only measure of allergic sensitivity that has a high precision is the CPT (Dreborg, 1985; Moller *et al.*, 1984). Changes in conjunctival sensitivity correlate well with changes in wheal area (Dreborg *et al.*, 2016b).

Ad. 3. Durham and Church (Durham and Church, 2001) have proposed estimating the allergen concentration eliciting a wheal with 6 mm diameter. This method does not correct for differences in SPT technique (Dreborg, 2015).

Ad. 4. Before the introduction of SPT and one concentration of allergen used for diagnosis, intra-dermal skin testing was used for end-point titration. Then the endpoint, a concentration of allergen, was used as a measure of skin sensitivity. In 1973, Aas and Belin (Aas and Belin, 1973) proposed relating the allergen wheal response to that of histamine. See above.

Ad. 5. The method involves histamine reflecting the reactivity of the skin. However, percent is not a concentration.

Ad. 6. Determining the concentration of allergen eliciting a wheal of the same size as that of histamine reduces the difference between testing personnel, centers and test occasions (Dreborg and Holgersson, 2015). Using the slope of the allergen dose-response relationship (Dreborg *et al.*, 1987) for calculation of the histamine equivalent allergen concentration, the allergen response can be expressed as a threshold concentration, histamine equivalent allergen concentration, C_{ah} (Dreborg and Holgersson, 2015). This measure is more useful and can be used for estimation of changes in skin sensitivity during therapy with, e.g., antihistamines or by immunotherapy (Dreborg *et al.*, 2016b; Dreborg, 2017a). However, when using the results of skin prick tests for this purpose, the technique must be optimal with a C.V. less than 20% (or best less than 10%) using the wheal diameter.

For calculation of the histamine equivalent allergen concentration (C_{ah}) the following formula should be used:

(2) $C_{ah} = \left[\dfrac{Dh}{Da}\right] 1/b) * C$ of allergen used, or with a slope b = 0.2 calculated using

the diameters,

$$C_{ah} = \left[\frac{Dh}{Da}\right] \frac{1}{0.2} * C \text{ of allergen used or } C_{ah} = \left[\frac{Dh}{Da}\right] 5 * C \text{ of allergen used}$$

(Dreborg and Holgersson, 2015), e.g., 4000 BAU or 10 HEP. Fresh food can be given the potency 1,000 "U" arbitrarily, or any other figure denoting non-diluted food. One thousand U makes it easy expressing the sensitivity of the skin in integer numbers and increase or decrease in skin sensitivity during the observation period.

The method can also be used to calculate the change in skin sensitivity between two time points. The data can describe the difference in concentration

(3) C_{ah} time one minus C_{ah} time two (Dreborg *et al.*, 2016b).

or as a ratio giving the times increase or decrease in skin sensitivity

(4) C_{ah} time one/C_{ah} time two (Dreborg *et al.*, 2016b).

These formulas are easy to introduce, e.g., in an Excel calculation sheet.

The larger the allergen wheal response, the lower the allergen threshold concentration, C_{ah}, causing an allergen wheal of the same size as that of the histamine wheal.

In Fig. 6.2a the allergen wheal sizes in % of the histamine wheals is shown (Formgren *et al.*, 1985). In Fig. 6.2b, the same data have been recalculated into C_{ah} before and after immunotherapy (Dreborg *et al.*, 2016b; Dreborg, 2017a).

Another theoretical example of results using C_{ah} before and after immunotherapy is shown in Table 6.2. One allergen is used for immunotherapy, the reactivity to the other is just observed as described by Dreborg *et al.* (Dreborg *et al.*, 2012).

It has been shown the histamine reaction is reduced during immunotherapy (Dreborg *et al.*, 2016b; Kuhn *et al.*, 1985). The calculated change in sensitivity to allergens is influenced by the change in general skin reactivity that is reflected by the histamine reactivity, as illustrated in Table 6.2. However, the difference in change between active and placebo does not change. The difference in change in relation to non-treatment or placebo is the crucial parameter.

There are several systems presenting skin prick test data based on the mean diameter or area of wheals.

To estimate the skin sensitivity at one time-point in terms of a threshold concentration formula (2) should be applied. Then results are minimally influenced by differences in skin test technique, and formula (3) and or (4) be used when investigating changes in skin sensitivity between groups, the change of skin sensitivity over time or by therapy of individuals.

Cutoff

The question when a test is positive or negative has been widely discussed since skin testing has been part of allergy diagnosis. In studies as well as in clinical practice, defining positive and negative results is important.

For decades, there was no agreement on how to define a positive SPT. In 1987, it was proposed ≥ 7 mm^2 ($\approx \geq 3$ mm D) (Dreborg *et al.*, 1987) to be the cutoff that was adopted by the Nordic Guidelines in 1989 (Registration of allergen preparations. Nordic Guidelines, 1989) and the EAACI position paper in 1993 (Dreborg *et al.*, 1993). However, there was no proper evidence-based documentation of that limit at that time.

There must be a clear definition of the background using the device, diluent and technique used in the office/study. The cutoff should be the upper limit of the background, i.e., the background mean + 3.3 standard deviations (s.d.) (Matsson *et al.*, 2009). The protocol for testing the background can be that used for proficiency testing using the negative solution (Dreborg, 2013) or using the instructions given by Bernstein *et al.* performing 80 tests, 5, 10 or 20 per patient (Bernstein *et al.*, 2008; Nelson *et al.*, 1998; Oppenheimer and Nelson, 2006). Bernstein *et al.* (Bernstein *et al.*, 2008) also defined the background and thereby the cutoff of a number of devices used in the US, using 80 tests with a negative control solution, Table 6.3.

For devices unique for Europe and other areas, data are missing. Therefore, until the background has been firmly established for European devices, the background should be calculated per assistant, office, device and diluent.

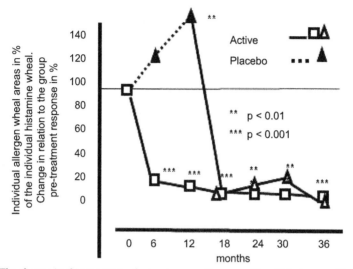

Fig. 6.2a: The change in skin reactivity during immunotherapy with a *D. farinae* purified, freeze-dried extract (major allergen content 100 µg/ml ± a factor 2 (Dreborg and Einarsson, 1992)) and placebo during three years, expressed as the allergen skin wheal response in percent of individual histamine wheal. The placebo group received active treatment after one year. Changes during three years in relation to skin sensitivity before immunotherapy (Formgren *et al.*, 1985). After (Dreborg, 2017a).

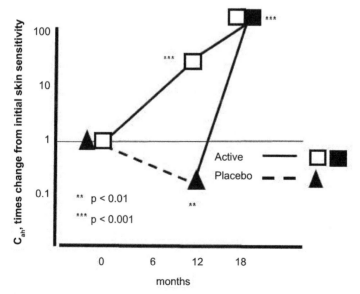

Fig. 6.2b: The same data recalculated using the C_{ah} *D. farinae* and placebo before and after one and one and a half year of immunotherapy expressed as C_{ah} (Dreborg and Holgersson, 2015), using the slope 0.2 for diameter. The placebo group received active treatment after one year. Changes in relation to skin sensitivity before immunotherapy. After (Dreborg, 2017a).

Note: The placebo group got placebo during the first year of treatment (non-filled triangles and broken lines). After 12 months, the placebo group received active treatment (Filled triangles and solid lines).

Table 6.2: One allergen is used for immunotherapy, the reactivity to the other is just observed. There are three examples. The response to histamine is the same or is reduced by 1 and 2 mm in diameter during immunotherapy. The calculated changes in sensitivity to the respective allergens are influenced by the change in histamine reactivity as illustrated by the three cases. However, the differences in change are the same in all three cases (Dreborg, 2017a; Dreborg and Holgersson, 2015). After (Dreborg, 2017a).

Allergen	Before immunotherapy			After immunotherapy			Times change within group	Times difference in change conc.
	D_h	D_a	C_{ah}	D_h	D_a	C_{ah}		
*Histamine wheal D **unchanged** during immunotherapy*								
Active	6	6	10	6	3	368	36.8	36.8
"Placebo"	6	6	10	6	6	10	1	
*Histamine wheal D **reduced by 1 mm** during immunotherapy*								
Active	6	6	10	5	3	142	14.2	36.8
Placebo	6	6	10	5	6	4	0.4	
*Histamine wheal D **reduced by 2 mm** during immunotherapy*								
Active	6	6	10	4	3	45	4.5	36.8
Placebo	6	6	10	4	6	1	0.1	

Table 6.3: The size of wheals that are larger than 99% of the wheals with saline, using the same device on subject's back by the same operator (n = 80) After Bernstein *et al.* (Bernstein *et al.*, 2008). There are no published data on European devices.

Device 1 Devices for which a 3-mm wheal would be significant	0.99 Quintile of reactions at the negative control sites, mm	Device 2 Devices for which a more than 3-mm wheal should be used as significant**	0.99 Quintile of reactions at the negative control sites, mm
Quintest (HS) puncture	0	DuoTip (Lincoln) twist	3.5
Smallpox needle (HS) prick	0	Bifurcated needle (ALO) prick	4.0
DuoTip (Lincoln) prick	1.5	MultiTest (Lincoln) puncture	4.0
Lancet (HS)	2.0	Bifurcated needle (ALO) puncture	4.5
Lancet (ALK)*	3.0	Quick Test (Pantrex)	4.0
DermaPICK II	0	Greer Track (Greer)	3.5

Abbreviations: HS, Hollister Steir; Greer, Greer Laboratories; ALO, Allergy Labs of Ohio; Lincoln, Lincoln Diagnostics; ALK, ALK.
*) Not the lancet used by ALK and other companies in Europe.
**) These devices have multiple tips.

These data are important factors that should be reported in clinical studies (Dreborg, 2017a).

The background using the device, diluent and technique used must be clearly defined and reported in all studies.

Precision

In vitro tests should always have a documented precision, C.V. The C.V. of *in vitro* tests is most often less than 10%. There are few reports on the precision of the SPT.

In 1980, Kjell Aas (Aas, 1980) reported the precision of SPT (Table 6.4). C.V. varied from 8% using the Pepys' method (Pepys, 1968; Pepys, 1975), using a short beveled fine needle, to 30% with a multi-test device.

In major European centers (Dreborg *et al.*, 1987), the C.V. varied from 15 up to 145% for allergens and from 12 to 65% for histamine, as calculated on wheal areas. Taudorf *et al.* found the C.V. of wheals, based on mean diameters, more than 15 mm^2 being between 20–30%, in contrast to figures between 30–60% with wheals less than 15 mm^2 (D = 4.1 mm) (Taudorf *et al.*, 1985). On the other hand, Dreborg *et al.* including many European centers found the mean C.V., based on areas, being 55% in the range 3–10 mm^2 and 30–40% for larger wheal sizes (Dreborg *et al.*, 1987). Both studies using the Østerballe needle with 1 mm point (Osterballe and Weeke, 1979).

The C.V. calculated on the diameter is half that of the C.V. calculated on the area, area = πr^2. Dreborg *et al.* (Dreborg *et al.*, 1987) used quadruplicate tests performed with each of three 10-fold concentrations of allergen (about 12,000 tests) and histamine dihydrochloride 1 and 10 mg/ml (about 8000 tests). However, duplicate tests are sufficient for calculation of the C.V. An example is shown in Fig. 6.3 and Table 6.5.

In clinical trials using SPT, the C.V. should be reported and in clinical practice the C.V. should be supervised regularly.

Table 6.4: Tests performed according to Pepys using a short beveled needle (Pepys, 1968; Pepys, 1975), with the Morrow-Brown needle (Morrow Brown, 1976) and with a multitest device, testing the same 80 patients with histamine dihydrochloride 1 mg/ml. After Aas (Aas, 1980). This assistant should obviously use the method of Pepys, causing the largest wheals, the lowest range of histamine weal sizes and the lowest C.V.

Device	n	D	s.d.	C.V.	Range
Short beveled needle	80	6.1	0.51	8	5–7
Morrow Brown needle	80	5.7	0.55	10	4.5–7
Multitest	80	4.5	1.35	30	2–7

D: The mean diameter, mean of the longest and the midpoint orthogonal diameters; s.d., the standard deviation; c.v., the coefficient of variation.

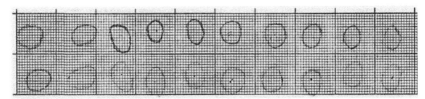

Fig. 6.3: Twenty wheals obtained by testing histamine dihydrochloride 10 mg/ml in one person using the Østerballe lancet with one 1 mm tip. From a center using duplicate tests in practice (permission by Professor Hans-Jörgen Malling) (Dreborg, 2017a). Data on individual wheal diameters, the mean and median diameters and C.V. are given in Table 6.5. Permission by patient and assistant (Dreborg, 2017a).

Table 6.5: Twenty (20) prick tests performed by one nurse on the volar aspect of the forearm of one atopic person, Fig. 6.3. The measured diameters (d1 and d2) and the mean of these (D) are given. Below are shown the mean and median of D of the 10 tests and the C.V. (Dreborg, 2017a).

d_1	d_2	$D = d_1 + d_2/2$
9.5	8	8.75
8	7.5	7.75
8,5	6	7.25
11	6.5	8.75
10	6	8
10	6	8
7	5	6
9	6.5	7.75
Mean		7.78
s.d.		0.88
C.V.%		11.32

Documentation of the Precision of SPT

In principle, there are two possibilities, to perform (at least) duplicate tests with histamine and all allergens used or in small children single tests in combination with proficiency testing at intervals (Bernstein *et al.*, 2008; Dreborg, 2013).

Duplicate tests. In most cases, it is easy to perform duplicate tests instead of single tests, since the extra time spent is limited. This includes the extra material needed, since the same device/needle/lancet can be used for the second test with the same allergen extract. To avoid transferal of infections via the fruit/food a new device should be used for each prick when performing prick-prick tests.

The precision is given by the coefficient of variation that is derived from the formula

(5) $\dfrac{sd*100}{mean}$ = C.V. percent.

When optically comparing two tests, the rule is that at normal levels between approximately 4 and 8 mm a difference in mean wheal diameter of 1 mm can be accepted. At the same time, it should be remembered, that the difference in strength of an extract causing a 4 mm mean wheal D to that causing a 8 mm wheal D differs 32 times (Dreborg and Holgersson, 2015). Thus, if an extract is labeled 10 U gives the 4 mm wheal D, then an extract labeled 320 U induces a wheal with 8 mm diameter in the same patient. Furthermore, it must be considered that in many diagnostic systems, the C.V. increases at lower response levels close to the cutoff concentration.

Proficiency tests. Proficiency tests should be considered for training of assistants to achieve high precision both for clinical trials and for improving the value of SPT in clinical practice.

The second indication for proficiency tests is to keep the precision high when using single tests, e.g., in young children.

The third indication for proficiency tests is to supervise the technique of the assistant by performing proficiency tests in adults at intervals.

Parts of a proficiency test is illustrated in Fig. 6.3 and Table 6.5

The AAAAI Practice parameter relates a proposal for proficiency testing, Table 6.6. However, there are no detailed proficiency test protocols published. Therefore, the protocol that has been utilized during workshops on skin testing during recent AAAAI Annual Meetings is shown as Table 6.7 (Dreborg, 2017a) after (Dreborg, 2013). It is proposed to perform 10 + 10 tests (Table 6.7) with the histamine reference on the volar aspect of the forearms on each of four

Table 6.6

Suggested Proficiency Testing and Quality Assurance
Technique for Prick/Puncture Skin Testing.
• Using desired skin test device, perform skin testing with positive (histamine 1–10) and negative controls (saline 1–10) in an alternate pattern on a subject's back.
• Record histamine results at 8 minutes by outlining wheals with a felt tip pen and transferring results with transparent tape to a blank sheet of paper.
• Record saline results at 15 minutes by outlining wheal and flares with a felt tip pen and transferring results with transparent tape to a blank sheet of paper.
• Calculate the mean diameter as $(D + d)/2$; D = largest diameter and d = orthogonal or perpendicular diameter at the largest width of D.
Histamine
• Calculate the mean diameter of each wheal
• Calculate the SD.
• Determine coefficient of variation (C.V.) = SD/mean
• Quality standard should be C.V. less than 30%
Saline
All negative controls should be ≤ 3-mm wheals and flares should be ≤ 10-mm in diameter

After the AAAAI Practice Parameter 2008, Bernstein *et al.* (1).

Table 6.7

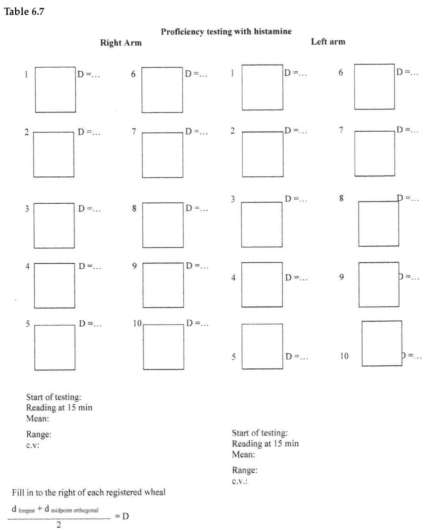

Proficiency testing with histamine

Start of testing:
Reading at 15 min
Mean:

Range:
c.v:

Start of testing:
Reading at 15 min
Mean:

Range:
c.v.:

Fill in to the right of each registered wheal

$$\frac{d_{longest} + d_{midpoint\ orthogonal}}{2} = D$$

Give the mean wheal diameter, the size of the **largest and the smallest mean wheal** diameters (**range**), should not be more than ± 1 mm.

The c.v. can be calculated per forearm, per patient and per testing personnel using data from four patients tested.

The mean diameter of the histamine wheal per tested person and testing personnel should be followed and changes be noted.

subjects at monthly intervals. Preferably, the same individuals should be used from time to time, and the C.V. and the median histamine wheal size recorded to supervise changes in testing technique (Dreborg, 2017a).

A drawback with single tests is the risk of negative tests due to low pressure on the lancet, causing false negative tests. In the above-mentioned study

(Dreborg *et al.*, 1987) tested about 500 patients with six allergen concentrations in quadruplicate (n 24) tests per patient, there was an incidence of accidental negative SPT up to 1/20 tests (non-published data) varying between centers (Dreborg, 2017a).

Formulas for calculation of mean weal diameter, C_{ah}, changes in C_{ah} are available on line (Dreborg, 2017a).

It is recommended to use duplicate tests in both scientific trials and clinical practice, and regularly calculate the C.V. In clinical practice, it is recommended inserting formulas (2), (3) and (4) in the registration program and in clinical trials comparing groups and or changes over time. The C.V. should be reported in papers using skin prick tests as a basis for reporting on atopy, skin sensitivity or changes in skin sensitivity (Dreborg, 2017a).

Recommendations for Clinical Trials

Allergen extracts (if used)

Allergen(s) extracts must be standardized with given composition and total allergenic potency.

Allergen extracts should be used in a form that assures stability, i.e., be glycerinated, or best, freeze-dried.

Food allergens

Food allergen extracts should in most cases be replaced by fresh or frozen food of defined source, Table 6.1.

Negative control

Possible irritating characteristics of the negative control solution should be documented in allergic individuals.

The negative control should be used to exclude dermographism.

In the case of prick-prick tests, the negative control should be a blank lancet, needle or multitest.

The background should be documented per device, and diluent.

Positive control

A positive control (histamine) should be used to register the reactivity of the skin.

The median histamine wheal size of the patient/patient sample should be documented per test occasion to document possible change in skin reactivity and or skin prick test technique.

Device(s)

Any device can be used, provided the background and the cut off of the device are known, and the precision of the testing personnel, is properly recorded.

Test location

Tests should be placed on the volar aspect of the forearms or, when more area is needed, on the back, avoiding sun-exposed skin.

The same location and test technique should be used throughout the study, in all patients, all participating centers and at all time-points.

Test technique

Any technique with documented precision and cut off can be used; provided data are specified.

Recording

The wheal contour should be carefully drawn with a fine filter tip pen or the like, preferably transferred to a record sheet.

The mean diameter or area of the histamine and allergen wheals should be measured and registered, and original data safely stored.

Evaluation

For evaluation, the histamine equivalent threshold concentration (C_{ah}) should be preferred that is minimally influenced by differences in skin test technique and changes in general skin reactivity.

The C_{ah} can be used to estimate the sensitivity at one point and changes in skin sensitivity over time and between locations.

Precision—Proficiency

The precision of assistants should be documented at intervals per assistant and per test technique.

The C.V. should be reported.

For regular training of personnel, proficiency testing is recommended, aiming at keeping the C.V. low and thereby data reliable.

In adults, adolescents and most schoolchildren the precision is best supervised by duplicate tests and regularly calculated and reported C.V.

In small children single tests can be accepted provided assistants perform proficiency tests at regular intervals, properly documented and reported in the publication.

To allow comparison with other studies, the C_{ah} should be presented and followed, i.e., formulas (1), (2), (3), and (4) being used.

Recommendations for Clinical Practice

Allergen extracts *if used*

Allergen(s) extracts should preferably be standardized with given composition and total allergenic potency.

Allergen extracts should be used in a form that assures stability, i.e., be glycerinated.

Food allergens

Food allergen extracts should in most cases be replaced by fresh or frozen food, Table 6.1.

Negative control

Possible irritating characteristics of the negative control solution should be documented.

The negative control should be used to exclude dermographism.

In the case of prick-prick tests, the negative control should be a blank lancet, needle or multitest.

Positive control

A positive control (histamine) should be used to register the reactivity of the skin.

The median histamine wheal size of the patients should be documented at intervals to document possible change in skin reactivity/skin prick test technique.

Device(s)

Any device can be used, provided the background and the cut off of the device/control solution are known, and the precision of the testing personnel, is properly recorded.

Test location

Tests should be placed on the volar aspect of the forearms, avoiding sun-exposed skin.

Test technique

Any technique with documented precision and cut off can be used.

Recording

The wheal contour should be carefully drawn with a fine filter tip pen or the like, preferably transferred to a record sheet.

The mean diameter or area of the histamine and allergen wheals should be measured and registered, and original data safely stored.

Evaluation

The mean diameter can be used for diagnosis of sensitization (wheal larger than the cut off limit).

The histamine equivalent threshold concentration (C_{ah}) should be preferred that is minimally influenced by differences in skin test technique and changes in general skin reactivity.

The C_{ah} can be used to estimate the sensitivity at one point and changes in skin sensitivity over time, when following up immunotherapy, cow's milk protein allergy and the like.

Precision—Proficiency

The precision, C.V. of assistants should be documented at intervals per assistant and test technique.

For regular training of personnel, proficiency testing is recommended, aiming at keeping the C.V. low and thereby data reliable.

The precision is best supervised in adults, adolescents and most school children using duplicate tests (± 1 mm).

In small children single tests can be accepted provided assistants perform proficiency tests at regular intervals.

Abbreviations

A	:	Area of the allergen or histamine wheal
AAAAI	:	American Academy of Allergy, Asthma and Immunology
ACAAI	:	American College of Allergy, Asthma, and Immunology
C	:	Concentration
C_{ah}	:	histamine equivalent allergen concentration
CPT	:	Conjunctival provocation test
C.V.	:	Coefficient of variation
D	:	Diameter of the allergen or histamine wheal
DBPCFC	:	Double blind, placebo controlled food challenge

EAACI : European Academy of Allergy and Clinical Immunology
NPT : Nasal Provocation test
OAS : Oral Allergy Syndrome
s-IgE : Allergen-specific IgE in serum
SPT : Skin prick/puncture test
s-IgE : Allergen IgE antibodies in serum

Keywords: skin prick test, prick-prick test, food allergen, precision, proficiency test, histamine equivalent allergen concentration, evaluation, registration, fresh fruit, fresh food, allergen

References

Aas, K., and Belin, L. (1973). Standardization of diagnostic work in allergy. International archives of Allergy and Applied Immunology 45(1): 57–60.

Aas, K., and Belin, L. (1974). Northern (Scandinavian) society for allergology. Standardization of diagnostic work in allergy. Acta Allergologica 29: 239–240.

Aas, K. (1980). Some variables in skin prick testing. Allergy 35(3): 250–252.

Allergen nomenclature. IUIS/WHO Allergen Nomenclature Subcommittee. (1994). Bulletin of the World Health Organization 72(5): 797–806.

Begin, P., Des Roches, A., Nguyen, M., Masse, M. S., Paradis, J., and Paradis, L. (2011). Freezing does not alter antigenic properties of fresh fruits for skin testing in patients with birch tree pollen-induced oral allergy syndrome. The Journal of Allergy and Clinical Immunology 127(6): 1624–1626 e1623.

Bernstein, I. L., Li, J. T., Bernstein, D. I., Hamilton, R., Spector, S. L., Tan, R., Sicherer, S., Golden, D. B., Khan, D. A., Nicklas, R. A., Portnoy, J. M., Blessing-Moore, J., Cox, L., Lang, D. M., Oppenheimer, J., Randolph, C. C., Schuller, D. E., Tilles, S. A., Wallace, D. V., Levetin, E., Weber, R., American Academy of Allergy, Immunology, American College of Allergy, and Immunology. (2008). Allergy diagnostic testing: an updated practice parameter. Annals of Allergy, Asthma and Immunology: Official Publication of the American College of Allergy, Asthma, & Immunology 100(3 Suppl 3): S1–148.

Bisgaard, H., and Kristensen, J. K. (1984). Quantitation of microcirculatory blood flow changes in human cutaneous tissue induced by inflammatory mediators. The Journal of Investigative Dermatology 83(3): 184–187.

Bjorksten, F., Halmepuro, L., Hannuksela, M., and Lahti, A. (1980). Extraction and properties of apple allergens. Allergy 35(8): 671–677.

cellSens. (2015) [Cell area scanning]. Munster: Olympus. Retrieved from http://www.olympus-lifescience.com/en/software/cellsens/

dos Santos, R. V., Titus, R. G., and Lima, H. C. (2007). Objective evaluation of skin prick test reactions using digital photography. Skin Research and Technology: Official Journal of International Society for Bioengineering and the Skin 13(2): 148–153.

dos Santos, R. V., Mlynek, A., Lima, H. C., Martus, P., and Maurer, M. (2008). Beyond flat weals: validation of a three-dimensional imaging technology that will improve skin allergy research. Clinical and Experimental Dermatology 33(6): 772–775.

Dreborg, S., and Foucard, T. (1983). Allergy to apple, carrot and potato in children with birch pollen allergy. Allergy 38(3): 167–172.

Dreborg, S. (1985). Conjunctival provocation test (CPT). Allergy 40(Suppl 4): 66–67.

Dreborg, S. (1987). The skin prick test. Methodological studies and clinical applications. (Ph.D. Dissertaion), Linköping University Medical Dissertation Linköping. 239pp.

Dreborg, S., Basomba, A., Belin, L., Durham, S., Einarsson, R., Eriksson, N., Frostad, A., Grimmer, O., Halvorsen, R., Holgersson, M., Kay, A. et al. (1987). Biological equilibration of allergen preparations: methodological aspects and reproducibility. Clinical Allergy 17(6): 537–550.

Dreborg, S. (1990). Bronchial provocation tests with biologically standardised allergenic preparations. pp. 185–191. *In*: G. Melillo, Norman.P.S., and M. P (Vol. Ed.), Clinical Immunology: Vol. 2. Philadelphia, Montreal: CW Decker.

Dreborg, S. (1991). Skin test in diagnosis of food allergy. Allergy Proceedings: The Official Journal of Regional and State Allergy Societies 12(4): 251–254.

Dreborg, S., and Einarsson, R. (1992). The major allergen content of allergenic preparations reflect their biological activity. Allergy 47(4 Pt 2): 418–423.

Dreborg, S., and Frew, A. (1993). Position Paper. Allergen standardisation and skin tests. Allergy 47(Suppl 14): 48–82.

Dreborg, S. (2001). Histamine reactivity of the skin. Allergy 56(5): 359–364.

Dreborg, S., Lee, T., Kay, A., and Durham, S. (2012). Immunotherapy is allergen-specific: a double-blind trial of mite or timothy extract in mite and grass dual-allergic patients. International Archives of Allergy and Immunology 158(1): 63–70.

Dreborg, S. (2013). Proficiency testing: Skin prick test. Paper presented at the AAAAI Anual Meeting 2013. San Antonio, USA. On line hand out retrieved from https://aaaai.confex.com/aaaai/2013/webprogramhandouts/Session1315.html.

Dreborg, S. (2015). Allergen skin prick test should be adjusted by the histamine reactivity. International Archives of Allergy and Immunology 166: 77–80.

Dreborg, S., and Holgersson, M. (2015). Evaluation of methods for estimation of threshold concentrations by the skin prick test. Proposal of two simple methods. International Archives of Allergy and Immunology 166: 71–76.

Dreborg, S., Holgersson, M., and Möller, C. (2016a). Evaluation of changes in skin reactivity by skin prick test titration. Immunotherapy: Open Access 2, 109, 102: doi 10.4172/2471-9552.1000116.

Dreborg, S., Basomba, A., Löfkvist, T., Holgersson, M., and Möller, C. (2016b). Evaluation of skin reactivity during (immuno-)therapy. Validation of methods for estimation of changes in skin reactivity and correlation to shock organ sensitivity. Immunotherapy Open Access 2: 109. doi:10.4172/imt.1000109.

Dreborg, S. (2017a). Evaluation of skin reactivity. The concept of histamine equivalent allergen threshold concentration. Submitted.

Dreborg, S. (2017b). The prick-prick test. In manuscript.

Durham, S. R., and Church, M. K. (2001). Principles of allergy diagnosis. *In*: S. Holgate, M.K. Church and L. Lichtenstein (eds.). Allergy 2nd ed. Mosby.

Einarsson, R., and Dreborg, S. (1987). Manufacturers' criteria for in-house references. Arbeiten aus dem Paul-Ehrlich-Institut, dem Georg-Speyer-Haus und dem Ferdinand-Blum-Institut zu Frankfurt am Main (80): 131–138.

Epstein, T. G., Liss, G. M., Murphy-Berendts, K., and Bernstein, D. I. (2016). Risk factors for fatal and nonfatal reactions to subcutaneous immunotherapy: National surveillance study on allergen immunotherapy (2008–2013). Annals of Allergy, Asthma and Immunology: Official Publication of the American College of Allergy, Asthma, & Immunology 116(4): 354–359 e352.

Formgren, H., Dreborg, S., Kober, A., Lanner, Å., and Olofsson, E. (1985). A controlled study of immunotherapy with Pharmalgen D. farinae mite extract. Annals Allergy 55: 312.

Genser, J. K., and Schmid-Grendelmeier, P. (2014). *In vivo* allergy diagnosis—skin tests. pp. 150–152. *In*: C.A. Akdis and I. Agache (eds.). Global Atlas of Allergy 1st ed. Zurich: European Academy of Allergy and Clinical Immunology, EAACI.

Heinzerling, L., Mari, A., Bergmann, K. C., Bresciani, M., Burbach, G., Darsow, U., Durham, S., Fokkens, W., Gjomarkaj, M., Haahtela, T., Bom, A. T., Wohrl, S., Maibach, H., and Lockey, R. (2013). The skin prick test—European standards. Clinical and Translational Allergy 3(1): 3.

Heinzerling, L. M., Burbach, G. J., Edenharter, G., Bachert, C., Bindslev-Jensen, C., Bonini, S., Bousquet, J., Bousquet-Rouanet, L., Bousquet, P. J., Bresciani, M., Bruno, A., Burney, P., Canonica, G. W., Darsow, U., Demoly, P., Durham, S., Fokkens, W. J., Giavi, S., Gjomarkaj, M., Gramiccioni, C., Haahtela, T., Kowalski, M. L., Magyar, P., Murakozi, G., Orosz, M., Papadopoulos, N. G., Rohnelt, C., Stingl, G., Todo-Bom, A., von Mutius, E., Wiesner, A., Wohrl, S., and Zuberbier, T. (2009). GA(2)LEN skin test study I: GA(2)LEN harmonization of skin prick testing: novel sensitization patterns for inhalant allergens in Europe. Allergy 64(10): 1498–1506.

Johansson, S. G. O., Hourihane, J. O., Bousquet, J., Bruijnzeel-Koomen, C., Dreborg, S., Haahtela, T., Kowalski, M. L., Mygind, N., Ring, J., van Cauwenberge, P., van Hage-Hamsten, M., and Wuthrich, B. (2001). A revised nomenclature for allergy. An EAACI position statement from the EAACI nomenclature task force. Allergy 56(9): 813–824.

Johansson, S. G. O., Bieber, T., Dahl, R., Friedmann, P. S., Lanier, B. Q., Lockey, R. F., Motala, C., Ortega Martell, J. A., Platts-Mills, T. A., Ring, J., Thien, F., Van, C. P., and Williams, H. C. (2004). Revised nomenclature for allergy for global use: Report of the nomenclature review committee of the World Allergy Organization, October 2003. The Journal of Allergy and Clinical Immunology 113(5): 832–836.

King, M. J., Phillips, S. E., and Lockey, R. F. (2014). Effect of photoaging on skin test response to histamine independent of chronologic age. Annals of Allergy, Asthma & Immunology: Official Publication of the American College of Allergy, Asthma, & Immunology 113(6): 647–651.

Konstantinou, G. N., Bousquet, P. J., Zuberbier, T., and Papadopoulos, N. G. (2010). The longest wheal diameter is the optimal measurement for the evaluation of skin prick tests. International Archives of Allergy and Immunology 151(4): 343–345.

Kuhn, W., Urbanek, R., Forster, J., Dreborg, S., and Burow, G. (1985). Hyposensibilizierung bei Pollnosis: dreijährige prospektive Vergleichsuntersuchung bei Kindern [Immunotherapy in pollinosis: A three year's prospective study in children]. Allergologie 8: 103–109.

Larsen, J. N., and Dreborg, S. (2008). Standardization of allergen extracts. pp. 133–145. In: A. Walker (ed.). Methods Mol Med Vol. 138 1 ed. Springer.

Lockey, R. F., Benedict, L. M., Turkeltaub, P. C., and Bukantz, S. C. (1987). Fatalities from immunotherapy (IT) and skin testing (ST). The Journal of Allergy and Clinical Immunology 79(4): 660–677.

Malling, H. J. (1984). Skin prick testing and the use of histamine references. Allergy 39(8): 596–601.

Matsson, P. N. J., Hamilton, R. G., Esch, R. E., Halsey, J. F., Homburger, H.A., Kleine-Tebbe, J., and Ownby, D. (2009). Analytical Performance Characteristics and Clinical Utility of Immunological Assays for Human Immunoglobulin E (IgE) Antibodies and Defined Allergen Specificities; Approved Guideline (Vol. 29, pp. 1–160). Philadelphia: Clinical and Laboratory Standards Institute.

Moller, C., Bjorksten, B., Nilsson, G., and Dreborg, S. (1984). The precision of the conjunctival provocation test. Allergy 39(1): 37–41.

Morrow Brown, H. (1976). Skin prick tests with a standardised puncture needle. Paper presented at the 2nd. Charles Blackley Symposium, Nottingham.

Nelson, H. S., Knoetzer, J., and Bucher, B. (1996). Effect of distance between sites and region of the body on results of skin prick tests. The Journal of Allergy and Clinical Immunology 97(2): 596–601.

Nelson, H. S., Lahr, J., Buchmeier, A., and McCormick, D. (1998). Evaluation of devices for skin prick testing. The Journal of Allergy and Clinical Immunology 101(2 Pt 1): 153–156.

Nyren, M., Ollmar, S., Nicander, I., and Emtestam, L. (1996). An electrical impedance technique for assessment of wheals. Allergy 51(12): 923–926.

Olsson, P., Hammarlund, A., and Pipkorn, U. (1988). Wheal-and-flare reactions induced by allergen and histamine: evaluation of blood flow with laser Doppler flow metry. The Journal of Allergy and Clinical Immunology 82(2): 291–296.

Oppenheimer, J., and Nelson, H. S. (2006). Skin testing. Annals of Allergy, Asthma & Immunology: Official Publication of the American College of Allergy, Asthma, & Immunology 96(2 Suppl 1): S6–12.

Ortolani, C., Ispano, M., Pastorello, E. A., Ansaloni, R., and Magri, G. C. (1989). Comparison of results of skin prick tests (with fresh foods and commercial food extracts) and RAST in 100 patients with oral allergy syndrome. The Journal of Allergy and Clinical Immunology 83(3): 683–690.

Osterballe, O., and Weeke, B. (1979). A new lancet for skin prick testing. Allergy 34(4): 209–212.

Pepys, J. (1968). Skin tests in diagnosis. In: Gell, R. and Coombs, R. (eds.), Clinical Aspects of Immunology (2nd ed., pp. 192). Oxford: Blackwell Scientific Publications.

Pepys, J. (1975). Skin testing. Br J Hosp Med 14: 412–417.

Phipatanakul, C. S., and Slavin, R. G. (1972). Use of thermography in clinical allergy. The Journal of Allergy and Clinical Immunology 50(5): 264–275.

Pijnenborg, H., Nilsson, L., and Dreborg, S. (1996). Estimation of skin prick test reactions with a scanning program. Allergy 51(11): 782–788.

Poulsen, L. K., Liisberg, C., Bindslev-Jensen, C., and Malling, H. J. (1993). Precise area determination of skin-prick tests: validation of a scanning device and software for a personal computer. Clinical and Experimental Allergy: Journal of the British Society for Allergy and Clinical Immunology 23(1): 61–68.

Radauer, C., Nandy, A., Ferreira, F., Goodman, R. E., Larsen, J. N., Lidholm, J., Pomes, A., Raulf-Heimsoth, M., Rozynek, P., Thomas, W. R., and Breiteneder, H. (2014). Update of the WHO/IUIS Allergen Nomenclature Database based on analysis of allergen sequences. Allergy 69(4): 413–419.

Rance, F., Juchet, A., Bremont, F., and Dutau, G. (1997). Correlations between skin prick tests using commercial extracts and fresh foods, specific IgE, and food challenges. Allergy 52(10): 1031–1035.

Registration of allergen preparations. Nordic Guidelines. (1989).

Rokita, E., Rok, T., and Taton, G. (2011). Application of thermography for the assessment of allergen-induced skin reactions. Medical Physics 38(2): 765–772.

Siebenhaar, F., Degener, F., Zuberbier, T., Martus, P., and Maurer, M. (2009). High-dose desloratadine decreases wheal volume and improves cold provocation thresholds compared with standard-dose treatment in patients with acquired cold urticaria: a randomized, placebo-controlled, crossover study. The Journal of Allergy and Clinical Immunology 123(3): 672–679.

Stuckey, M., Witt, C., Schmitt, L., Warlow, R., Lattimore, M., and Dawkins, R. (1985). Histamine sensitivity influences reactivity to allergens. The Journal of Allergy and Clinical Immunology 75: 373–376.

Taudorf, E., Malling, H. J., Laursen, L. C., Lanner, A., and Weeke, B. (1985). Reproducibility of histamine skin prick test. Inter- and intravariation using histamine dihydrochloride 1, 5, and 10 mg/ml. Allergy 40(5): 344–349.

Uematsu, T., Takiguchi, Y., Mizuno, A., Sogabe, K., and Nakashima, M. (1987). Application of thermography to the evaluation of the histamine skin test in man. Journal of Pharmacological Methods 18(2): 103–110.

Varjonen, E., Bjorksten, F., and Savolainen, J. (1996). Stability of cereal allergens. Clinical and Experimental Allergy: Journal of the British Society for Allergy and Clinical Immunology 26(4): 436–443.

Witt, C. S., Stuckey, M. S., and Dawkins, R. L. (1987). Extreme cutaneous histamine sensitivity with hay fever and increased IgE concentrations in an unselected population. Br Med J (Clin Res Ed) 295(6596): 461–463.

Yuenyongviwat, A., Koonrangsesomboon, D., and Sangsupawanich, P. (2012). Comparison of skin test reactivity to histamine on back and forearm in young children. Asian Pacific Journal of Allergy and Immunology/Launched by the Allergy and Immunology Society of Thailand 30(4): 301–305.

CHAPTER 7

Immunotherapy for Food Allergy

Bright I. Nwaru and *Aziz Sheikh**

Introduction

The incidence and prevalence of food allergy have risen over the past 10–15 years (Boyce *et al.*, 2010; Nwaru *et al.*, 2014a, 2014b), and this has been described as the second wave of the allergy epidemic (Prescott and Allen, 2011). Globally, depending on the definition used and population group studied, up to 10% of the population may be affected by food allergy at some point in their lives (Zuberbier *et al.*, 2004; Rona *et al.*, 2007; Chafen *et al.*, 2010). With increased morbidity, poor quality of life, substantial healthcare and societal burden, and in some cases deaths resulting from food-triggered anaphylaxis, food allergy is now being seen as a growing public health problem (Sampson, 2005; Boyce *et al.*, 2010; Burks *et al.*, 2012; Longo *et al.*, 2013; Muraro *et al.*, 2014a). Some food allergies, such as cow's milk, hen's egg, wheat and soy tend to resolve over time, but some—particularly, peanut, tree nuts and seafood allergies—may remain lifelong disorders. The majority of food allergy reactions are primarily mediated by immunoglobulin E (IgE), resulting from an imbalance in the T helper cell 1 (Th1)/Th2 ratio, with a skewing towards Th2, allowing for excessive IgE production and relative deficiency of Th1 (Sabra *et al.*, 2003; Burks *et al.*, 2012; Muraro *et al.*, 2014b; Sampson *et al.*, 2014). IgE-mediated reactions to foods typically have rapid onset of symptoms after consumption of even very small amounts of the offending food, and reactions generally involve the skin, gastrointestinal tract, cardiovascular system and respiratory tract (Burks *et al.*, 2012; Muraro *et al.*, 2014a; Sampson *et al.*, 2014).

Asthma UK Centre for Applied Research, Centre for Medical Informatics, Usher Institute of Population Health Sciences and Informatics, The University of Edinburgh, Old Medical School, Teviot Place, EH8 9AG, UK.

Email: bright.nwaru@ed.ac.uk

* Corresponding author: aziz.sheikh@ed.ac.uk

There is currently no definitive therapy or cure for IgE-mediated food allergy, hence current efforts have targeted possible preventive and management strategies (De Silva *et al.*, 2014a; Muraro *et al.*, 2014a; Sampson *et al.*, 2014). The first option for the management of acute, life-threatening reactions from food allergy, i.e., anaphylaxis, is the use of intramuscular epinephrine (adrenaline) (Burks *et al.*, 2012; De Silva *et al.*, 2014b; Muraro *et al.*, 2014b; Sicherer and Sampson, 2014). At-risk individuals should have their injectable epinephrine at hand in case of accidental exposure to foods to which they are allergic, which can subsequently trigger off anaphylaxis (Boyce *et al.*, 2010; Muraro *et al.*, 2014a; Sampson *et al.*, 2014). Other second- and third-line treatments may also need to be employed in the management of anaphylaxis, but the priority is always the prompt administration of epinephrine (Sheikh *et al.*, 2011; Burks *et al.*, 2012; Muraro *et al.*, 2014a).

Strict avoidance of offending foods is of paramount importance in the long-term management of food allergy (De Silva *et al.*, 2014b; Muraro *et al.*, 2014a; Sampson *et al.*, 2014). Whilst the strategy of food avoidance is straightforward in principle, it can prove very challenging in practice, particularly in the context of foods that are used in a range of food products (e.g., milk, eggs and peanuts) (De Silva *et al.*, 2014b; Muraro *et al.*, 2014a; Sampson *et al.*, 2014). It is for this reason that across several countries and regions, including the United States, European Union, Australia, Canada, Japan and Singapore, food-labeling laws have been implemented, which require food manufacturers to state in a simple language, the ingredients used to prepare foods that might have come from allergenic food sources. This strategy can help food allergy sufferers to navigate through food choices when, for example, traveling, in a restaurant and at school (Sheikh *et al.*, 2011; Burks *et al.*, 2012; Muraro *et al.*, 2014a).

Given the risk of accidental exposure to a culprit food and the resulting risk of triggering anaphylaxis, there is a need to identify alternative management strategies and, if possible, curative treatments (Boyce *et al.*, 2010; De Silva *et al.*, 2014b; Muraro *et al.*, 2014a; Sampson *et al.*, 2014). In this regard, immunotherapy, the carefully controlled incremental administration of small amounts of native or modified allergens to patients with food allergy in order to induce desensitization and immune tolerance (see Box 7.1), is a potential disease modifying treatment approach (Scadding, 2013; De Silva *et al.*, 2014b; Muraro *et al.*, 2014a). Although allergen immunotherapy has been used in the management of other allergic disorders (e.g., hay fever) for many decades, it is only recently that the underlying biological mechanisms underpinning this treatment approach have begun to be understood (Wang and Sampson, 2013; McGowan and Wood, 2014; Narisety and Keet, 2012). Whilst its efficacy has been established for disorders such as allergic rhinitis and venom allergy (Boyle *et al.*, 2012), its role in food allergy remains an area of vigorous research and debate (Calderon *et al.*, 2007; Nurmatov *et al.*, 2012; Nurmatov *et al.*, 2014; Romantsik *et al.*, 2014; Jutel *et al.*, 2015).

Box 7.1: Meaning of desensitization and tolerance in allergen-specific immunotherapy.

Desensitization	Tolerance
Desensitization refers to the ability to achieve a temporal antigen hypo-responsiveness through regular increase in the amount of a food protein that is needed to achieve a clinical reaction. Subjects are usually given the offending food starting with very low dose, which are then gradually increased over time. Desensitization is only a temporary state, therefore if dosing is discontinued, its protection is lost.	Tolerance refers to the ability to achieve a permanent antigen hypo-responsiveness, which allows safe consumption of large amounts of a food protein after treatment with immunotherapy has been discontinued. It is therefore a much more permanent state of immunologic change than that achieved by desensitization.

Historical Perspectives to Allergen-Specific Immunotherapy

The first successful trial of allergen-specific immunotherapy (subcutaneous) in humans is credited to the seminal work undertaken by Leonard Noon and reported in the Lancet in 1911 (Noon, 1911; Scadding, 2013) in which he injected hay fever patients with extract of grass pollen; this followed by John Freeman's continuation of the procedure later that year at the death of Noon (Freeman, 1911; Freeman, 1930). According to the procedure, Noon prepared grass pollen-derived allergen extract, and by finding the right dilution in skin tests, he injected hay fever patients with allergen extract in increasing doses. He used conjunctival provocation tests (before and after the treatment) to measure the effect of the treatment through administering droplets of different extract dilutions into the eye of the hay fever patients and then evaluating the redness and possible inflammatory reactions. He later called the conjunctival provocation "prophylactic inoculation" (Noon, 1911; Freeman, 1911; Freeman, 1930; Ring and Gutermuth, 2011; Fitzhugh and Lockey, 2011). Noon died early from tuberculosis, but his work was continued by his colleague, Freeman, who applied the procedure in a larger sample of cases (Freeman, 1911; Freeman, 1930; Ring and Gutermuth, 2011; Fitzhugh and Lockey, 2011). Across the world, this landmark procedure was taken up by physicians as it established several clinical principles that remain relevant in practice till today, although with some refinements: these include having a protocol of increasing extract dosage; an initial interval of 1–2 weeks for injection; and taking a caution against overdose that might result from anaphylaxis (Fitzhugh and Lockey, 2011).

Although Noon and Freeman's trials were the first formal experimentation in humans, overarching principles of their procedure were based on earlier works and observations made by Charles Blackley and William Dunbar. In the 1870s, Blackley conducted the first investigations into the nature of pollen allergy and its treatment by instilling rye grass pollen into his own nostril and later performed the same procedure on his skin in order to observe whether his allergic symptoms would bring relief (Fitzhugh and Lockey, 2011). Dunbar, in 1903, performed a passive immunization with anti-pollen extract, which he prepared as an ointment and applied to the eyes, nose, and mouth in order to relieve rhinitis symptoms (Fitzhugh and Lockey, 2011). In 1908, Alfred Schofield described an egg allergy case in a boy who developed tolerance to egg after several months of constant incremental administration of egg with some calcium lactate added to halt any transudation (Schofield, 1908; Lack, 2013). Robert Cooke introduced the therapy by Noon and Freeman to the United States, which he coined "active immunization" in 1914 and later proposed the use of the term "hyposensitization" in its place in 1922 (Ring *et al.*, 2011). Further progress was made in 1954 when William Frankland and Rosa Augustin published results of the first double-blind, placebo-controlled trial on the efficacy of allergen-specific immunotherapy (Frankland and Augustin, 1954; Fitzhugh and Lockey, 2011). Rapid developments continue to take place around the world on the efficacy of allergen-specific immunotherapy until the World Health Organization (WHO) validated the evidence that had so far accumulated on the efficacy, safety, and tolerability of subcutaneous immunotherapy (SCIT) as a therapy for allergy, which was the time indicated for allergic rhinitis, Hymenoptera hypersensitivity, and asthma, although risk of adverse events (anaphylaxis) was noted (Bousquet *et al.*, 1998; Fitzhugh and Lockey, 2011).

Types of Immunotherapy Approaches for Food Allergy

As described in the preceding historical perspective to immunotherapy, SCIT, also sometimes known as allergy shots, was the first immunotherapy approach used, and although widely used in other forms of allergy, such as allergic rhinitis, it is not now used in the context of food allergy, largely because of safety concerns (Cox *et al.*, 2012; Kulis *et al.*, 2015; Khoriaty and Umetsu, 2013). In addition to SCIT, subsequent investigations into allergen-specific immunotherapy for food allergy have focused on the following specific routes of administration: epicutaneous, sublingual and oral immunotherapies (Beyer, 2012; Kulis *et al.*, 2015; Chiang and Yang, 2014) (see Box 7.2). Epicutaneous immunotherapy (EPIT) provides an alternative route of administration that involves the placement of dried allergen extract using a circular disk onto intact skin, especially on the uttermost layer of the skin, epidermis (Senti *et al.*, 2011; Yang and Chiang, 2014). Moisture from the skin solubilizes the allergen, which is then taken up by dendritic cells on the outer layer of the skin (Khoriaty and Umetsu, 2013; Kulis *et al.*, 2015; Yang and Chiang, 2014). EPIT is non-invasive, safe, self-administrable, and appears promising for the treatment of food allergy, particularly peanut and cow's milk allergy (Khoriaty and Umetsu, 2013; Kulis *et al.*, 2015). However, its efficacy has been shown primarily in animal models and a small number of studies in humans (Sampson *et al.*, 2015); there are currently ongoing clinical trials investigating its efficacy (Kulis *et al.*, 2015; Senti *et al.*, 2011; Yang and Chiang, 2014).

Box 7.2: Types of allergen-specific immunotherapy approaches for food allergy.

SCIT	EPIT	SLIT	OIT
SCIT, also known as allergy shots, is the first approach to allergen-specific immunotherapy ever used. However, due to safety concerns, it is no longer used for food allergy. It involves weekly injection of the allergen extract during a build-up stage, which is followed by monthly injection for a period of 3–5 years (Cox *et al.*, 2012; Kulis *et al.*, 2015; Khoriaty and Umetsu, 2013).	EPIT involves the placement of dried allergen extract of the specific food on the uttermost layer of the skin, allowing moisture from the skin to solubilize the allergen. EPIT has the advantage of being self-administrable, non-invasive and safe. However, it has so far been evaluated in animals studies and few studies in humans, and appears promising particularly for peanut and cow's milk allergy (Kulis *et al.*, 2015; Senti *et al.*, 2011; Yang and Chiang, 2014).	In SLIT, drops of extracts of the specific allergen are placed under the tongue, held for 2 minutes and then swallowed. During the build-up phase, very low doses of the allergen are started with, then increased over weeks until a maintenance dose is achieved and continued daily for several years (Wang and Sampson, 2013; Moran *et al.*, 2013; Nowak-Wegrzyn and Albin, 2015; McGowan and Wood, 2014).	As the name suggests, OIT involves giving the allergen extracts by mouth—small amounts of the allergen extracts are ingested in a powder form or mixture of the extracts with a food vehicle. The build-up and maintenance phases for OIT are similar to those of SLIT, but OIT usually starts with higher dosages than SLIT (Khoriaty and Umetsu, 2013; Nowak-Wegrzyn and Albin, 2015; McGowan and Wood, 2014).

Sublingual immunotherapy (SLIT) involves the placement of drops of allergen extracts under the tongue, held for 2 minutes, and then swallowed (Wang and Sampson, 2013; Moran *et al.*, 2013; Nowak-Wegrzyn and Albin, 2015; McGowan and Wood, 2014). Although different protocols have been used across different studies and settings, in essence the procedure involves a build-up phase and a maintenance phase. The build-up phase involves starting with extremely low doses of food allergen, which are then increased over several weeks until a maintenance dose is reached; the maintenance dose is then typically taken daily for several years (Wang and Sampson, 2013; Moran *et al.*, 2013; Nowak-Wegrzyn and Albin, 2015; McGowan and Wood, 2014). The dose usually starts with micrograms and gradually increased to milligram amounts; thus by allowing smaller doses to be given at a time, SLIT may allow food proteins to bypass gastric digestion by taking advantage of the tolerogenic antigen-presenting cells in the oral mucosa (Khoriaty and Umetsu, 2013; Nowak-Wegrzyn and Albin, 2015; McGowan and Wood, 2014).

Oral immunotherapy (OIT) involves ingestion of small amounts of allergen extracts from culprit foods in a powder form or mixture of culprit foods with a food vehicle (Khoriaty and Umetsu, 2013; Nowak-Wegrzyn and Albin, 2015; McGowan and Wood, 2014). The schedules for dose escalation and maintenance in OIT are similar to those described for SLIT, however, OIT typically starts with milligram amounts, which are increased to several grams for maintenance dose; the duration of treatment for OIT is usually longer than SLIT (Khoriaty and Umetsu, 2013; Nowak-Wegrzyn and Albin, 2015; McGowan and Wood, 2014).

Amongst the various approaches highlighted above, OIT and SLIT have been the most studied, and, in the context of food allergy, they appear to be the most promising therapies for food allergy; however issues of safety and tolerability of treatment remain key concerns (Nariety and Keet, 2012; Wang and Sampson, 2013; Moran *et al.*, 2013). In this chapter, drawing from our recent rigorously conducted systematic reviews and those of other groups in the field (Nurmatov *et al.*, 2012; Nurmatov *et al.*, 2014; Yepes-Nunez *et al.*, 2015; Yeung *et al.*, 2012; Sun *et al.*, 2014; Romantsik *et al.*, 2014), we present an overview of the current evidence on the efficacy of allergen-specific immunotherapy for food allergy, and discuss future research directions. Given that their clinical efficacy is the most established, in comparison to other routes of administration, we focus on the potentials of OIT and SLIT. So far, the majority of studies on the efficacy of OIT and SLIT have focused on cow's milk, egg, and peanut allergy, but they have also been investigated in relation to a variety of other foods, including hazelnut, peach, orange, apple, corn, fish, bean, wheat and lettuce (Nurmatov *et al.*, 2014). However, our discussion focuses on the evidence so far with respect to cow's milk, egg, and peanut allergy as the main food allergies studied. In this regard, we describe the current evidence for each of these food allergies in terms of clinical efficacy, safety and tolerability (see Box 7.1 above).

OIT/SLIT for cow's milk allergy

In our recent systematic review (Nurmatov *et al.*, 2014), results of eight studies (Randomized Controlled Trials [RCT] and Controlled Clinical Trials [CCT]) that investigated the efficacy of OIT/SLIT for cow's milk allergy showed a substantial reduction in the risk of desensitization in cow's milk allergy (relative risk [RR] 0.14, 95% confidence interval [95% CI] 0.04–0.44), reduction in the magnitude in skin prick test mean wheal diameter by –3.42 (95% CI –6.18 to –0.66) mm, but while no significant effect was observed for allergen-specific IgE; as anticipated, allergen-specific IgG4 was increased (Nurmatov *et al.*, 2014). Only two studies reported on long-term tolerance but with inconsistent findings, indicating that long-term effect on tolerance is unclear at this point. With respect to safety, both systemic and local (minor oropharyngeal/gastrointestinal) reactions were more commonly associated with OIT/SLIT (Nurmatov *et al.*, 2014). In an earlier Cochrane systematic review that included five trials, the pooled effect of OIT for desensitization in cow's milk allergy was RR 6.61 (95% CI 3.51–12.44) compared to a control group (Yeung *et al.*, 2012). In that review, none of the studies evaluated the effect of

OIT on long-term tolerance in cow's milk allergy, but there was generally an improvement in serologic endpoints (allergen-specific IgE and IgG4) across studies (Yeung *et al.*, 2012). However, adverse effects were frequently reported across studies in that review, including oral pruritis, abdominal pain and, in some cases, anaphylactic reactions; the majority of these symptoms were however mild and self-limiting (Yeung *et al.*, 2012).

OIT/SLIT for hen's egg allergy

In our systematic review, four trials examined the effect of OIT for egg allergy and a pooled estimate demonstrated substantial reduction in risk of egg allergy as assessed by double-blind placebo-controlled food challenge (RR 0.19, 95% CI 0.04–0.99) (Nurmatov *et al.*, 2014). With respect to long-term effect on tolerance, two studies investigated this, while one study reported that about 28% of children undergoing OIT sustained unresponsiveness after cessation of OIT, one study found no evidence of difference in long-term tolerance between OIT and control patients (Nurmatov *et al.*, 2014). There was also no clear effect on serologic endpoints (allergen-specific IgE and IgG4). In a recent Cochrane systematic review, compared to no therapy (11.9%), egg allergy patients receiving OIT/SLIT (39%) were more likely to be desensitized (RR 3.39, 95% CI 1.74–6.62); patients receiving OIT/SLIT were also more favorably partially desensitized compared to patients on no therapy (RR 5.73, 95% CI 3.13–10.50); and overtime, the magnitude of their SPT wheal size were more significantly reduced compared to patients in the no therapy group (Romantsik *et al.*, 2014). Although included studies were heterogeneous with regards to definition, mild-to-severe adverse effects were greater in the OIT/SLIT group compared to the no therapy group (RR 6.06, 95% CI 3.11–11.83). With regards to serologic endpoints (allergen-specific IgE and IgG4), included studies used different laboratory methods with varying cut-offs, consequently findings were conflicting, with some studies reporting increased concentration of IgE and IgG4 concentrations, while others reported no significant differences between the two groups (Romantsik *et al.*, 2014).

OIT/SLIT for peanut allergy

We found three trials that have investigated the effect of OIT/SLIT on peanut allergy and our pooled estimates showed a significant reduction in risk (RR 0.16, 95% CI 0.06–0.41) in children undergoing OIT/SLIT compared to those in control arm (Nurmatov *et al.*, 2014). There were no data on the effect of OIT/SLIT on long-term tolerance in peanut allergy and data on immunologic outcomes were reported differently across studies (Nurmatov *et al.*, 2014). A related systematic review that included the three trials we found also reported that OIT/SLIT significantly improved peanut allergy (odds ratio [OR] 38.44, 95% CI 6.01–245.81) in patients treated with the intervention compared to control group, but the estimates were very imprecise (Sun *et al.*, 2014). The authors reported that adverse outcomes were common in the OIT/SLIT across the trials included but the use of epinephrine during the study did not differ between the OIT/SLIT patients and the control group (Sun *et al.*, 2014). In a previous Cochrane review that included only one small trial, we found that peanut OIT resulted in reductions in SPT wheal size, interleukin-5, interleukin-13, and an increase in peanut-specific IgG4 (Nurmatov *et al.*, 2012). In comparison to the placebo group, adverse events were more common in the OIT patients including use of medications (Nurmatov *et al.*, 2012).

Summary of Efficacy of OIT and SLIT

Overall, synthesis of results from studies of both OIT and SLIT for desensitization in allergy to cow's milk, hen's egg and peanut are encouraging; however, effect on long-term tolerance is uncertain. Both OIT and SLIT achieved desensitization to varying degrees and differed in doses, duration of treatment and safety profile. Studies comparing OIT and SLIT show that OIT appears to be more efficacious than SLIT in inducing desensitization, at least to cow's milk and peanut, and while overall safety appears to be similar between OIT and SLIT, reactions from OIT appear more likely to involve multiple systems, upper and lower respiratory tracts and the gastrointestinal tract (McGowan and Wood, 2014). Overall, the quality and strength of the available evidence is limited by the small size of the trials and concerns about the methodological quality of some studies (Yeung *et al.*, 2012). Comparison of findings across studies has also been limited due to varying protocols used across studies. Apart from effect on clinical efficacy, so far, there are no data on the effect of OIT and SLIT on other outcomes of cow's milk, hen's egg and peanut, such as quality of life of patients and their families, healthcare utilization, including emergency hospital admissions and cost-effectiveness (Nurmatov *et al.*, 2014). Since the publication of our systematic review, few clinical trials have now reported further findings on the effect of OIT on atopy (Zolkipli *et al.*, 2015), effect of SLIT on peanut allergy (Burks *et al.*, 2015), OIT vs. SLIT on peanut allergy (Narisety *et al.*, 2015) and OIT on peanut allergy. Whilst the results of these trials are favorable with regards to improving investigated outcomes, a cumulative synthesis is required to integrate their findings to previous studies in order to more comprehensively evaluate the current evidence.

Conclusions and Future Directions

Developments in immunotherapy for food allergies are showing encouraging results for patients, particularly OIT and SLIT, which appear very promising for cow's milk allergy, hen's egg allergy and peanut allergy. However, before their wider application in clinical practice, issues of safety and effect on long-term tolerance need to be clarified. Further studies, with sufficient power and improved design, are required to address the issues of optimal dosage of each administration approach, duration, age-dependent efficacy and level of severity across food allergy outcomes. Given the lack of cost-effectiveness studies, it is presently unclear whether, in comparison to conventional food avoidance, immunotherapy is more cost-effective; additional studies are needed to address this issue. Ongoing efforts now need to be intensified with regards to standardization of safe and easy to use protocols across studies, which will then enhance comparability of findings and facilitate quicker application of findings into clinical practice.

Keywords: allergen immunotherapy, anaphylaxis, cow's milk allergy, desensitization, egg allergy, epicutaneous immunotherapy, hypo-responsiveness, IgE-food allergy, oral immunotherapy, peanut allergy, subcutaneous immunotherapy, sublingual immunotherapy, tolerance

References

Anagnostou, K., Islam, S., King, Y., Foley, L., Pasea, L., Bond, S. *et al.* (2014). Assessing the efficacy of oral immunotherapy for the desensitization of peanut allergy in children (STOP II): a phase 2 randomized controlled trial. Lancet 383: 1297–1304.

Beyer, K. (2012). A European perspective on immunotherapy for food allergies. The Journal of Allergy and Clinical Immunology 129: 1179–1184.

Bousquet, J., Lockey, R., and Malling, H. J. (eds.). (1998). Allergen immunotherapy: therapeutic vaccines for allergic diseases: a WHO position paper. The Journal of Allergy and Clinical Immunology 102: 558–562.

Boyce, J. A., Assa'ad, A., Burks, A. W., Jones, S. M., Sampson, H. A., and Wood, R. A. (2010). Guidelines for the diagnosis and management of food allergy in the United States: report of the NIAD-Sponsored expert panel. The Journal of Allergy and Clinical Immunology 126: S1–S58.

Boyle, R. J., Elremeli, M., Hockenhull, J., Cherry, M. G., Bulsara, M K., and Daniels, M. (2012). Venom immunotherapy for preventing allergic reactions to insect stings. Cochrane Database Syst Rev 10: CD008838.

Burks, A. W., Tang, M., Sicherer, S., Muraro, A., Eigenmann, P. A., Ebisawa, M. *et al.* (2012). ICON: food allergy. The Journal of Allergy and Clinical Immunology 129: 906–920.

Burks, A. W., Wood, R. A., Jones, S. M., Sicherer, S. H., Fleischer, D. M., Scurlock, A. M. *et al.* (2015). Sublingual immunotherapy for peanut allergy: long-term follow-up of a randomized multicenter trial. The Journal of Allergy and Clinical Immunology 135: 1240–1248.

Chafen, J. J., Newberry, S. J., Riedl, M. A., Bravata, D. M., Maglione, M., Suttorp, M. J. *et al.* (2010). Diagnosing and managing common food allergies: a systematic review. JAMA 303: 1848–1856.

Cox, L., Calderon, M., and Pfaar, O. (2012). Subcutaneous allergen immunotherapy for allergic disease: examining efficacy, safety and cost-effectiveness of current and novel formulations. Immunotherapy 4: 601–616.

De Silva, D., Geromi, M., Halken, S., Host, A., Panesar, S. S., Muraro, A. *et al.* (2014a). Primary prevention of food allergy in children and adults: systematic review. Allergy 69: 581–589.

De Silva, D., Geromi, M., Panesar, S. S., Muraro, A., Werfel, T., Hoffmann-Sommergruber, K. *et al.* (2014b). Acute and long-term management of food allergy: systematic review. Allergy 69: 159–167.

Fitzhugh, D. J., and Lockey, R. F. (2011). Allergen immunotherapy: a history of the first 100 years. Current Opinion in Allergy and Clinical Immunology 11: 554–559.

Freeman, J. (1911). Further observations on the treatment of hay fever by hypodermic inoculations of pollen vaccine. Lancet 178: 814–817.

Freeman, J. (1930). Rush inoculation with special reference to hay fever treatment. Lancet 215: 744–747.

Jutel, M., Agache, I., Bonini, S., Burks, A. W., Calderon, M., Canonica, W. *et al.* (2015). International consensus on allergy immunotherapy. The Journal of Allergy and Clinical Immunology 136: 556–568.

Khoriaty, E., and Umetsu, D. T. (2013). Oral immunotherapy for food allergy: towards a new horizon. Allergy, Asthma & Immunology Research 5: 3–15.

Kulls, M., Wright, B. L., Jones, S. M., and Burks, A. W. (2015). Diagnosis, management, and investigational therapies for food allergies. Gastroenterology 148: 1132–1142.

Lack, G. (2013). An innovative treatment for food allergy. pp. 25–27. *In*: A. Sheikh, T. Platts-Mills and A. Worth (eds.). Landmark Papers in Allergy: Seminal Papers in Allergy with Expert Commentaries. Oxford: Oxford University Press.

Longo, G., Berti, I., Burks, A. W., Kraus, B., and Barbi, E. (2013). Ige-mediated food allergy in children. Lancet 382: 1656–1664.

McGowan, E. C., and Wood, R. A. (2014). Sublingual (SLIT) versus oral immunotherapy (OIT) for food allergy. Current Allergy Asthma and Reports 14: 486.

Moran, T. P., Vickery, B. P., and Burks, A. W. (2013). Oral and sublingual immunotherapy for food allergy: current progress and future directions. Current Opinion Immunology 25: 781–787.

Muraro, A., Werfel, T., Hoffman-Sommergruber, K., Roberts, G., Beyer, K., Bindsley-Jensen, C. *et al.* (2014a). EAACI food allergy and anaphylaxis guidelines: diagnosis and management of food allergy. Allergy 69: 1008–1025.

Muraro, A., Halken, S., Arshad, S. H., Beyer, K., Dubois, A. E., Du Toit, G. *et al.* (2014b). EAACI food allergy and anaphylaxis guidelines. Primary prevention of food allergy. Allergy 69: 590–601.

Narisety, S. D., and Keet, C. A. (2012). Sublingual vs. oral immunotherapy for food allergy: identifying the right approach. Drugs 72: 1977–1989.

Narisety, S. D., Frischmeyer-Guerrerio, P. A., Keet, C. A., Gorelik, M., Schroeder, J., Hamilton, R. G. *et al.* (2015). A randomized, double-blind, placebo-controlled pilot study of sublingual versus oral immunotherapy for the treatment of peanut allergy. The Journal of Allergy and Clinical Immunology 135: 1275–1282.

Noon, L. (1911). Prophylactic inoculation against hay fever. Lancet 177: 1572–1573.

Nowak-Wegrzyn, A., and Fiocchi, A. (2010). Is oral immunotherapy the cure for food allergies? Current Opinion in Allergy and Clinical Immunology 10: 214–219.

Nurmatov, U., Venderbosch, I., Devereux, G., Simons, F. E., and Sheikh, A. (2012). Allergen-specific oral immunotheraöy for peanut allergy. Cochrane Database Syst Rev 11: CD009014.

Nurmatov, U., Devereux, G., Worth, A., Healy, L., and Sheikh, A. (2014). Effectiveness and safety of orally administrered immunotherapy for food allergies: a systematic review and meta-analysis. British Journal of Nutrition 111: 12–22.

Nwaru, B. I., Hickstein, L., Panessar, S. S., Muraro, A., Werfel, T., Cardona, V. *et al.* (2014a). The epidemiology of food allergy in Europe: a systematic review and meta-analysis. Allergy 69: 62–75.

Nwaru, B. I., Hickstein, L., Panessar, S. S., Roberts, G., Muraro, A., Sheikh, A. *et al.* (2014b). Prevalence of common food allergies in Europe: a systematic review and meta-analysis. Allergy 69: 992–1007.

Prescott, S., and Allen, K. J. (2011). Food allergy: riding the second wave of the allergy epidemic. Pediatric of Allergy Immunology 22: 155–160.

Ring, J., and Gutermuth, J. (2011). 100 years of hyposensitization: history of allergen-specific immunotherapy (ASIT). Allergy 66: 713–724.

Romantsik, O., Bruschettini, M., Tosca, M. A., Zappettini, S., Della Casa Alberighi, O., and Calevo, M. G. (2014). Oral and sublingual immunotherapy for egg allergy. Cochrane Database Syst Rev 11: CD010638.

Rona, R. J., Keil, T., Summers, C., Gislason, D., Zuidmeer, L., Sodergren, E. *et al.* (2007). The prevalence of food allergy: a meta-analysis. The Journal of Allergy and Clinical Immunology 120: 638–646.

Sabra, A., Bellani, J. A., Rais, J. M., Castro, H. J., de Inocencio, J. M., and Sabra, S. (2003). IgE and non-IgE food allergy. Annals of Allergy Asthma and Immunology 90: 71–76.

Sampson, H. A. 2005. Food allergy—accurately identifying clinical reactivity. Allergy 60: 19–24.

Sampson, H. A., Agbotounou, W., Thebault, C., Thebault, C., Charles, R., Martin, L. *et al.* (2015). Epicutaneous immunotherapy (EPIT) is effective and safe to treat peanut allergy: a multinational double-blind placebo-controlled randomized phase IIb trial. The Journal of Allergy and Clinical Immunology 135: AB390.

Scadding, G. (2013). Laying the foundation for specific immunotherapy. pp. 28–32. *In*: A. Sheikh, T. Platts-Mills and A. Worth (eds.). Landmark Papers in Allergy: Seminal Papers in Allergy with Expert Commentaries. Oxford: Oxford University Press.

Schofield, A. (1908). A case of egg poisoning. Lancet 171: 716.

Senti, G., von Moos, S., and Kundig, T. M. (2011). Epicutaneous allergen administration: is this the future of allergen-specific immunotherapy? Allergy 66: 798–809.

Sheikh, A., Worth, A., and Gallagher, M. (2011). Allergic problems. pp. 585–592. *In*: A. Khot and A. Polmear (eds.). Practical General Practice: Guidelines for Effective Clinical Management. Edinburgh: Elsevier.

Sicherer, S. H., and Sampson, H. A. (2014). Food allergy: epidemiology, pathogenesis, diagnosis, and treatment. The Journal of Allergy and Clinical Immunology 133: 291–307.

Sun, J., Hui, X., Ying, W., Liu, D., and Wang, X. (2014). Efficacy of allergen-specific immunotherapy for peanut allergy: a meta-analysis of randomized controlled trials. Allergy & Asthma Proceedings 35: 171–177.

Wang, J., and Sampson, H. A. (2013). Oral and sublingual immunotherapy for food allergy. Asian Pacific Journal of Allergy and Immunology 31: 198–209.

Yang, Y. H., and Chiang, B. L. (2014). Novel approaches to food allergy. Clinical Reviews in Allergy & Immunology 46: 250–257.

Yepes-Nunez, J. J., Zhang, Y., Figuls, R. I., Bartra Tomas, J., Reyes, J. M. *et al.* (2015). Immunotherapy (oral and sublingual) for food allergy to fruits. Cochrane Database Syst Rev 11: CD010522.

Yeung, J. P., Kloda, L. A., McDevitt, J., Ben-Shoshan, M., and Alizadehfar, R. (2012). Oral immunotherapy for milk allergy. Cochrane Database Syst Rev 11: CD009542.

Zolkipli, Z., Roberts, G., Cornelius, V., Clayton, B., Pearson, S., and Michaelis, L. (2015). Randomized controlled trial of primary prevention of atopy using house dust mite allergen oral immunotherapy in early childhood. The Journal of Allergy and Clinical Immunology 136: 1541–1547.

Zuberbier, T., Edenharter, G., Worm, M., Ehlers, I., Reimann, S., Hantke, T. *et al.* (2004). Prevalence of adverse reactions to food in Germany—a population study. Allergy 59: 338–345.

CHAPTER 8

Allergenomics–A Strategy for Food Allergen Discovery

Anas M. Abdel Rahman

Introduction

As soon as somebody eats a certain food and it is followed by an adverse and reducible immune-mediated reaction, then it is known as a food allergy. Regardless of the amount of allergy-causing food, the allergy symptoms are triggered such as digestive problems, hives or swollen airways. The severe symptoms of food allergy could be a life-threatening reaction known as anaphylaxis. An estimated 6–8% of children (< 3 years) and up to 3% of adults are affected by food allergy, with no direct cure, where the symptoms are absent during avoidance of the specific trigger (O'Keefe *et al.*, 2014). The immune responses in food allergy can be classified as IgE-mediated, non-IgE-mediated or a combination of them, where the pathogenesis is still not completely understood.

In the last couple of decades, the food allergies prevalence has tremendously risen worldwide in both developed and developing countries, going upto 8% in children and infants.

Allergenic food proteins (allergens) are heterogeneous due to its genetic variations (polymorphism), Post-Translational Modifications (PTMs), and native structure in the moiety (van Hengel, 2007). These allergens can be classified as plant food allergens with and without pollen allergen cross-reactivity, or animal-derived food allergens (Carrard *et al.*, 2015). Although hundreds of allergens have been identified so far, only a few major of them occur in regular foods such as cow's milk and egg. Food labeling came to provide consumers access to the required information to implement their

---
Department of Genetics, Research Center, King Faisal Specialist Hospital and Research Center (KFSHRC), and College of Medicine, Al-Faisal University, Riyadh, Saudi Arabia.
Email: aabdelrahman46@kfshrc.edu.sa

food avoidance strategy. Particular legislations have been established in the most developed countries such as the USA and Canada to protect sensitive people from undesirable allergic reactions. An analytical strategy has to be set up to give proper information about the allergen content in any food, in qualitative and quantitative manner. This chapter covers the main principles of allergenomics strategy in food allergen discovery and monitoring in several food matrices from the author's laboratory experience. In addition, a review of using either allergenomics or mass spectrometry in food allergy research will be addressed in this chapter.

Allergen Discovery

Allergenicity evaluation

Characterization of food allergen requires profiling the food proteome against human serum of sensitized individuals to a particular kind of food. The proteome has to be extracted globally from the food sample, and then separated in two-dimension gel electrophoresis (2DE). The high resolution of 2DE makes it the key technique in the allergen discovery, where the first dimension separates the crude extract proteins based on their isoelectric point (pI) and the second dimension based on their size using regular sodium dodecyl sulfate-polyacrylamide gel electrophoresis (SDS-PAGE).

Food allergens are usually detected using antibody-based assays, without any primary structure knowledge (amino acid sequence). The IgE is typically collected from sensitized patients for allergen detection through direct binding. Immunoblotting is the ideal technique for allergenicity evaluation that follows separation of food extract in gel electrophoresis. The protein bands (or spots) are transferred to a membrane and then incubated with the human serum sample. The allergenic proteins bind specifically to the patients' IgE. The protein-IgE complex is incubated with a secondary antibody, attached to an enzyme such as Horseradish peroxidase (HRP), that binds specifically to the human IgE. The reactive band visualization is performed by developing color through the adding substrates reacted with HRP.

Allergen characterization

Once the allergenicity of the proteome is evaluated, the identity of the individual proteins has to be figured out at several stages. The N-terminal amino acid of food allergens used to be identified using Edman degradation. The Edman reaction is performed on the protein N-terminus, where the amine side reacts with phenylisothiocyanate (PITC) to form a phenylthiocarbamyl (PTC) protein (Edman, 1950). The PTC is cleaved with trifluoroacetic acid to give Phenylthiohydantoin (PTH). The structure of PTH depends on the terminal amino acids that have a particular retention time once separated by the High-Performance Liquid chromatography (HPLC). The same procedure will be repeated for the next amino acid and for further information about the sequence of the protein.

The primary structure of the allergenic food protein is used to be mainly identified using the molecular genetics technique. From the N-terminal sequence of the target protein, a specific primer is designed for its corresponding gene and amplified using Polymerase Chain Reaction (PCR) and the DNA product is identified by the Sanger sequencer. The complementary amino acid sequence is deduced from the DNA sequence of the corresponding gene. A recombinant protein is engineered from the extracted DNA of the target gene and evaluated with the patient's sera for structure identification and allergenicity.

Protein mass spectrometry

Mass Spectrometry (MS) is a technique used for molecular structure characterization in gas-phase. These chemicals become ionized using several chambers based on the chemistry, size of the compound, and based on the nature of the solution. For example, small and volatile compounds are separated by gas chromatography and ionized either by Chemical Ionization (CI) or Electron Impact (EI). Most of the biochemical molecules are ionized by either electrospray ionization (ESI) or Matrix-Assisted Laser Desorption Ionization (MALDI). Historically, proteins used to be ionized by the Fast Atom Bombardment (FAB) and analyzed by sector-type MS. Nowadays, proteins are introduced to MS in liquid or solid phase and can be ionized in ESI or MALDI, respectively. In protein analysis, the ESI usually generates multiply charged ion with low m/z value, while the MALDI singly charged ion, which requires the mass analyzer to be set up differently to be able to deal with the various size of ions in highly resolved matter. Two MS-based approaches, *Bottom-up* and *Top-down*, are used for protein primary structure determination as shown in Fig. 8.1. These two strategies referred to the protein sample handling before the MS analysis on one side, and the data analysis and level of information obtained from the experiment on another side. The *top-down* approach is an emerging technique that involves gas-phase ionization of intact protein, which is required for high-resolution MS with ion trapping features such as Fourier Transform Ion Cyclotron Resonance (FTICR) or Orbitrap (Fig. 8.1).

The *bottom-up* strategy, at least, requires a high-resolution linear MS such as QToF. In the *bottom-up* approach, the protein amino acid sequence is figured out from the combination of its peptides' sequences together. These peptides are generated by cleaving the target protein using either chemical (e.g., Cyanogen Bromide) or enzymatic (e.g., Trypsin, Pepsin) digestion methods or a combination of more than one method to increase the sequence coverage as summarized in Table 8.1. Trypsin, the most common protease, has the aspartic residue at the active site that attracts the charged amino acids mainly arginine or lysine from the target protein, and then prominently cleaves proteins at the c-terminus of arginine (R) and lysine (K), except when either of them is bound to proline. The tryptic peptides, generated from the trypsin digestion, are analyzed in

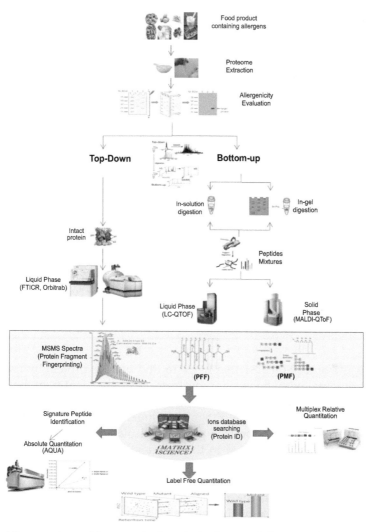

Fig. 8.1: Allergenomics workflow; starting from the food source of allergen ended by the quantity of allergens in different matrices.

Liquid Chromatography tandem mass spectrometry (LC-MSMS or MALDI-ToF) for protein identification using peptide mass fingerprinting (PMF) approach without any speculative Amino Acid (AA) sequence information. The PMF creates a set of peptide' ions that is unique for each protein, and the MS spectrum of these ions is used as a protein fingerprint to identify the novel protein.

In silico MS spectra are generated to the available proteins in the public databases such as National Center for Biotechnology Information (NCBI) and SwissProt databases. These databases are interfaced with search engines such

Table 8.1: List of enzymes and chemicals used for protein digestion in MS analysis.

	Protein digestion method	Cleavage sites
Enzyme (Class)	Trypsin (Serine Protease)	Carboxyl side of arginine and lysine
	Endoproteinase Glu-C (Serine Endoproteinase)	Carboxyl side of glutamate. Ammonium bicarbonate buffers (pH 7.8) Carboxyl side of glutamine and asparagine Phosphate buffers (pH 4.0)
	Pepsin (Digestive Protease)	Carboxyl side of tyrosine, tryptophan, phenylalanine, and leucine
	Chymotrypsin (Digestive Protease)	Carboxyl side of tyrosine, phenylalanine, and tryptophan
	Endoproteinase Arg-C (Sulfhydryl Proteinase)	Carboxyl side of arginine
Chemical cleavage reaction (Crimmins et al., 2005)	Cyanogen bromide (CNBr)	Carboxyl side of methionine
	2-(2-nitrophenylsulfonyl)-3-methyl-3-bromoindolenine (BNPS)	Carboxyl side of tryptophan
	Formic Acid (FA)	Asp-Pro Peptide Bonds
	Hydroxylamine (HA)	Asn-Gly Peptide Bonds
	2-nitro-5-thiocyanobenzoate (NTCB)	N-terminus of Cys

as MASCOT and SEQUEST that helps to find out the protein by matching the experimental with the *in-silico* spectrum. Once the identity of the protein is unveiled, the amino acid sequence for each peptide has to be confirmed experimentally using Peptide Fragment Fingerprinting (PFF). In the gas-phase, the precursor ion for each peptide is isolated in the first mass filter (e.g., quadrupole), fragmented in the collision cell (e.g., Collision-Induced Dissociation (CID)), and the fragment ions are separated in the second mass filter (e.g., Time of Flight (TOF)). The product-ion spectra for the proteolytic peptides are aligned with the *in-silico* spectra to find out the identity and the primary structure of its belonging protein. It is worth mentioning that *bottom-up* rarely achieves complete sequence information, which makes it limited to the ability to find site-specific mutation and PTMs of proteins.

Food Allergenomics

The significant development of biotechnology has contributed to shifting the attention of the scientist from studying single protein to a detail examination of the proteome (Koeberl *et al.*, 2014). The invention of ESI and MALDI sources was a key development for analyzing proteins by MS. The advancement and combination of the technology of protein separation, immunoblotting, and MS have given a powerful analytical strategy for allergenomics analysis as described and detailed in Fig. 8.1. The functional proteomic techniques have to be highly sensitive, resolution, throughput and high confidence for protein identification. The protein's PTM could be globally identified and quantified as part of the protein identity.

Proteomics separation

The species food proteome is commonly extracted and purified from non-protein compounds, to reduce the sample complexity prior MS analysis. Usually, the extract is separated on 2DE and Liquid Chromatography (LC). Separation of intact proteins is the key element in proteomics analysis, where the primary questions strictly determine the choice of separation. 2DE is the most reliable and efficient technique for separating intact proteins from complex samples, and powerful to separate and quantify protein with same molecular weight. However, it is labor-intensive and time-consuming. Also, 2DE has limitations for separating hydrophobic and alkaline proteins and suffers from low dynamic range and reproducibility. The 2DE differential protein expression and the PTM quantity could be evaluated using radioactive or fluorescence differential in-gel (DIGE) in an accurate and sensitive manner (Linda Monaci, 2009). Separation plays a crucial role in both *top-down* and *bottom-up* proteomics approaches, wherein "shotgun" proteomics, a complex mixture of digested proteins and their peptides are chromatographly separated and introduced to the MS with minimal ion-suppression. The compatibility with the electrospray MS, high resolving power, reproducibility of liquid chromatography has attracted the LC to become the best alternative to the 2DE for the protein and peptide separation. Liquid chromatography has several types of stationary phase (Reversed Phase (RP), Ion-Exchange (IE), Affinity Chromatography (AC) and Size-Exclusion (SE)), and mobile phases that make it the tool of choice for proteomics analysis. The sample preparation and handling in LC is the minimal compared to 2DE. Multidimensional chromatography is very useful for complex proteome, for instance combining the RP-HPLC with the IE-HPLC, increases the resolution of the peptides and enriches peptides with low abundant ions, which reduces the ion suppression effect for better sensitivity (Abdel Rahman *et al.*, 2012b; Shi *et al.*, 2004).

In general, the proteomics strategy has been demonstrated to identify the global food species' allergens to what is referred to as "allergenomics" (Fig. 8.1). The food species total proteins, including allergens, are extracted out and efficiently resolved by 2DE. The protein allergencity is evaluated using the immunoblotting technique, where the protein spots are electrotransferred to a nitrocellulose membrane, and subsequently incubated with sera from of allergic patients. The reactive spot/protein, bound to human IgE, is targeted as a potential allergen and identified by analyzing the digested peptides of the protein using MS, and then find the sequence by database searching. This approach has become the master tool for allergen discovery in several food species such as wheat, apple, crab and shrimp.

Allergenomics studies

Food allergenomics is an emerging analytical tool for globally studying the allergenic proteins contained in certain foods. These proteins are developing individualistic adverse reactions and mediated by abnormal responses of the immune system. Plants, crustacean, shellfish, fish, milk, eggs, soybeans and wheat are the most common causes of IgE-mediated food allergies.

Plants may develop allergic reactions in some people after inhalation of plant pollens or consumption of foods derived from plants and animal materials. The allergic symptoms range from mild to severe and life-threatening. Allergens usually bind to specific IgE antibody and cause cross-linking of IgE receptor on mast cells and evoke degranulation of these cells. These cells store chemical mediators such as histamines, proteases and cytokines in their granules, which consequently realised extracellularly to cause allergenic reactions in local tissue. As some species can contain several allergens and the main allergen causing a more personalized allergic reaction, studying these allergen requires the allergenomics strategy as described before and shown in (Fig. 8.1). Allergenomics have become central tools for global allergen analysis in plants compared to the conventional method that targets one protein at the time.

Food allergens are functionally and structurally different from each other, some of them are stored proteins (e.g., globulin), some are enzymatic (e.g., α-amylase) and the others are structural proteins (e.g., Profilin) (Nakamura and Teshima, 2013). Epitopes, the binding site of allergen to patients' IgE, have either a linear (6–20 amino acid) or conformational structures, where those allergens with a linear epitope are most likely cross-reacted with another species' protein that have the same amino acid sequence. Since, several allergic reactions, such as hypotension and anaphylaxis could be developed from several species, the food labeling with allergenic ingredient is required by most of the developed countries. Therefore, it is very crucial to have accurate methods to quantify trace amounts of allergens as discussed before. Nakamura and Teshima in 2013 reviewed the most important and novel plant allergens and the method of identification (Nakamura and Teshima, 2013). In the last decade, amino acid sequencing was the only way to identify the targeted allergen for instance identification of the hazelnuts allergen (Cor a9) using 2DE followed by amino acid sequencing (Beyer *et al.*, 2002). The MS, the technique of choice for identification of plant allergens, has been used to identify the elongation factor 2 allergen (EF-2) in grass pollen, and in many other studies Table 8.2 (Bassler *et al.*, 2009; Boldt *et al.*, 2005; D'Amato *et al.*, 2009; Kao *et al.*, 2005; Sotkovsky *et al.*, 2008).

The limitations of using allergenomics for plant allergen identification are the incomplete databases used for searching peptide ions using MS, and the difficulty of estimation the allergencity of the protein without using patients' IgE. Even, if the target protein is bound to the patient IgE, it has to

Table 8.2: A summary table showing the most common food allergens and the latest mass spectrometric method of analysis. ID: Identification, PTM: Post Translation Modification, PMF: Peptide Mass Fingerprinting.

Group	Species	Allergen	Reference	MS Technique	The purpose of the study
	Hazelnuts	2S albumin	(Calvano et al., 2014)	MALDI-QTOF	ID
			(Nitride et al., 2013)	LCMSMS	*De novo* Sequencing
	Sesame	7S Vicilin (Ses i 3) 2S albumin (Ses i 2)	(Nitride et al., 2013)	LCMSMS	Cross-reactivity
		2S albumin (Ses i 1)	(Moreno et al., 2005)	MALDI-TOF	Thermostability
Plants		Lipid transfers protein Defensin	(Boldt et al., 2005)	MALDI-TOF	N-Terminal Sequencing, and PTM identification
		Oleosin Profilin	(Liang et al., 2006)	LC-QTOF	N-Terminal Sequencing
	Peanuts	A-amylase Conglutin Agglutinin Cupin	(Chassaigne et al., 2007)	LC-QTOF	ID
			(Hebling et al., 2012)	LCQTOF	ID
		Phospholipidase Conarachin A-arachin	(Guo et al., 2008)	LC-QTOF	ID
		Der p 1 Der p 2	(Raftery et al., 2003)	LC-QTOF MALDI-TOF	PMF
	Grass pollen	Der f 1	(De Canio et al., 2009)	MALDI-TOF/TOF	ID
		Der f 2 Panallergens (Bet v 1)	(Halim et al., 2015)	HR FTMS CID, HCD, and ETD	Glycoproteomics, PTM
		CCD-bearing Protein (Phl p 1) Phl p 5	(Kao et al., 2005)	MALDI-TOF, LC-MSMS	N-Terminal Sequencing and ID

Table 3.1 contd. ...

Table 3.1 contd.

Group	Species	Allergen	Reference	MS Technique	The purpose of the study
Plants	Tomato	Profilin	(Sheoran et al., 2007)	MALDI-TOF	PMF
		β-Fructofuranosidase	(Sheoran et al., 2007; Wilson et al., 2001)	MALDI-TOF	Glycomics
		Lipid Transfer Protein 2	(Bassler et al., 2009)	LCMSMS	ID
	Soybeans	Defensin	(Houston et al., 2011)	LCMSMS	Quantitative (MRM), and Label-free
		Profilin			
		Hydrophobic protein	(Batista et al., 2007)	LCMSMS	ID
		Glycinin			
		β-conglycinin	(Cucu et al., 2012)	MALDI-TOF	ID
		Biotinylated protein			
	Wheat	Serpin	(Picariello et al., 2015)	LC-ESI MS/MS	ID
		α-amylase inhibitor			
		γ-gliadin	(Akagawa et al., 2007)	MALDI-TOF	ID
		LMW-glutenin	(Sotkovsky et al., 2008)	MALDI-TOF MALDI-QTOF LC-ESI MS/MS	ID and allergen discovery
		β-amylase			
		profilin			
		β-D-glucan exco hydrolase	(Uvackova et al., 2013)	LCQTOF	Quantitative, food quality
	Maize	LTP	(Kuppannan et al., 2011)	LC-ESI MS/MS	Quantitation (MRM)
		Vicilin			
		globulin-2	(Calvano et al., 2014)	MALDI-QTOF	ID
		γ-zein	(Pastorello et al., 2000)	LC-MSMS	ID, N-terminal Sequencing
		trypsin inhibitor			
		Endochitinase	(Krishnan et al., 2010)	MALDI-TOF	ID (PMF)
		thioredoxin			

				LCMSMS	Protein expression
		globulin	(Emami et al., 2010; Lin et al., 2005)		
	Rice	trypsin-alpha amylase inhibitor	(Taiyoji et al., 2009)	MALDI-TO/TOF	ID
		RA17 seed	(Zhang et al., 2015)	MALDI-TOF/TOF	Allergen descovery
	Sweet orange Fruit	Cit s 1	(Zhang et al., 2015)	MALDI-TOF	N-terminal Sequencing
	Date palm	Putative β-galactosidase	(Postigo et al., 2009)	MALDI-TOF/MS-MS	ID
		Type IIa membrane protein			
Milk	Cow	Caseins	(Natale et al., 2004)	MALDI-TOF	ID
		beta-lactoglobulin bovine alpha S1	(Fenaille et al., 2005)	MALDI-TOF	monitoring milk protein oxidative modifications
		Whey alpha-lactalbumin, beta-lactoglobulin, bovine serum albumin (BSA) lactoferrin	(D'Amato et al., 2009)	LCQTOF	Allergenomics
			(Coscia et al., 2012; Orru et al., 2013)	LCQTOF	ID, Secretion of cow's milk allergens in human milk (Colostrum)
			(Monaci et al., 2013; Parker et al., 2015)	LCMSMS	Quantitation
Egg	Chicken	White Eggs: Ovalbumin, ovomucoid, ovotransferrin, lysozyme ovomucin	(Suzuki et al., 2010)	LCMSMS MALDI-QTOF	ID and Characterization
			(Lee and Kim, 2010)	MALDIQTOF LCQTOF	ID. detect hidden egg allergens in foods
			(Heick et al., 2011a; Heick et al., 2011b; Monaci et al., 2013; Parker et al., 2015)	LCMSMS	Quantitation, food screening
			(Monaci et al., 2014; Pilolli et al., 2014)	Orbitrap	

Table 3.1 contd. ...

Table 3.1 contd.

Group	Species	Allergen	Reference	MS Technique	The purpose of the study
	Crustacean Shrimp	Tropomyosin Arginine kinase Sarcoplasmic calcium-binding protein Myosin light chain Troponin C Triosephosphate Isomerase	(Abdel Rahman et al., 2010a; Abdel Rahman et al., 2013; Abdel Rahman et al., 2011; Ayuso et al., 2008; Garcia-Orozco et al., 2007; Khanaruksombat et al., 2014; Yu et al., 2003) (Abdel Rahman et al., 2013; Nagai et al., 2015) (Bauermeister et al., 2011)	LCQTOF MALDI-QTOF LCMSMS	ID Quantitation
Shellfish	Crustacean Crab	Tropomyosin Arginine kinase Troponin Sarcoplasmic calcium-binding protein	(Abdel Rahman et al., 2011; Abdel Rahman et al., 2010b; Misnan et al., 2012; Rosmilah et al., 2012; Shen et al., 2011)	LCQTOF MALDI-QTOF	ID, AA Sequencing
			(Abdel Rahman et al., 2012a; Abdel Rahman et al., 2010c)	LCMSMS	Quantitation, Air samples
	Crustacean Lobster	Tropomyosin Arginine kinase Myosin light chain 2 Troponin C Sarcoplasmic calcium-binding	Unpublished work (Kamath et al.,)	LCMSMS, MALDIQToF ID	Amino Acid Sequencing

	Crustacean Crayfish	Tropomyosin Arginine Kinase Sarcoplasmic calcium-binding protein Troponin I	(Chen et al., 2013a; Chen et al., 2013b; Gonzalez-de-olano et al., 2011)	LCMSMS, MALDIQToF	ID
	Crustacean Krill	Tropomyosin	(Nagai et al., 2015)	LCMSMS	Quantitative
	Mollusks Octopus	Arginine Kinase	(Shen et al., 2012)	MALDI-TOF	ID
	Mollusks Squid	Tropomyosin	(Yadzir et al., 2012)	LCQTOF	Allergenomics
	Gilthead sea bream		(Piovesana et al., 2015; Rosmilah et al., 2013)	LCQTOF	Proteomics
	The longtail tuna	Parvalbumin	(Aiello et al., 2015)	MALDI-QTOF	ID, complete AA Sequencing
	Rainbow trout Merlucciidae	B-enolase Aldolase A	(Carrera et al., 2010)	FTICR	ID, Isoform detection
Fish	Nile perch cod		(Tomm et al., 2013)	Orbitrap	ID

be administered orally or dermatologically to confirm its cross-reactivity the Fc epsilon receptor I on mast cells.

The regulations in most of the developed countries require the food companies to list the allergenic ingredient on a food label because the trace amount of allergens can cause anaphylaxis in susceptible patients. This process requires accurate methods for quantifying trace amount of allergen in different food matrices. ELISA was an excellent standard method for allergen quantification before having the MS on board. Production of a specific antibody for each allergen is one of the major limitations in using ELISA for allergen quantification. The enormous sensitivity of MS and its specificity for allergen quantitation make it the right approach for studying the exposure level of allergen in high throughput scale.

Targeted and absolute quantitation MS-based methods such as MRM and SRM are often used for trace allergen analysis. This approach is almost unique to detect the contamination of non-allergic food with allergens. Several studies attempt to measure the level of allergens in different food matrices by targeting the allergen's signature peptide using MS. Examples of those studies are quantifying the major peanut allergens Ara h 2 and Ara h 3/4 (Careri *et al.*, 2007), nuts (Chassaigne *et al.*, 2007; Pedreschi *et al.*, 2012), milk (Ansari *et al.*, 2011; Lutter *et al.*, 2011; Newsome and Scholl, 2013), egg (Lee and Kim, 2010) and soybean (Houston *et al.*, 2011). A multiplex analysis for many allergens from several foods (egg, milk, soy, etc.) in food matrices, and several allergens from the same seafood species such as shrimp or crab (Abdel Rahman *et al.*, 2011; Abdel Rahman *et al.*, 2012a; Abdel Rahman *et al.*, 2013; Heick *et al.*, 2011a).

The advancement of the mass spectrometry techniques reveals the capability of analyzing precisely the food allergen qualitatively and quantitatively for the purpose of protecting the consumers from potential threat particularly in the mixed and processed food as will be discussed in details in Chapter 10.

Keywords: Allergenomics, Mass Spectrometry, Allergenic proteins, Food allergy, Allergen Discovery, allergen characterization, Food allergenome, Proteomics, Seafood allergen, Allergencity Evaluation

References

Abdel Rahman, A. M., Kamath, S., Lopata, A. L., and Helleur, R. J. (2010a). Analysis of the allergenic proteins in black tiger prawn (Penaeus monodon) and characterization of the major allergen tropomyosin using mass spectrometry. Rapid Communications in Mass Spectrometry: RCM 24(16): 2462–2470.

Abdel Rahman, A. M., Lopata, A. L., O'Hehir, R. E., Robinson, J. J., Banoub, J. H., and Helleur, R. J. (2010b). Characterization and *de novo* sequencing of snow crab tropomyosin enzymatic peptides by both electrospray ionization and matrix-assisted laser desorption ionization QqToF tandem mass spectrometry. Journal of Mass Spectrometry: JMS 45(4): 372–381.

Abdel Rahman, A. M., Lopata, A. L., Randell, E. W., and Helleur, R. J. (2010c). Absolute quantification method and validation of airborne snow crab allergen tropomyosin using tandem mass spectrometry. Analytica Chimica Acta 681(1-2): 49–55.

Abdel Rahman, A. M., Kamath, S. D., Lopata, A. L., Robinson, J. J., and Helleur, R. J. (2011). Biomolecular characterization of allergenic proteins in snow crab (Chionoecetes opilio) and *de novo* sequencing of the second allergen arginine kinase using tandem mass spectrometry. Journal of Proteomics 74(2): 231–241.

Abdel Rahman, A. M., Gagne, S., and Helleur, R. J. (2012a). Simultaneous determination of two major snow crab aeroallergens in processing plants by use of isotopic dilution tandem mass spectrometry. Analytical and Bioanalytical Chemistry 403(3): 821–831.

Abdel Rahman, A. M., Helleur, R. J., Jeebhay, M. F., and Lopata, A. L. (2012b). Characterization of seafood proteins causing allergic diseases. pp. 107–140. *In*: P.C. Pereira (ed.). Allergic Diseases—Highlights in the Clinic, Mechanisms and Treatment (1 ed.). InTech Croatia.

Abdel Rahman, A. M., Kamath, S. D., Gagne, S., Lopata, A. L., and Helleur, R. (2013). Comprehensive proteomics approach in characterizing and quantifying allergenic proteins from northern shrimp: toward better occupational asthma prevention. Journal of Proteome Research 12(2): 647–656.

Aiello, D., Materazzi, S., Risoluti, R., Thangavel, H., Di Donna, L., Mazzotti, F., Casadonte, F., Siciliano, C., Sindona, G., and Napoli, A. (2015). A major allergen in rainbow trout (Oncorhynchus mykiss): complete sequences of parvalbumin by MALDI tandem mass spectrometry. Molecular BioSystems 11(8): 2373–2382.

Akagawa, M., Handoyo, T., Ishii, T., Kumazawa, S., Morita, N., and Suyama, K. (2007). Proteomic analysis of wheat flour allergens. Journal of Agricultural and Food Chemistry 55(17): 6863–6870.

Ansari, P., Stoppacher, N., Rudolf, J., Schuhmacher, R., and Baumgartner, S. (2011). Selection of possible marker peptides for the detection of major ruminant milk proteins in food by liquid chromatography-tandem mass spectrometry. Analytical and Bioanalytical Chemistry 399(3): 1105–1115.

Ayuso, R., Grishina, G., Bardina, L., Carrillo, T., Blanco, C., Ibanez, M. D., Sampson, H. A., and Beyer, K. (2008). Myosin light chain is a novel shrimp allergen, Lit v 3. The Journal of Allergy and Clinical Immunology 122(4): 795–802.

Bassler, O. Y., Weiss, J., Wienkoop, S., Lehmann, K., Scheler, C., Dolle, S., Schwarz, D., Franken, P., George, E., Worm, M., and Weckwerth, W. (2009). Evidence for novel tomato seed allergens: IgE-reactive legumin and vicilin proteins identified by multidimensional protein fractionation-mass spectrometry and *in silico* epitope modeling. Journal of Proteome Research 8(3): 1111–1122.

Batista, R., Martins, I., Jeno, P., Ricardo, C. P., and Oliveira, M. M. (2007). A proteomic study to identify soya allergens—the human response to transgenic versus non-transgenic soya samples. International Archives of Allergy and Immunology 144(1): 29–38.

Bauermeister, K., Wangorsch, A., Garoffo, L. P., Reuter, A., Conti, A., Taylor, S. L., Lidholm, J., Dewitt, A. M., Enrique, E., Vieths, S., Holzhauser, T., Ballmer-Weber, B., and Reese, G. (2011). Generation of a comprehensive panel of crustacean allergens from the North Sea Shrimp Crangon crangon. Molecular Immunology 48(15-16): 1983–1992.

Beyer, K., Grishina, G., Bardina, L., Grishin, A., and Sampson, H. A. (2002). Identification of an 11S globulin as a major hazelnut food allergen in hazelnut-induced systemic reactions. The Journal of Allergy and Clinical Immunology 110(3): 517–523.

Boldt, A., Fortunato, D., Conti, A., Petersen, A., Ballmer-Weber, B., Lepp, U., Reese, G., and Becker, W. M. (2005). Analysis of the composition of an immunoglobulin E reactive high molecular weight protein complex of peanut extract containing Ara h 1 and Ara h 3/4. Proteomics 5(3): 675–686.

Calvano, C. D., De Ceglie, C., and Zambonin, C. G. (2014). Proteomic analysis of complex protein samples by MALDI-TOF mass spectrometry. Methods in Molecular Biology 1129: 365–380.

Careri, M., Costa, A., Elviri, L., Lagos, J. B., Mangia, A., Terenghi, M., Cereti, A., and Garoffo, L. P. (2007). Use of specific peptide biomarkers for quantitative confirmation of hidden allergenic peanut proteins Ara h 2 and Ara h 3/4 for food control by liquid chromatography-tandem mass spectrometry. Analytical and Bioanalytical Chemistry 389(6): 1901–1907.

Carrard, A., Rizzuti, D., and Sokollik, C. (2015). Update on food allergy. Allergy.

Carrera, M., Canas, B., Vazquez, J., and Gallardo, J. M. (2010). Extensive *de novo* sequencing of new parvalbumin isoforms using a novel combination of bottom-up proteomics, accurate molecular mass measurement by FTICR-MS, and selected MS/MS ion monitoring. Journal of Proteome Research 9(9): 4393–4406.

Chassaigne, H., Norgaard, J. V., and Hengel, A. J. (2007). Proteomics-based approach to detect and identify major allergens in processed peanuts by capillary LC-Q-TOF (MS/MS). Journal of Agricultural and Food Chemistry 55(11): 4461–4473.

Chen, H. L., Cao, M. J., Cai, Q. F., Su, W. J., Mao, H. Y., and Liu, G. M. (2013a). Purification and characterisation of sarcoplasmic calcium-binding protein, a novel allergen of red swamp crayfish (Procambarus clarkii). Food Chemistry 139(1-4): 213–223.

Chen, H. L., Mao, H. Y., Cao, M. J., Cai, Q. F., Su, W. J., Zhang, Y. X., and Liu, G. M. (2013b). Purification, physicochemical and immunological characterization of arginine kinase, an allergen of crayfish (Procambarus clarkii). Food and Chemical Toxicology: An International Journal Published for the British Industrial Biological Research Association 62: 475–484.

Coscia, A., Orru, S., Di Nicola, P., Giuliani, F., Rovelli, I., Peila, C., Martano, C., Chiale, F., and Bertino, E. (2012). Cow's milk proteins in human milk. Journal of Biological Regulators and Homeostatic Agents 26(3 Suppl): 39–42.

Crimmins, D. L., Mische, S. M., and Denslow, N. D. (2005). Chemical cleavage of proteins in solution. Current Protocols in Protein Science/Editorial Board, John E. Coligan ... [et al.], Chapter 11, Unit 11 14.

Cucu, T., De Meulenaer, B., and Devreese, B. (2012). MALDI based identification of soybean protein markers—possible analytical targets for allergen detection in processed foods. Peptides 33(2): 187–196.

D'Amato, A., Bachi, A., Fasoli, E., Boschetti, E., Peltre, G., Senechal, H., and Righetti, P. G. (2009). In-depth exploration of cow's whey proteome via combinatorial peptide ligand libraries. Journal of Proteome Research 8(8): 3925–3936.

De Canio, M., D'Aguanno, S., Sacchetti, C., Petrucci, F., Cavagni, G., Nuccetelli, M., Federici, G., Urbani, A., and Bernardini, S. (2009). Novel IgE recognized components of Lolium perenne pollen extract: comparative proteomics evaluation of allergic patients sensitization profiles. Journal of Proteome Research 8(9): 4383–4391.

Edman, P. (1950). Method for determination of the amino acid sequence in peptides. Acta Chemica Scandinavica 4: 283–293.

Emami, K., Morris, N. J., Cockell, S. J., Golebiowska, G., Shu, Q. Y., and Gatehouse, A. M. (2010). Changes in protein expression profiles between a low phytic acid rice (Oryza sativa L. sp. japonica) line and its parental line: a proteomic and bioinformatic approach. Journal of Agricultural and Food Chemistry 58(11): 6912–6922.

Fenaille, F., Parisod, V., Tabet, J. C., and Guy, P. A. (2005). Carbonylation of milk powder proteins as a consequence of processing conditions. Proteomics 5(12): 3097–3104.

Garcia-Orozco, K. D., Aispuro-Hernandez, E., Yepiz-Plascencia, G., Calderon-de-la-Barca, A. M., and Sotelo-Mundo, R. R. (2007). Molecular characterization of arginine kinase, an allergen from the shrimp Litopenaeus vannamei. International Archives of Allergy and Immunology 144(1): 23–28.

Gonzalez-de-olano, D., Pastor-Vargas, C., Gandolfo-Cano, M., Gonzalez-Mancebo, E., Melendez-Baltanas, A., Morales-Barrios, M. P., Perez-Gordo, M., Vivanco, F., and Bartolome, B. (2011). Allergy to crayfish. Journal of Investigational Allergology and Clinical Immunology 21(4): 318–319.

Guo, B., Liang, X., Chung, S. Y., Holbrook, C. C., and Maleki, S. J. (2008). Proteomic analysis of peanut seed storage proteins and genetic variation in a potential peanut allergen. Protein and Peptide Letters 15(6): 567–577.

Halim, A., Carlsson, M. C., Madsen, C. B., Brand, S., Moller, S. R., Olsen, C. E., Vakhrushev, S. Y., Brimnes, J., Wurtzen, P. A., Ipsen, H., Petersen, B. L., and Wandall, H. H. (2015). Glycoproteomic analysis of seven major allergenic proteins reveals novel post-translational modifications. Molecular and Cellular Proteomics: MCP 14(1): 191–204.

Hebling, C. M., Ross, M. M., Callahan, J. H., and McFarland, M. A. (2012). Size-selective fractionation and visual mapping of allergen protein chemistry in Arachis hypogaea. Journal of Proteome Research 11(11): 5384–5395.

Heick, J., Fischer, M., Kerbach, S., Tamm, U., and Popping, B. (2011a). Application of a liquid chromatography tandem mass spectrometry method for the simultaneous detection of seven allergenic foods in flour and bread and comparison of the method with commercially available ELISA test kits. Journal of AOAC International 94(4): 1060–1068.

Heick, J., Fischer, M., and Popping, B. (2011b). First screening method for the simultaneous detection of seven allergens by liquid chromatography mass spectrometry. Journal of Chromatography A 1218(7): 938–943.

Houston, N. L., Lee, D. G., Stevenson, S. E., Ladics, G. S., Bannon, G. A., McClain, S., Privalle, L., Stagg, N., Herouet-Guicheney, C., MacIntosh, S. C., and Thelen, J. J. (2011). Quantitation of soybean allergens using tandem mass spectrometry. Journal of Proteome Research 10(2): 763–773.

Kao, S. H., Su, S. N., Huang, S. W., Tsai, J. J., and Chow, L. P. (2005). Sub-proteome analysis of novel IgE-binding proteins from Bermuda grass pollen. Proteomics 5(14): 3805–3813.

Khanaruksombat, S., Srisomsap, C., Chokchaichamnankit, D., Punyarit, P., and Phiriyangkul, P. (2014). Identification of a novel allergen from muscle and various organs in banana shrimp (Fenneropenaeus merguiensis). Annals of Allergy, Asthma & Immunology: Official Publication of the American College of Allergy, Asthma, & Immunology 113(3): 301–306.

Koeberl, M., Clarke, D., and Lopata, A. L. (2014). Next generation of food allergen quantification using mass spectrometric systems. Journal of Proteome Research 13(8): 3499–3509.

Krishnan, H. B., Kerley, M. S., Allee, G. L., Jang, S., Kim, W. S., and Fu, C. J. (2010). Maize 27 kDa gamma-zein is a potential allergen for early weaned pigs. Journal of Agricultural and Food Chemistry 58(12): 7323–7328.

Kuppannan, K., Albers, D. R., Schafer, B. W., Dielman, D., and Young, S. A. (2011). Quantification and characterization of maize lipid transfer protein, a food allergen, by liquid chromatography with ultraviolet and mass spectrometric detection. Analytical Chemistry 83(2): 516–524.

Lee, J. Y., and Kim, C. J. (2010). Determination of allergenic egg proteins in food by protein-, mass spectrometry-, and DNA-based methods. Journal of AOAC International 93(2): 462–477.

Liang, X. Q., Luo, M., Holbrook, C. C., and Guo, B. Z. (2006). Storage protein profiles in Spanish and runner market type peanuts and potential markers. BMC Plant Biology 6: 24.

Lin, S. K., Chang, M. C., Tsai, Y. G., and Lur, H. S. (2005). Proteomic analysis of the expression of proteins related to rice quality during caryopsis development and the effect of high temperature on expression. Proteomics 5(8): 2140–2156.

Linda Monaci, A. V. (2009). Mass spectrometry-based proteomics methods for analysis of food allergens. Trends in Analytical Chemistry 28(5): 581–591.

Lutter, P., Parisod, V., and Weymuth, H. (2011). Development and validation of a method for the quantification of milk proteins in food products based on liquid chromatography with mass spectrometric detection. Journal of AOAC International 94(4): 1043–1059.

Misnan, R., Murad, S., Yadzir, Z. H., and Abdullah, N. (2012). Identification of the major allergens of Charybdis feriatus (red crab) and its cross-reactivity with Portunus pelagicus (blue crab). Asian Pacific Journal of Allergy and Immunology/Launched by the Allergy and Immunology Society of Thailand 30(4): 285–293.

Monaci, L., Losito, I., De Angelis, E., Pilolli, R., and Visconti, A. (2013). Multi-allergen quantification of fining-related egg and milk proteins in white wines by high-resolution mass spectrometry. Rapid Communications in Mass Spectrometry: RCM 27(17): 2009–2018.

Monaci, L., Pilolli, R., De Angelis, E., Godula, M., and Visconti, A. (2014). Multi-allergen detection in food by micro high-performance liquid chromatography coupled to a dual cell linear ion trap mass spectrometry. Journal of Chromatography A 1358: 136–144.

Moreno, F. J., Maldonado, B. M., Wellner, N., and Mills, E. N. (2005). Thermostability and *in vitro* digestibility of a purified major allergen 2S albumin (Ses i 1) from white sesame seeds (Sesamum indicum L.). Biochimica et Biophysica Acta 1752(2): 142–153.

Nagai, H., Minatani, T., and Goto, K. (2015). Development of a method for crustacean allergens using liquid chromatography/tandem mass spectrometry. Journal of AOAC International 98(5): 1355–1365.

Nakamura, R., and Teshima, R. (2013). Proteomics-based allergen analysis in plants. Journal of Proteomics 93: 40–49.

Natale, M., Bisson, C., Monti, G., Peltran, A., Garoffo, L. P., Valentini, S., Fabris, C., Bertino, E., Coscia, A., and Conti, A. (2004). Cow's milk allergens identification by two-dimensional immunoblotting and mass spectrometry. Molecular Nutrition and Food Research 48(5): 363–369.

Newsome, G. A., and Scholl, P. F. (2013). Quantification of allergenic bovine milk alpha(S1)-casein in baked goods using an intact (1)(5)N-labeled protein internal standard. Journal of Agricultural and Food Chemistry 61(24): 5659–5668.

Nitride, C., Mamone, G., Picariello, G., Mills, C., Nocerino, R., Berni Canani, R., and Ferranti, P. (2013). Proteomic and immunological characterization of a new food allergen from hazelnut (Corylus avellana). Journal of Proteomics 86: 16–26.

O'Keefe, A. W., De Schryver, S., Mill, J., Mill, C., Dery, A., and Ben-Shoshan, M. (2014). Diagnosis and management of food allergies: new and emerging options: a systematic review. Journal of Asthma and Allergy 7: 141–164.

Orru, S., Di Nicola, P., Giuliani, F., Fabris, C., Conti, A., Coscia, A., and Bertino, E. (2013). Detection of bovine alpha-S1-casein in term and preterm human colostrum with proteomic techniques. International Journal of Immunopathology and Pharmacology 26(2): 435–444.

Parker, C. H., Khuda, S. E., Pereira, M., Ross, M. M., Fu, T. J., Fan, X., Wu, Y., Williams, K. M., DeVries, J., Pulvermacher, B., Bedford, B., Zhang, X., and Jackson, L. S. (2015). Multi-allergen quantitation and the impact of thermal treatment in industry-processed baked goods by ELISA and liquid chromatography-tandem mass spectrometry. Journal of Agricultural and Food Chemistry 63(49): 10669–10680.

Pastorello, E. A., Farioli, L., Pravettoni, V., Ispano, M., Scibola, E., Trambaioli, C., Giuffrida, M. G., Ansaloni, R., Godovac-Zimmermann, J., Conti, A., Fortunato, D., and Ortolani, C. (2000). The maize major allergen, which is responsible for food-induced allergic reactions, is a lipid transfer protein. The Journal of Allergy and Clinical Immunology 106(4): 744–751.

Pedreschi, R., Norgaard, J., and Maquet, A. (2012). Current challenges in detecting food allergens by shotgun and targeted proteomic approaches: a case study on traces of peanut allergens in baked cookies. Nutrients 4(2): 132–150.

Picariello, G., Mamone, G., Cutignano, A., Fontana, A., Zurlo, L., Addeo, F., and Ferranti, P. (2015). Proteomics, peptidomics, and immunogenic potential of wheat beer (Weissbier). Journal of Agricultural and Food Chemistry 63(13): 3579–3586.

Pilolli, R., De Angelis, E., Godula, M., Visconti, A., and Monaci, L. (2014). Orbitrap monostage MS versus hybrid linear ion trap MS: application to multi-allergen screening in wine. Journal of Mass Spectrometry: JMS 49(12): 1254–1263.

Piovesana, S., Capriotti, A. L., Caruso, G., Cavaliere, C., La Barbera, G., Zenezini Chiozzi, R., and Lagana, A. (2015). Labeling and label free shotgun proteomics approaches to characterize muscle tissue from farmed and wild gilthead sea bream (Sparus aurata). Journal of Chromatography A.

Postigo, I., Guisantes, J. A., Negro, J. M., Rodriguez-Pacheco, R., David-Garcia, D., and Martinez, J. (2009). Identification of 2 new allergens of Phoenix dactylifera using an immunoproteomics approach. Journal of Investigational Allergology and Clinical Immunology 19(6): 504–507.

Raftery, M. J., Saldanha, R. G., Geczy, C. L., and Kumar, R. K. (2003). Mass spectrometric analysis of electrophoretically separated allergens and proteases in grass pollen diffusates. Respiratory Research 4: 10.

Rosmilah, M., Shahnaz, M., Zailatul, H. M., Noormalin, A., and Normilah, I. (2012). Identification of tropomyosin and arginine kinase as major allergens of Portunus pelagicus (blue swimming crab). Tropical Biomedicine 29(3): 467–478.

Rosmilah, M., Shahnaz, M., Meinir, J., Masita, A., Noormalin, A., and Jamaluddin, M. (2013). Identification of parvalbumin and two new thermolabile major allergens of Thunnus tonggol using a proteomics approach. International Archives of Allergy and Immunology 162(4): 299–309.

Shen, H. W., Cao, M. J., Cai, Q. F., Ruan, M. M., Mao, H. Y., Su, W. J., and Liu, G. M. (2012). Purification, cloning, and immunological characterization of arginine kinase, a novel allergen of Octopus fangsiao. Journal of Agricultural and Food Chemistry 60(9): 2190–2199.

Shen, Y., Cao, M. J., Cai, Q. F., Su, W. J., Yu, H. L., Ruan, W. W., and Liu, G. M. (2011). Purification, cloning, expression and immunological analysis of Scylla serrata arginine kinase, the crab allergen. Journal of the Science of Food and Agriculture 91(7): 1326–1335.

Sheoran, I. S., Ross, A. R., Olson, D. J., and Sawhney, V. K. (2007). Proteomic analysis of tomato (Lycopersicon esculentum) pollen. Journal of Experimental Botany 58(13): 3525–3535.

Shi, Y., Xiang, R., Horvath, C., and Wilkins, J. A. (2004). The role of liquid chromatography in proteomics. Journal of Chromatography A 1053(1-2): 27–36.

Sotkovsky, P., Hubalek, M., Hernychova, L., Novak, P., Havranova, M., Setinova, I., Kitanovicova, A., Fuchs, M., Stulik, J., and Tuckova, L. (2008). Proteomic analysis of wheat proteins recognized by IgE antibodies of allergic patients. Proteomics 8(8): 1677–1691.

Suzuki, M., Fujii, H., Fujigaki, H., Shinoda, S., Takahashi, K., Saito, K., Wada, H., Kimoto, M., Kondo, N., and Seishima, M. (2010). Lipocalin-type prostaglandin D synthase and egg white cystatin react with IgE antibodies from children with egg allergy. Allergology International: Official Journal of the Japanese Society of Allergology 59(2): 175–183.

Taiyoji, M., Shitomi, Y., Taniguchi, M., Saitoh, E., and Ohtsubo, S. (2009). Identification of proteinaceous inhibitors of a cysteine proteinase (an Arg-specific gingipain) from Porphyromonas gingivalis in rice grain, using targeted-proteomics approaches. Journal of Proteome Research 8(11): 5165–5174.

Tomm, J. M., van Do, T., Jende, C., Simon, J. C., Treudler, R., von Bergen, M., and Averbeck, M. (2013). Identification of new potential allergens from Nile perch (Lates niloticus) and cod (Gadus morhua). Journal of Investigational Allergology and Clinical Immunology 23(3): 159–167.

Uvackova, L., Skultety, L., Bekesova, S., McClain, S., and Hajduch, M. (2013). MS(E) based multiplex protein analysis quantified important allergenic proteins and detected relevant peptides carrying known epitopes in wheat grain extracts. Journal of Proteome Research 12(11): 4862–4869.

van Hengel, A. J. (2007). Food allergen detection methods and the challenge to protect food-allergic consumers. Analytical and Bioanalytical Chemistry 389(1): 111–118.

Wilson, I. B., Zeleny, R., Kolarich, D., Staudacher, E., Stroop, C. J., Kamerling, J. P., and Altmann, F. (2001). Analysis of Asn-linked glycans from vegetable foodstuffs: widespread occurrence of Lewis a, core alpha1,3-linked fucose and xylose substitutions. Glycobiology 11(4): 261–274.

Yadzir, Z. H., Misnan, R., and Murad, S. (2012). Identification of tropomyosin as major allergen of white squid (Loligo edulis) by two-dimensional immunoblotting and mass spectrometry. The Southeast Asian Journal of Tropical Medicine and Public Health 43(1): 185–191.

Yu, C. J., Lin, Y. F., Chiang, B. L., and Chow, L. P. (2003). Proteomics and immunological analysis of a novel shrimp allergen, Pen m 2. Journal of Immunology 170(1): 445–453.

Zhang, J., Wu, L. S., Fan, W., Zhang, X. L., Jia, H. X., Li, Y., Yin, Y. F., Hu, J. J., and Lu, M. Z. (2015). Proteomic analysis and candidate allergenic proteins in Populus deltoides CL. "2KEN8" mature pollen. Frontiers in Plant Science 6: 548.

CHAPTER 9

Proteomics in Food Allergy

Pasquale Ferranti,[1,*] *Anas M. Abdel Rhaman,*[2]
Maria Adalgisa Nicolai[1] and *Monica Gallo*[3]

Introduction

Allergic reactions can be caused by a variety of environmental challenges, including inhalation of dust or pollen, and by ingestion of foods. They are a consequence of an inappropriate immune response, which may result in tissue inflammation and damage and, in most cases, involve generation of an IgE-mediated response towards the offending environmental agent, defined as allergen. Although the search for clinically relevant allergens has drastically progressed, structural characterization of allergens still requires extensive efforts and large amounts of starting material. Therefore, methods which may allow simultaneous identification of multiple proteins are invaluable for allergen screening in food matrices. Today, these challenging issues are being addressed by use of integrated, up-to-date analytical approaches which constitute the platform of modern food proteomics, and where a pivotal role is played by mass spectrometry (MS). Recently, MS-based approaches for food peptide and protein characterization are proving to be essential at various levels in the study of food allergy, from the structural characterization of novel food allergens to the controversial issue of the resistance to digestion of allergenic proteins or to the efficiency of removal of epitopes from a food destined to allergic subjects. Over the next years, the integrated omic-based

[1] Department of Agricultural Sciences, University of Naples Federico II, Parco Gussone, Portici I-80055, Italy.
[2] Newborn Screening & Biochemical Genetics Laboratory, Department of Genetics, Research Center King Faisal Specialist Hospital and Research Center (KFSHRC), MBC#03 P.O. Box 3354, Riyadh 11211, Kingdom of Saudi Arabia.
[3] Department of Molecular Medicine and Medical Biotechnology, University of Naples Federico II, via Pansini, 5 - 80131 Naples, Italy.
* Corresponding author

approaches are expected to greatly expand our knowledge on the mechanisms that form the basis of food allergy and to assist the development of novel ingredients and more efficient technological processes for production of effectively safe foods.

Food Allergy: Definition and Diagnosis

Food Allergy (FA) is an abnormal adverse reaction against an offending food component, generally a protein, sustained by an immunological mechanism (Fig. 9.1). Despite the surprising advances in biochemical and clinical research, the issue of FA still remains one of the most controversial and debated in the scientific community, primarily due to the uncertain boundaries of the disease. Similarly, a precise estimation of social costs and of the impact FA has on the quality of life is still missing. For its deep health and social impact, several ambitious research projects aimed at improving knowledge on FA have been launched in the last couple of years by governmental and international agencies.

The self-perception of food reactions tends to overestimate the prevalence of FA highly in comparison with studies that make use of objective evaluation tools, particularly those including a Double-Blind Placebo-Controlled Food Challenge (DBPCFC) oral test which is considered the "golden standard"

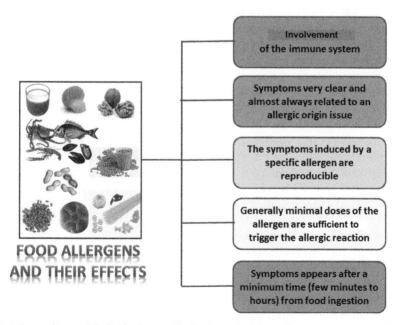

Fig. 9.1: In predisposed individuals, specific foods or food ingredients may cause an allergic reaction, recognized by reproducible and objective symptoms.

of diagnosis. Recent estimations appear to agree about a prevalence range of 3.2–4% of confirmed FA during the first year of life. According to recent studies, FA could be under-diagnosed, and its prevalence would reach 6–7.5% (Kagan, 2003; Ramesh, 2008; Sicherer and Sampson, 2006).

An operating IgE-mediated mechanism of FA can be clinically evidenced by a positive IgE test, as well as by the measurement of chemical mediators released in the blood. Although detection of allergens-specific IgE in blood serum is the most straightforward screening method, double-blind placebo controlled challenges constitute the reference procedure for the diagnosis of allergy, due to a strong overlapping between pollinosis and food allergy (Bousquet *et al.*, 2006). In any case, since the specificity of all diagnostic approaches depends on the purity of the allergens applied, the attention of investigators has been focused on the identification and employment of well-defined allergens in diagnosis. However, these determinations are mostly based on immunological evidence, whereas only a few of the suspected causative wheat allergens have been structurally characterized or cloned to allow functional analysis (Constantin *et al.*, 2008; Palacin *et al.*, 2009; Snegaroff *et al.*, 2007). Therefore, the reliability of current diagnostic procedures is still insufficient.

FA diagnosis always starts with a clinical history and a dietetic survey. If clinical investigation suggests an FA, it is necessary to pass to the diagnostic phase. The main obstacle in this diagnostic process is that today no test *in vivo* or *in vitro* is able to diagnose FA with absolute specificity and sensitivity. It is, therefore, necessary to distinguish between sensitization and allergy itself. The sensitization is defined as the presence of a specific IgE response that occurs following exposure of the immune system to a particular allergen. The tests currently available for the study of sensitization are represented by the Skin Prick Test (SPT) (*in vivo*) and by the IgE-specific test (*in vitro*), none of which is able, by itself, to unequivocally predict the occurrence of FA (see Chapter 6).

SPT is frequently used to screen for FA. The diagnostic accuracy of SPT depends on the quality of the extracts of food allergens used; unlike what happens to inhalant allergens, many available food extracts are not standardized. In children with atopic dermatitis and allergy to eggs, milk, hazelnut and fish, SPT has excellent sensitivity and negative predictive value (over 90%) but a low specificity and positive predictive value (50–85%). Thus, a negative skin test is an excellent method to exclude the Ig-E mediated FA, but a positive test is not able to ensure the effective clinical reactivity of the patient and the final FA diagnosis should always be based on an oral test. On the other hand, many vegetal foods extracts available on the market today for the SPT show a low sensitivity and therefore a high rate of false negatives. This is due to the limited stability of many plant allergens. In these cases, a skin test with native foods clearly shows superior performance (prick-prick test). Prick-prick-test is also useful when there is a discrepancy between the patient's medical history and a negative SPT with a commercial extract or when a specific food extract is not commercially available. The main limitations of the prick-prick tests are the low specificity (high rate of false positives), the inability to standardize the food source and, of course, the dependence of its execution by the fresh food availability. The low specificity can be ascribed to food-pollen cross-reactivity (i.e., cross-reaction triggered by sensitization to pollen and occurring during ingestion of one or more foods) and the presence of common allergens in many vegetables; the poor repetitiveness is due to the not uniform allergen distribution in the plant. Ultimately, the only way to check the actual clinical relevance of the skin prick-prick test is to carry out an oral test.

The oral test is excellent for the diagnosis of FA, and provides solid information for assigning elimination diet. The oral test can be performed in as open, single-blind or double-blind mode, controlled with placebo. DBPCFC is currently considered the golden standard for FA, but is not free of risks besides being technically laborious.

Food Allergens and Epitopes. New Food Allergens

Allergens have been classified by similarity (Fig. 9.2) in plant allergens (four superfamilies named prolamins, cupins, profilins and bet v1) and animal allergens (essentially from milk, egg, fish and shellfish). This categorization has been made on the basis of primary sequence similarities, but the story is much more complex. For instance allergens of profilins and Bet V1 super-families arise from their close similarity to aeroallergens of pollen. Panallergens are proteins that share a high similarity between them, even if they are not

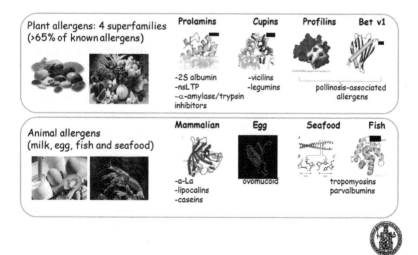

Fig. 9.2: Classification of food allergens in the two general groups: plant allergens and animal allergens.

perfectly identical to each other. They are present in different plants or animal families, either taxonomically related or not (Ledesma *et al.*, 2006). They can be stable allergens (such as lipid transfer proteins) or labile (like Bet V1 or as profilin); stability or lability refers to the ability to resist or less to the digestive proteolysis and/or to the heat treatment.

Bet V1 is the major allergen of birch and is the protein to which more than 95% of allergic to birch pollen is sensitive. It is a highly conserved protein belonging to the pathogenesis-related family of protein type 10 (PR-10). Many Bet v1-related food allergen has been identified so far: the birch proteins expose risks of Oral Allergy Syndrome (OAS) upon ingestion of apple, pear, cherry, apricot, celery, carrot, hazelnuts and chestnuts. The symptoms do not occur however when foods are eaten cooked as Bet V1 is a weak allergen.

Profilins are proteins that are found in the cytoplasm of all nucleated cells. Their function consists mainly in binding, polymerize or depolymerize the actin monomer. Through this function, the profilin regulate the intrinsic cell motility, cell elongation, and, ultimately, their shape (profile). Given their functional significance, it is not surprising that the amino acid sequences of the profilin are well preserved in plant species that are very different and evolutionarily distant. Many contain pollen allergen profilin and among them also *Graminaceae* and artemisia. The profilin is also contained in the latex, very heat labile, and the gastric digestion and therefore allergic symptoms are manifested only when the responsible foods are eaten raw (i.e., apple, pear, cherry, peach, hazelnut, celery, banana, melon, peanut, tomato, soybean, pineapple and latex).

Lipid Transport Proteins (LTPs) are typically located below the peel of some fruit types which perform defensive functions against plant pathogens. These stable allergens can sensitize the subject through ingestion and subsequently induce severe systemic reactions even when foods have been cooked or subjected to industrial treatment (as occurs for fruit juice, beer, wine, hazelnut and peanut). The Mediterranean area of allergy to *Rosaceae* (especially the peach) is related to sensitization to LTP, which is present in many *Rosaceae* as well as in other fruits, grains, vegetables. Foods that cause allergic symptoms in LTP-positive subjects are the *Rosaceae* (peach, apple, pear, apricot, cherry, strawberry), nuts, corn, rice, beer, grapes.

A food matrix may contain different potential allergens, and this is actually the most common occurrence, which also makes it more difficult to establish a clear FA diagnosis and therefore also to trace a reliable epidemiological picture of the frequency of an allergy to a given allergen in a given population or worldwide. An example is a hazelnut, a powerful allergenic food, which presents allergens from all four vegetal allergen super-families. Nine main allergens have been identified so far in hazelnut. The case of hazelnut is not the exception but rather the rule. Allergens of soy, the most studied legume species, are reported in Table 9.1.

An allergic response is triggered in a vulnerable subject when an allergenic protein form crosslinks with the IgE antibodies on the surface of mast cells,

Table 9.1: Soy (Glycine max) allergens.

Allergen	Function/Type	Length (aa)	Notes
Gly m 1	Hydrophobic seed protein from hull	80	
Gly m 2	Hydrophobic seed protein from hull	–	Birch-related pollen antigens
Gly m 3.0102	Homolog to Bet v2 (profilin)	131	
Gly m 4	Bet v1-related PR-10 protein, SAM22	158	
Gly m 5.0101	α subunit beta conglycinin (7S vicilin)	605	
Gly m 5.0201	α′ subunit beta conglycinin (7S vicilin)	639	
Gly m 5.0301	β subunit beta conglycinin (7S vicilin)	439	
Gly m 6.0101	glycinin (11S legumin)	495	
Gly m 6.0201	glycinin (11S legumin)	485	Cupins
Gly m 6.0301	glycinin (11S legumin)	481	
Gly m 6.0401	glycinin (11S legumin)	562	
Gly m 6.0501	glycinin (11S legumin)	516	
Gly m 6.0301	glycinin (11S legumin)	481	
Gly m 8	Napin-tye 2S albumin 1	155	Prolamin
Gly m Bd 28K	Vicilin-like glycoprotein	473	Cupin
Gly m Bd 30K	P34/seed vac. thiol prot., oil body ass.	247	Cupin
Gly Major 50K	Vicilin-like	517	Cupin
Kunitz tr. in.			Prolamin

causing the release of histamine or other substances such as leukotrienes and prostaglandins (Sicherer and Sampson, 2006). The portion of the protein responsible for the formation of cross-links with immunoglobulin E is called epitope. An epitope can be a simple structure, as a sequence of few amino acids along the primary structure (linear epitopes) or more complex three-dimensional structures (conformational epitope).

In linear epitopes, the primary amino acid sequence of the allergen is the exclusive structural feature affecting IgE-binding affinity. In contrast, secondary or tertiary structure elements are required for the bind of conformational epitopes to IgE. Due to the thermal-induced conformational transitions, the antigenic potential of conformational epitopes can be reduced or completely annulled upon protein denaturation by cooking or thermal processing. The role of conformational IgE-binding epitopes is relevant to the aetiology of aeroallergen-mediated allergic reactions. Considering that the access of food allergens cross-reactive with aeroallergens may occur across oral or nasal mucosa, the stability to digestion is a not a critical factor of conformational epitopes. The major apple allergens Mal d 1 is an example of extremely digestion-labile proteins which can prime allergic symptoms due to the cross-reactivity with the birch pollen allergen Bet v 1 (Son *et al.*, 1999).

Although genetic factors undoubtedly contribute to the development of food allergies, the available data indicate that the latter is not the only one responsible. In some studies, it was found that populations with a similar genetic background may have a different prevalence of food allergies, and vice versa (Du Toit *et al.*, 2008). Therefore, it appears that the prevalence is related to a plethora of genetic, environmental and demographic factors (Ben-Shoshan *et al.*, 2012), such as greater exposure to new foods, geographical differences, changes in food processing and changes in food technology. For example, to examine the effects of food processing on food allergens, it is important to understand the interaction between the allergenic protein and IgE antibodies. Under certain circumstances, food processing can alter the epitope, thereby altering the allergenicity of the foods themselves (Nowak-Wegrzyn and Fiocchi, 2009; Paschke, 2009; Sathe and Sharma, 2009; Sathe *et al.*, 2005). This process can lead to the destruction, modification, masking or unmasking, resulting in a decrease or increase, epitope or may not have consequences on allergenicity (Sathe *et al.*, 2005). The consequences depend not only on the molecular properties of the allergen but also on the type of processing and interaction between the allergen and other food components (Sathe and Sharma, 2009).

Some thermal processes (such as baking, grilling, drying and sterilization) can have effects on allergenicity. High temperatures can cause the destruction epitope due to protein denaturation. However, some allergenic proteins, such as allergen Ara h 1 present in peanuts, can be thermostable (Koppelman *et al.*, 1999). Although the type of heat process is important: for example, it has been shown that peanut allergenicity is lower in boiled peanuts than roasted ones. This has been attributed to the loss in water of the low-molecular weight allergens (Mondoulet *et al.*, 2005). The interaction with other proteins, fats and carbohydrates in the food matrix may also influence on allergenicity. One example is the Maillard reaction, that is, the chemical interaction between amino acids and sugars during heating (or storage). In milk, the interaction between the beta-lactoglobulin protein and lactose sugar causes a higher allergenicity (Bleumink and Berrens, 1966).

Proteolysis can deeply impact on allergenicity. The proteolysis can be produced thanks to enzymes such as proteases and has been employed for reducing the allergenicity of soybean seeds (Yamanishi *et al.*, 1996). The physical elimination of the allergenic component is another way to reduce the allergenicity of foods. For certain foods, it uses a set of techniques. The treatment of milk with protease followed by ultrafiltration is used, for example, to prepare hypoallergenic products such as formulated for infants;

the combination of enzyme and heat treatment has instead demonstrated its ability to reduce the allergenic potential of 100 times in hen egg (Paschke, 2009).

These findings highlight opportunities and challenges for manufacturers of foodstuffs as regards the reduction and elimination of food allergens. Numerous publications in addition to their widespread use in clinical practice show that the dosage of specific IgE is the best scorer available in the routine for the diagnosis of allergies. Allergy is a progressive disorder in which awareness is the early stage, and the appearance of disease symptoms represent the late stage. It follows that the presence of a detectable awareness with laboratory tests can be detected in patients who have not yet manifested the clinical signs of allergy; on the other hand the dosage of specific IgE shows the inherent limitations, largely attributable to the presence of cross-reactivity that provides false positive results; Another limitation is represented by the fact that the extracts used for the production of allergens to be tested are often unstable and/or present in very low amounts and then exposing to the risk of false negative results. Ultimately, as already said previously, the positive predictive value of diagnostic methods based on IgE assay is generally lower than the negative predictive power. The two main lines of development of allergy tests are represented by the use of recombinant allergens and the use of arrays for the simultaneous analysis of hundreds of different allergens. The possibilities offered by technology now make it possible to study and isolate allergens under represented from a wide range of different food sources. Consequently, it will soon be possible to use recombinant allergens directly, thus overcoming the problems caused by the low amounts or the instability of allergens derived from natural extracts. Furthermore, the possibility offered by the technology of today have in a known order thousands of molecules on a single support of limited dimensions which have analytical tools that allow simultaneously to analyze hundreds or thousands of such recombinant allergens. Of course, it is expected that recombinant allergens may be used, as well as for the diagnosis, also to achieve targeted immunotherapies.

These considerations lead to the fact that the core problems of FA remain unresolved under several standpoints that include:

- clinical evidence suggests that many of the suspected allergens present in food have not been identified or characterized yet.
- the structural traits which make a protein an allergen and the relationship between allergenic determinants and disease patterns still remain substantially unknown.
- the mechanisms through which allergenic proteins and their derived peptides elicit the adverse reactions to food ingestion awaits to be completely explained yet. These knowledge gaps also slow down the development novel and sensitive screening and confirmatory tests for diagnosis and prognosis of allergy as well as more efficient therapeutic protocols.

These issues could be addressed only by the development of novel high-throughput analytical approaches having their core on the "omic" sciences.

The Proteomic Approach to Study Food Allergy

The need for reliable methods allowing accurate structural identification and dosage of the offending allergens has prompted researchers to develop new methods for the unambiguous characterization of food allergens (Table 9.2). Over the last years, the integrated approaches based on the various "-omics" for food peptide and protein characterization (proteomics, peptidomics, metabolomics), all of which rely on Mass Spectrometry (MS) analysis, are proving to be essential at various levels in the study of FA, from the structural characterization of novel food allergens to the controversial feature of the resistance to digestion of allergenic proteins or to the efficiency of removal of epitopes from a food destined to patients. This integrated approach for studying allergy was introduced as allergenomics in 2007 by Akagawa's group (Akagawa *et al.*, 2007).

Since the late 90's, proteomics has found applications in many medical disciplines and the early work in the field of FA date back to 2001. Since then, proteomics has been applied to allergen characterization of virtually all types of food of both animal and vegetable origin, often contributing to the discovery of new food allergens. Those species which show a remarkable complexity at the protein level are intensely studied, including the major allergens of sesame, lupine, pistachio, the protein isoforms of peanut. New egg, crustaceans, fruit and nut allergens were discovered and characterized (Nitride *et al.*, 2013).

In 2004 the term *allergenomics* was coined to enter the omics world in the study of food allergens. In addition to the discovery of novel food allergens, proteomic techniques are also finding application in the verification of new genetically modified foods, control of allergens in purified or recombinant products due to the search for trace allergens in foods, in the assessment of chemical modifications on food allergens by industrial treatments. With the progress of technology and the ever increasing range of tools easier to use, MS-based proteomics has become over time an important tool for the study of food allergens (Fig. 9.3).

MS allows the simultaneous identification and quantification of allergens in food, which is independent from individual sensitivity. To achieve this, MS-based proteomics makes large use of the MALDI (Matrix-Assisted Laser Desorption Ionization) and ESI (electrospray ionization) ion sources, which allow mass spectral acquisition with minimal analyte requirement. Interestingly, ESI is easily coupled to upstream high resolution separation techniques such as HPLC and UPLC. In the basic proteomic approach to protein structural characterization, identification is achieved using a strategy

Table 9.2: Analytical techniques for physico-chemical characterization of allergens.

Technique	Analytical parameter and information provided	Detection limit (LOD/ LOQ)	Relevance for allergen risk assessment	References
CD	Changes in protein 2D and 3D structure. Structure of linear and conformational epitopes. Identity of cloned with native allergens.	1–2 nmol/5– 10 nmol	Structural epitope definition may improve design of screening and diagnostic tests.	(Mihajlovic *et al.*, 2016) (Wangorsch *et al.*, 2016)
FTIR	Changes in protein 2- and 3-D structure. Structure of epitopes. Process inactivation of allergens.	0.1–0.5 nmol/1–2 nmol	Design of novel sensors for allergen detection. Development of immunotherapy approaches.	(Jiang *et al.*, 2015) (Plundrich *et al.*, 2014)
X-ray diffraction	Allergen 2- and 3-D structure. Structure of epitopes. Process inactivation of allergens.	1–10 mmol	Structural definition of epitopic structures may improve design of screening and diagnostic tests.	(Offermann *et al.*, 2015) (Pomes *et al.*, 2015)
Computational methods	Prediction of allergens structure. Location of epitopes.	–	Structural definition of epitopic structures may improve design of screening and diagnostic tests.	(Herman *et al.*, 2015) (Gonzalez-Fernandez *et al.*, 2014)
NMR	Allergen 2- and 3-D structure. Structure of epitopes. Process inactivation of allergens.	1–10 mmol	Structural definition of epitopic structures may improve design of screening and diagnostic tests.	(Alessandri *et al.*, 2012) (Berkner *et al.*, 2014)
Electron microscopy (SEM, TEM)	Imaging of food structure. Location of allergens in food compartments. Interaction of allergens with food components.	1–10 mmol	High sensitivity sensors for detection and prediction of allergens in foodstuffs.	(Johnson *et al.*, 2015) (Jiang *et al.*, 2015)

known as shotgun proteomics. It involves, as a first step, the digestion of the target proteins into small peptides, which, by means of their uniqueness, allow the identification of the protein from which they are derived (peptide mass fingerprint). In order to increase the method specificity, the amino acid sequence of specific peptides is determined by MS/MS through peptide fragmentation using CID (Collision Induced Dissociation).

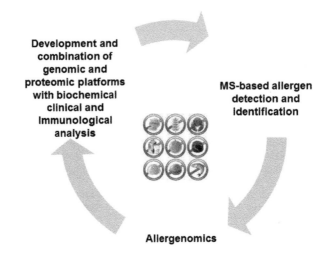

Fig. 9.3: Integrated approaches of the various omic sciences led to the birth of allergenomics for the study of food allergy.

Because of its technical capabilities, MS is increasingly supporting the investigations about the fate of food proteins and, in the specific case, of food allergens (Table 9.3). For instance, MS techniques, including Multiple Reaction Monitoring (MRM), have been exploited to detect and quantify the snow crab airborne allergens that are responsible for asthma of people occupationally exposed to seafood (Abdel Rahman *et al.*, 2010; Abdel Rahman *et al.*, 2012).

For a more precise functional identification, allergen characterization requires the combination of proteomic with clinical, immunological and genomic approaches (Fig. 9.4). In this respect, the application of proteomic technologies to the identification of new allergens has been convenient in a number of instances. In these cases, the proteomic analytical strategy consists of the 2D-PAGE separation of the protein extracts and subsequent staining of the IgE-reactive spots by immunoblotting with sera of the allergic individuals. IgE-binding proteins can be identified by MS-based techniques after in-gel tryptic digestion.

Pre-fractionation of proteins from complex samples prior to MS analysis are the most common strategies applied to perform proteomic investigations (Stasyk and Huber, 2004). To date, two-dimensional electrophoresis (2DE) has proven to be a reliable and efficient method to separate a large number of proteins is a single step. By this technique proteins are usually separated by gel electrophoresis according to their pI (isoelectric focusing, IEF) and subsequently to their molecular weight (SDS-PAGE). 2DE is extremely powerful and can achieve the separation of several thousand different proteins spots in one gel. Stains such as Coomassie blue, silver, SYPRO Ruby can be employed to visualize the proteins (Candiano *et al.*, 2004). Once stained, protein

Table 9.3: MS-based techniques for allergen characterization.

Technique	Information	Strength	Pitfall	References
MALDI-MS	Allergen molecular weight. Effective presence of PTMs. Effects of food processing. Allergen presence in complex food ingredient and products.	Fast, allows straightforward allergen detection with minimal sample preparation. Tolerance to complex mixtures and to salt and detergent contamination.	Non-quantitative or semi-quantitative only. Necessity of proper matrix selection. Difficulty of on-line combination with LC, but possibility of automation for fast gel based-proteomic analysis.	(Picariello *et al.*, 2011) (Steinhart *et al.*, 2001)
MALDI imaging	Definition of allergen location within the food tissues or compartments.	Direct identification of allergen presence and location.	Long and laborious sample preparation, influence of matrix effects, difficult automation, poor inter-sample reproducibility.	(Bencivenni *et al.*, 2014) (Cavatorta *et al.*, 2009)
ESI Tandem MS	Structural identification of allergens. Epitope mapping. PTMs and effects of food processing. Allergen presence in complex food ingredient and products.	Easy combination to LC for shotgun analysis of complex food matrices. High sensitivity structural identification. Possibility of untargeted analysis.	Difficulty of managing huge amounts of data.	(Johnson *et al.*, 2016b) (Picariello *et al.*, 2015)
Selected reaction monitoring (SRM)	Quantification of several allergens in mixture.	Multiplexed allergen quantification.	Necessity of labeled synthetic standard. Necessity of appropriate analytical software tools.	(Posada-Ayala *et al.*, 2015) (Monaci *et al.*, 2014)
HR-MS	Identification and quantification of allergens.	Fast and straightforward.	Cost of instrumentation. Possibility of false positives, depending on matrix complexity and sample preparation method.	(Monaci *et al.*, 2011)
Ion mobility MS	Allergen composition of raw and processed food ingredients.	Label-free semi-quantitative analysis.	Targeted analysis only. Instrumentation still poor diffuse.	(Johnson *et al.*, 2016b)

Table 9.3 contd. ...

... Table 9.3 contd.

Technique	Information	Strength	Pitfall	References
H/D exchange	Identification of epitopes and of Ig-binding regions.	Fast and straightforward.	Strong influence of experimental conditions. Difficulty in reproducing native physiological parameters. Poor reproducibility.	(Guan *et al.*, 2015) (Zhang *et al.*, 2013)
Chemical cross-linking	Identification of epitopes and of Ig-binding regions. Protein digestibility.	Precise and fine identification of epitopic regions.	Analytical conditions still to be set up.	No relevant applications existing yet.

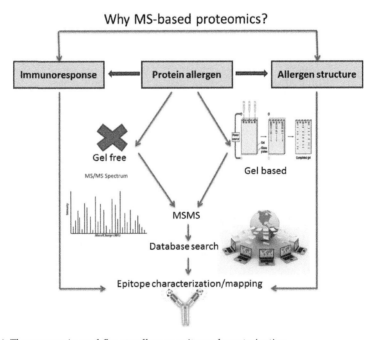

Fig. 9.4: The proteomic workflow to allergen epitope characterization.

spots excised from the gel are in-gel digest with a protease (i.e., trypsin) and identified by MS or MS/MS experiment (Timperman and Aebersold, 2000). The first approach, typically obtained by MALDI-TOF, allows the identification by Peptide Mass Fingerprinting (PMF), and the set of masses is then compared to the theoretically expected tryptic peptide masses for each entry in the database. On the other hand, MS/MS analysis (e.g., MALDI-TOF-TOF or ESI-MS/MS) determines structural information related to the sequence of peptides, rather than only their mass (Suckau *et al.*, 2003), making these searches more specific and discriminating.

A common feature of all strategies applied in the proteomic analysis is the availability of a tool for the interpretation of a huge amount of MS/MS spectra produced. The identifications are usually administered automatically via powerful, commercially accessible software such as Mascot mass (Johnson *et al.*, 2016a), SEQUEST mass (Deutsch *et al.*, 2008) in combination with continually updated public databases such as the ones held in the NCBI-Pubmed and UniProt.

The large range of strategies in which MS has a key role requires the extensive knowledge of potentiality and pitfalls of each approach and a careful case-by-case analysis as a function of the needed analytical response. Thus, MS enables analytical access starting from a simple qualitative or quantitative monitoring of an established peptide/protein allergen up to the "profiling" of the entire repertoire of MHC-binding peptides (Hillen and Stevanovic, 2006) or to the structural conformational characterization and the hydrogen/deuterium exchange-based epitope mapping (Hager-Braun and Tomer, 2005). Obviously, enhanced instrumental performances and gradually increasing skills of the operators are required for more sophisticated experiments.

2DE gels coupled with MS analysis can also be integrated with antibodies assay in the classical blotting setup. In this case, the immunoblotting step is used to assign the protein(s) of interest on a reference 2DE mass, and a subsequent 2DE gel is run to perform the identification and characterization of the protein(s) of interest (Cox *et al.*, 2016). The pioneer study of Sander *et al.* combining PAGE, immunoblotting, and MS to identify water-soluble wheat enzymes involved in respiratory allergy traced the proteomic strategy followed since then for allergen identification (exemplified in Fig. 9.2) (Sander *et al.*, 1997). With a similar approach, wheat allergens—AAI (Alpha-Amylase Inhibitors), peroxidase I, thaumatin-like protein and Lipid Transfer Protein (LTP)—were identified in baker's asthma patients using 1D-SDS PAGE combined with Tandem MS.

Food Allergen Detection and Characterization using Mass Spectrometry

Labeling regulations for allergens in the various nations and EU have been set, but they are hardly comprehensive (see Chapter 10). In the US, the Food Allergen Labeling and Consumer Protection Act dated 2004 requires manufacturers to include a "contains" statement, a clear list of ingredients that are defined as allergens by the "big eight" list. Similar directives have been provided by the EU law. However, the problem arises when allergens are not intentional ingredients. If food is produced in the same facility and on the same equipment as food containing allergens, some of these potentially dangerous ingredients may wind up cross-contaminating other foods. To warn consumers of possible cross-contamination, companies often adopt advisory statements revealing that food was produced in a facility that also processes allergens. But these statements are completely voluntary; they are not required by labeling laws.

Undeclared food allergens account for 30–40% of food recalls in the United States. Compliance with ingredient labeling regulations and the implementation of effective manufacturing allergen control plans require the use of reliable methods for allergen detection and quantitation in complex food matrices.

However, allergens constitute a very heterogeneous class of compounds, which may vary in molecular weight (from a few thousand to tens of thousands of daltons), isoelectric point, amount and type of post-translational modifications, and the variety of which is increased by the presence, for a number of allergenic proteins, of different isoforms. In addition, the technological treatment of foods may change the protein structure, increasing the molecular diversity and affecting their potential allergenic (van Hengel, 2007).

Currently, there are several technical possibilities for the detection of potential allergens in food products. Methods based on the analysis of proteins, typically, provide for the immunochemical detection protocols such as radio allergosorbent test (RAST), enzyme allergosorbent test (EAST), and enzyme-linked immunosorbent assay (ELISA). Methods are not routinely used the rocket immunoelectrophoresis (RIE) and immunoblotting, while RIE and immunoblotting only provide qualitative or semi-quantitative results, RAST, EAST and ELISA can be used as quantitative methods (Poms *et al.*, 2004). Screening for allergens in food is generally based on ELISA, which is based on the use of antibodies (Abs) specifically raised against proteins. These Abs are specifically targeted for the allergenic food. Numerous ELISA methods have been developed for the detection of different food allergens, and several commercial kits have become available in recent years (Schubert-Ullrich *et al.*, 2009). The results obtained with the ELISA test can be expressed as whole food, such as total or soluble proteins or as specific protein. For example, in the case of peanut the results are usually expressed as peanut, or as total soluble protein or as a specific allergenic protein (e.g., Ara h 1); in the case of milk as skimmed milk powder or as beta-lactoglobulin or casein. Obviously, the results expressed as claimed in one of these bases substantially differ from the others. From the point of view of the protection of public health, the expression of the results as mg of allergenic food per kg of foodstuff is probably the most appropriate since the threshold values are usually studied as the tolerable amount of food. The method is fast and easy to perform. However, a series of qualitative and quantitative analyses regularly generate variable results, together with false positives and false negatives, constituting a severe limitation of this technique; additionally, each target allergen requires a separate ELISA test kit. Consequently, companies often do not test products for the presence of all possible allergens. Therefore, they perform a cost-effectiveness analysis and select the top one, two, or three allergens most likely to be present. Any others can go undetected.

Another approach is based on Real-Time Polymerase Chain Reaction (RT-PCR). To date, commercial kits are available for almost all foods included in the EU allergen list (cereals, shellfish, eggs, fish, peanuts, soy, cow's milk, almond, hazelnut, walnut, cashew, pistachio, celery, mustard, sesame, lupine, mollusks) as well as for other allergens not included in the legislation list (buckwheat, peach, tomato). As in the case of ELISA, the sensitivity achieved by PCR is normally expressed as mg allergenic food/kg of foodstuff. Although the method can identify DNA of milk, peanuts, soy, walnuts, hazelnuts, fish and crustaceans, there are several pitfalls that can determine an allergen to remain undetected. The most notable is that PCR detects the presence of DNA, but not of proteins. Egg white and several milk products, significant allergenic foods, contain little DNA, but high quantities of protein. Therefore, this method is not reliable in these cases. A further drawback is that it is an indirect method where the presence of the allergen is not monitored, but only the presence of material from the organism, and this can produce false negatives and positives. Furthermore, the method does not discriminate between different proteins from the same food matrix, which can have very different allergenic potential.

Among the methods developed to identify allergenic proteins in food, in recent years, mass spectrometry (MS) has played an increasingly central role, due to its specificity and sensitivity. MS-based analytical approaches for detecting food allergenic proteins follow essentially two approaches (Poms *et al.*, 2004) (a) chromatographic separation followed by MS detection and quantification of intact proteins (direct approach); (b) protein digestion with specific enzymes, followed by LC-MS detection and quantification of characteristic marker (proteotypic) peptides of the searched protein (indirect approach). The second method is very convenient, due to the fact that peptides are more easily separable than the parent protein and, more importantly, they can be detected with much higher sensitivity.

Application of the direct detection of intact allergens proteins is therefore scarce. A LC-ESI-IT-MS/MS method has been published for the detection of milk whey protein in fruit juice, after a solid phase extraction step. The detection limit was quite high (1 mg/l) (Monaci and van Hengel, 2008). MALDI-TOF MS has also been applied to the detection of lysozyme (a potential allergen) added in some dairy products such as Grana Padano hard cheese, as antimicrobial agent to avoid undesired fermentation. In this method lysozyme, previously purified by immunocapture with magnetic particles coated with a specific anti-lysozyme antibody, was detectable at 5 ppm sensitivity (Schneider *et al.*, 2010).

The examples of detection of specific peptides derived from allergenic proteins are instead uncountable. The only requirement to this method is the absolute reproducibility of the enzymatic digestion process, which ideally should be perfectly controlled, so that the prototypic peptide can be reliably quantified.

In one of the first published examples, the method has been applied to LC-ESI-MS detection and quantification of the peanut allergen Ara h 1, in an ice cream model matrix. Detection of proteotypic peptides allowed to uniquely identify and quantify Ara h 1 at 20 mg/kg (Shefcheck and Musser, 2004). The method was then implemented with LC-ESI-MS/MS, for Ara h 1 detection in chocolate. The use of a triple quadrupole instrumentation allowed to lower the sensitivity down to 2 mg/kg (Shefcheck *et al.*, 2006). With a more sophisticated instrumentation, a capLC/nano-ESI/Q-TOF MS/MS instrument, it was possible to detect the Ara h 1, Ara h 2 and Ara h 3 in either raw or roasted peanuts. This improvement is very important in order to extend allergen detection in processed products (Chassaigne *et al.*, 2007). Similarly, a LC/ESI-MS/MS method has been proposed for detection of milk casein through the analysis of proteotypic peptides in tryptic digests. The sensitivity of the method was estimated to 5 mg/kg of protein (Weber *et al.*, 2006). A semiquantitative method based on LC/ESI-MS/MS has been proposed for the detection of peptides derived from casein present in wine (Monaci *et al.*, 2010). Also the use of purification techniques, digestion and analysis of the most innovative, such as immunomagnetic extraction procedures combined with tryptic digestions assisted by microwave, in combination with MS/MS analysis, have confirmed the sensitivity levels presented previously, on the order of low ppm.

Also LC-ESI-Q-TRAP MS/MS technology has been recently proposed for detection of allergens in foods [*http://sciex.com/Documents/brochures/Allergens-QTRAP4k_1830610.pdf*], allowing the simultaneous detection of four major food allergens peanut, milk, wheat and egg at ppm levels.

Two very recent studies (Gomaa and Boye, 2015; Parker *et al.*, 2015) have been recently tested on industry-processed model foods incurred with egg, milk and peanut allergens, with the objective to compare analytical method performance for allergen quantitation in thermally processed bakery products, and to determine the effects of thermal treatment on allergen detection. Quantitation of egg, milk and peanut in incurred baked goods was compared at various processing stages using commercial ELISA kits and a multi-allergen LC-MS/MS method based on Multiple-Reaction Monitoring (MRM). Thermal processing was determined to negatively affect the recovery and the quantitation of egg, milk, and peanut to different extents depending on the allergen, matrix and analytical test method. Importantly, the LC-MS/MS quantitative method allowed the highest recovery across all monitored allergens, whereas the ELISA systems under performed in the determination of allergen content of industry-processed bakery products.

In other recent studies, marker proteins to peanuts and various tree nuts were extracted, subjected to trypsin digestion and analysis by either LC-Q/TOF MS/MS (Sealey-Voyksner *et al.*, 2016) or Orbitrap (Monaci *et al.*, 2015) in order to find highly conserved peptides that can be used as target peptides to detect peanuts and tree nuts in food. The target peptides chosen (at least two for any allergen) were those found to be present in both native (unroasted) and thermally processed (roasted) forms of peanuts and tree nuts (peanut, almond, pecan, cashew, walnut, hazelnut, pine nut, Brazil nut, macadamia nut, pistachio nut, chestnut and coconut) to determine the presence of trace levels of peanut and tree nuts in food by these multiplexed LC-MS methods.

Potentialities of MS have been recently compared to DNA and ELISA approaches for hen egg proteins (Lee and Kim, 2010) and for beer (Tanner *et al.*, 2013). An exhaustive overview of the existing methods for the detection of allergens in food products, which also includes the detailed analysis of advantages and pitfalls of the single strategies, has recently been published (Picariello *et al.*, 2011). The urgency of structural confirmation based on MS to provide unambiguous identification and quantification of allergen arises from the limitations of the classically used methods.

Quantitation of Food Allergenome

Food allergens are traditionally quantified by ELISA. There are a couple of ELISA techniques for protein quantification; competitive and sandwich, where the sandwich technique is more accurate and precise as two antibodies involved in the experiment. In the sandwich technique, the microtiter plate well is coated with a primary antibody that binds specifically to the food extract protein. The bound protein will be detected through an enzyme attached to the secondary antibody, and then the color developed in a quantitative manner. This technique minimizes the non-specific binding for better sensitivity.

The ultimate goal of allergens discovery is to find a way for detecting this allergen in several matrices. Understanding the level of food allergens is very crucial to help allergic people from avoiding any unpleasant exposure. For the purpose of food safety, absolute quantitation is highly demanded to replace the nonspecific and insensitive immune-assay techniques such as ELISA. Food allergenome takes advantage of the enormous development of the proteomics field. Essentially, the quantitative proteomics is used to study the live cellular regulatory processes in an absolute or relative fashion. The relative quantitation is mainly used to investigate the differences in protein expression between at least two different proteomes while the absolute quantitation is used to quantify the amount of protein in the sample independently.

Relative quantitation

The food allergenome could be relatively quantified using 2DE to compare the protein expression between two or more gels. The 2D-DIGE can compare between few samples run on the same gel (Unlu *et al.*, 1997). The relative MS-based quantitation method is classified into two main groups; stable-isotope labeling and label-free.

The label-free method is less reproducible than the stable-isotopic with the relative standard deviation (RSD) 30 and 10%, respectively. The label-free approach requires high-resolution MS, as the principle of the quantitation based on the signal of the tryptic peptides' precursor ion. This method is less expensive than the others, as no reference material is required. Any existent protein has a peptidic precursor ion; thus, this method is highly comprehensive within the sample proteins and universal for a different type of samples (Anas M. Abdel Rahman, 2012). The label-free can be performed using either protein-based method (spectral count or derived indices) to study the protein expression or peptide-based method for the identified ones (ion intensities and protein correlation profile).

Absolute quantitation

The allergens' absolute quantification (AQUA) is usually performed using the stable-isotopic-labeled technique (Desiderio and Kai, 1983). Using Selected Reaction Monitoring (SRM) in the triple-quadruple tandem mass spectrometer, the AQUA became a standard protocol in the quantification of characterized allergens. The signature peptide represents its protein stoichiometrically, which is supposed to have a distinctive combination of precursor ion, product ion and chromatographic retention time (Rt). The signal-to-noise (s/n) ratio of the SRM is an additional value to the AQUA approach, where the linear dynamic range might go up to five orders of magnitude for the most of the peptides.

The native protein concentration is calculated by the molar ratio of the signature peptide to its protein. Sample loss during the preparation requires an internal standard for better representation. In detail, the representative signature peptide is selected from the pool of digested protein. The stable-isotopic labeled (heavy) and natural (light) forms of the signature peptide are chemically synthesized to be used for method development and controls as internal standard and standards, respectively. In the "isotope dilution" strategy, the labeled signature peptide is added deliberately to the sample in known amounts. Proteins with size < 15 kDa can also be quantified using the top-down approach, where the internal standard, in this case, is a recombinant labeled protein has the same sequence as the target analyte. The light and heavy recombinant proteins are developed inside the bacterial system (*E. coli*) using the metabolic labeling strategy in labeled-culture media (Brun *et al.*, 2011).

The isobaric mass tags strategies such as Isobaric Tag for Relative and Absolute Quantitation (iTRAQ) and Tandem Mass Tage (TMT) are used for global allergenomics discovery, where the strategies give the qualitative and quantitative of the allergens in the sample. The relative abundance of the tags ions represents the level of allergen in the combined samples while the rest of the product ion spectrum give the identity of the protein to the databases such as MASCOT.

Food Digestion and Food Allergy. Food Digestion Analysis, Development of Models to Study of Protein Digestion. Digestion of Allergens and Epitopes Identification

The antigenic potential of allergen epitopes can be reduced or completely annulled upon protein denaturation by cooking, heat processing and especially by the process of gastrointestinal digestion.

Several food digestion models have been developed in the last years, as recently reviewed (Picariello, 2016). They may be *in vivo* or *in vitro* and all try to reproduce the events occurring during food digestion with the aim of characterizing the products and determining their functional properties. Several research groups have developed an *in vitro* model mimicking the sequential phases of food digestion (gastric, duodenal and intestinal) which includes the action of purified enzymes of brush border membrane of the intestine. These enzymes have the most intense proteolytic action to reach the final products of digestion.

The mixture of proteins, peptides and amino acids produced during food protein digestion is the greatest complexity. It includes proteins and polypeptides which survive digestion and may be constituted by hundreds or even more components depending on the food matrix, and our allergens and epitopes are among them. As for allergen detection in raw matrices, the study of these processes requires the development of efficient omic strategies which conjugate biochemical, cellular and MS tools (see Chapter 8). For this reason, complementary MALDI and ESI-MS have been to identify the regions of milk proteins that survive an *in vitro* multi-phasal model of the gastrointestinal digestion (Picariello *et al.*, 2010).

Design of Novel Food Destined to People Affected by Allergy: The Role of Proteomics

The food sector is exposed to numerous problems related to the allergenic risk management; for example, the lack of normative nature orientations about the threshold values and the quantities and the absence of analytical methods adopted to identify the allergens. Nowadays, the food industry standards are critical in helping companies in the industry to be compliant or even exceed the requirements of the law in many cases. They also enable companies in the sector to ensure a degree of consistency in terms of safety and product quality.

An exemplary application of proteomics in this field is in the analysis of the products of the starch hydrolysis, obtained industrially through chemical and/or enzymatic methods. In this products gluten determination by immunological tests is made unreliable by several factors, including the low amount of gluten to be detected, dispersed in a high amount of interfering compounds (low and high mass sugars, other by-products of the process). Gluten semi-quantitative measurement in these products by combining procedures of extraction and isolation with MALDI–TOF–MS analysis made it possible to detect and identify low quantities of protein (estimated sensitivity 1–10 ppm), thus allowing to verify whether these products exceeded the 20 ppm limit required for foods "rendered" gluten-free (Ferranti *et al.*, 2007). The pattern of proteins/peptides present in samples was found to vary either qualitatively or quantitatively, depending on the sample type. This also meant that the MS approach may allow to identify the differences and quantify the protein/peptide level in different industrial products of the same category.

As pointed out, FA is treated symptomatically and through the strict exclusion of the allergen from the diet. On the other hand, serious nutritional, psychological and compliance-related implications arise from its substitution when the foods in question are important components of the diet. Furthermore, because of the increasing number of persons affected by FA, efforts have been made to produce hypoallergenic foods, characterized by a limited allergen content, which should prevent sensitization and alleviate clinical symptoms (Fig. 9.5).

Basically, there are two ways for producing hypoallergenic foods. The genetic approach is based on the selection or production of alternative materials without or with minor allergen content (Johansson *et al.*, 2004). For instance, the use of kamut (*T. polonicum*) or of the diploid *T. monococcum* (einkorn) species has been proposed upon the hypothesis that these ancient Triticum species have a low allergen content (Nakamura *et al.*, 2005). DNA recombinant techniques have been used to inhibit production of the a-amylase-like allergen in rice (Tada *et al.*, 1996).

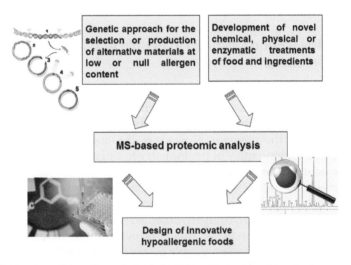

Fig. 9.5: Production of hypoallergenic foods is achieved by means of two basic approaches: the genetic approach based on the selection or production of alternative materials without or with minor allergen content, and the approach based on the application of chemical, physical or enzymatic treatments.

The second approach is based on the application of chemical, physical or enzymatic treatments. The real question is whether these treatments are effective in eliminating the immunoreactive sequences. Therefore, the consequences of these processes on immunogenicity and allergenicity can be evaluated only by the combination of proteomic, peptidomic and immunological approaches, for which the term allergomics has been recently introduced (Akagawa *et al.*, 2007). As an example, proteomic analysis has recently shown that deamidation of glutamine residues produced contradictory results: deamidation of the allergenic epitope QQQPP lowered IgE reactivity of patients, whereas deamidation of wheat protein isolates commonly used as additives in food industry apparently induced the appearance of novel antigens (Leduc *et al.*, 2003; Leszczynskaa, 2006). Hydrolytic treatment with actinase suppressed allergic reactions in tested patients, whereas hydrolyzed wheat proteins, used as food additives, lost IgE-binding capacity when cleaved by acid treatment but not if obtained by enzymatic reaction (Akiyama *et al.*, 2006).

The major technological problem faced in the development of hypoallergenic baked products is that modifications of potential allergens is likely to induce also a loss of functional properties of dough. Efficient methods to produce hypoallergenic flour need to be also supported by technological advances in order to obtain satisfying if not optimal sensory quality products. Probiotic preparation used as a starter culture allowed preparing sourdough bread with elevated acceptability scores. MS was in this specific case instrumental to ensure degradation of allergenic epitopes following the entire technological production process of bread and also to monitor protein modifications during pepsin and pancreatin digestion mimicking physiological-like conditions of food digestion.

Conclusions

The remarkable instrumental developments of the last years have boosted omics disciplines and molecular profiling approaches. Thanks to this innovative platform and integration between the different skills of researchers, scientific activity topics range from food to life sciences. In particular the use of MS methods can address problems inherent to innovative fields of chemistry, biochemistry and food technology, and develop rapid, accurate and reliable analytical tools for quality control and safety. These approaches are rapidly supplementing or even replacing the previously consolidated methods. Over the next years, the integrated omics-based approaches are expected to accelerate the development of novel functional foods and ingredients. This meets the ever-increasing demands of both consumers, producers and supervisory authorities, due to new issues introduced by the liberalization and globalization of markets. Despite the variety of sample preparation methods and of the proteomic approach used, ranging from the simplest to the most sophisticated, the detection limits the settling in all cases around values of a few ng/g.

Importantly, MS has been entrusted the task of challenging the issue of (food) allergen standardization (Reuter *et al.*, 2009), that is related to diagnosis and treatment of allergies besides the analytical aspect of the identification and quantification of allergens. It is therefore reasonable to assume that if standards procedures are adopted based on the MS for use in control laboratories, the sensitivity limits are within the same order of magnitude. MS, thanks to its identifying power, will virtually reduce to zero the possibility of false negatives and false positives, even in very harshly treated food samples (e.g., toasted) or in the presence of complex food matrices.

Furthermore, in the perspective of understanding what food components become after ingestion, proteomics will relevantly contribute to unravel some of the routes through which food components interact one another to generate novel immune-determinants or to potentiate those already existent. Food allergy and intolerance are fields in which MS are proving to be essential at various levels, including the issue of the allergen resistance to digestion or the efficiency of removal of epitopes from a food destined to allergic people. Therefore, large cost- and health-saving results are being achieved by application of the MS-based efficient monitoring procedures. Also the advances and future developments of protein array technology, which will be largely driven by MS-derived structural information, will ensure more rapid and accurate detection of food composition for the safety of intolerant consumers. For all these reasons, employment of the novel MS techniques in food proteomics is expected to increase during the next years, due to their emerging potentiality in the molecular characterization of food products.

Keywords: Food Allergy, Mass Spectrometry, Proteomics, Allergenomics, Epitope mapping, Allergen Monitoring, Allergen Quantification

References

Abdel Rahman, A. M., Lopata, A. L., Randell, E. W., and Helleur, R. J. (2010). Absolute quantification method and validation of airborne snow crab allergen tropomyosin using tandem mass spectrometry. Analytica Chimica Acta 681(1-2): 49–55.

Abdel Rahman, A. M., Gagne, S., and Helleur, R. J. (2012). Simultaneous determination of two major snow crab aeroallergens in processing plants by use of isotopic dilution tandem mass spectrometry. Analytical and Bioanalytical Chemistry 403(3): 821–831.

Akagawa, M., Handoyo, T., Ishii, T., Kumazawa, S., Morita, N., and Suyama, K. (2007). Proteomic analysis of wheat flour allergens. Journal of Agricultural and Food Chemistry 55(17): 6863–6870.

Akiyama, H., Sakata, K., Yoshioka, Y., Murata, Y., Ishihara, Y., Teshima, R., Sawada, J., and Maitani, T. (2006). Profile analysis and immunoglobulin E reactivity of wheat protein hydrolysates. International Archives of Allergy and Immunology 140(1): 36–42.

Alessandri, S., Sancho, A., Vieths, S., Mills, C. E., Wal, J. M., Shewry, P. R., Rigby, N., and Hoffmann-Sommergruber, K. (2012). High-throughput NMR assessment of the tertiary structure of food allergens. PloS One 7(7): e39785.

Anas M. Abdel Rahman, R. J. H., Mohamed F. Jeebhay, and Andreas L. Lopata. (2012). Characterization of seafood proteins causing allergic diseases. pp. 107–140. *In*: P.C. Pereira (ed.). Allergic Diseases—Highlights in the Clinic, Mechanisms and Treatment (1 ed.). InTech.

Ben-Shoshan, M., Harrington, D. W., Soller, L., Fragapane, J., Joseph, L., Pierre, Y. S., Godefroy, S. B., Elliott, S. J., and Clarke, A. E. (2012). Demographic predictors of peanut, tree nut, fish, shellfish, and sesame allergy in Canada. Journal of Allergy 2012: 858306.

Bencivenni, M., Faccini, A., Zecchi, R., Boscaro, F., Moneti, G., Dossena, A., and Sforza, S. (2014). Electrospray MS and MALDI imaging show that non-specific lipid-transfer proteins (LTPs) in tomato are present as several isoforms and are concentrated in seeds. Journal of Mass Spectrometry 49(12): 1264–1271.

Berkner, H., Seutter von Loetzen, C., Hartl, M., Randow, S., Gubesch, M., Vogel, L., Husslik, F., Reuter, A., Lidholm, J., Ballmer-Weber, B., Vieths, S., Rosch, P., and Schiller, D. (2014). Enlarging the toolbox for allergen epitope definition with an allergen-type model protein. PloS One 9(10): e111691.

Bleumink, E., and Berrens, L. (1966). Synthetic approaches to the biological activity of beta-lactoglobulin in human allergy to cows' milk. Nature 212(5061): 541–543.

Bousquet, J., Anto, J. M., Bachert, C., Bousquet, P. J., Colombo, P., Crameri, R., Daeron, M., Fokkens, W., Leynaert, B., Lahoz, C., Maurer, M., Passalacqua, G., Valenta, R., van Hage, M., and Van Ree, R. (2006). Factors responsible for differences between asymptomatic subjects and patients presenting an IgE sensitization to allergens. A GA2LEN project. Allergy 61(6): 671–680.

Brun, M. A., Griss, R., Reymond, L., Tan, K. T., Piguet, J., Peters, R. J., Vogel, H., and Johnsson, K. (2011). Semisynthesis of fluorescent metabolite sensors on cell surfaces. Journal of the American Chemical Society 133(40): 16235–16242.

Candiano, G., Bruschi, M., Musante, L., Santucci, L., Ghiggeri, G. M., Carnemolla, B., Orecchia, P., Zardi, L., and Righetti, P. G. (2004). Blue silver: a very sensitive colloidal Coomassie G-250 staining for proteome analysis. Electrophoresis 25(9): 1327–1333.

Cavatorta, V., Sforza, S., Mastrobuoni, G., Pieraccini, G., Francese, S., Moneti, G., Dossena, A., Pastorello, E. A., and Marchelli, R. (2009). Unambiguous characterization and tissue localization of Pru P 3 peach allergen by electrospray mass spectrometry and MALDI imaging. Journal of Mass Spectrometry 44(6): 891–897.

Chassaigne, H., Norgaard, J. V., and Hengel, A. J. (2007). Proteomics-based approach to detect and identify major allergens in processed peanuts by capillary LC-Q-TOF (MS/MS). Journal of Agricultural and Food Chemistry 55(11): 4461–4473.

Constantin, C., Quirce, S., Grote, M., Touraev, A., Swoboda, I., Stoecklinger, A., Mari, A., Thalhamer, J., Heberle-Bors, E., and Valenta, R. (2008). Molecular and immunological characterization of a wheat serine proteinase inhibitor as a novel allergen in baker's asthma. Journal of Immunology 180(11): 7451–7460.

Cox, J. M., Berna, M. J., Jin, Z., Cox, A. L., Sloop, K. W., Gutierrez, J. A., and Ackermann, B. L. (2016). Characterization and quantification of oxyntomodulin in human and rat plasma using high-resolution accurate mass LC-MS. Bioanalysis 8: 1579–1595.

Desiderio, D. M., and Kai, M. (1983). Preparation of stable isotope-incorporated peptide internal standards for field desorption mass spectrometry quantification of peptides in biologic tissue. Biomedical Mass Spectrometry 10(8): 471–479.

Deutsch, E. W., Lam, H., and Aebersold, R. (2008). Data analysis and bioinformatics tools for tandem mass spectrometry in proteomics. Physiological Genomics 33(1): 18–25.

Du Toit, G., Katz, Y., Sasieni, P., Mesher, D., Maleki, S. J., Fisher, H. R., Fox, A. T., Turcanu, V., Amir, T., Zadik-Mnuhin, G., Cohen, A., Livne, I., and Lack, G. (2008). Early consumption of peanuts in infancy is associated with a low prevalence of peanut allergy. The Journal of Allergy and Clinical Immunology 122(5): 984–991.

Ferranti, P., Mamone, G., Picariello, G., and Addeo, F. (2007). Mass spectrometry analysis of gliadins in celiac disease. Journal of Mass Spectrometry: JMS 42(12): 1531–1548.

Gomaa, A., and Boye, J. (2015). Simultaneous detection of multi-allergens in an incurred food matrix using ELISA, multiplex flow cytometry and liquid chromatography mass spectrometry (LC-MS). Food Chemistry 175: 585–592.

Gonzalez-Fernandez, J., Rodero, M., Daschner, A., and Cuellar, C. (2014). New insights into the allergenicity of tropomyosin: a bioinformatics approach. Molecular Biology Reports 41(10): 6509–6517.

Guan, X., Noble, K. A., Tao, Y., Roux, K. H., Sathe, S. K., Young, N. L., and Marshall, A. G. (2015). Epitope mapping of 7S cashew antigen in complex with antibody by solution-phase H/D exchange monitored by FT-ICR mass spectrometry. Journal of Mass Spectrometry 50(6): 812–819.

Hager-Braun, C., and Tomer, K. B. (2005). Determination of protein-derived epitopes by mass spectrometry. Expert Review in Proteomics 2(5): 745–756.

Herman, R. A., Song, P., and Kumpatla, S. (2015). Percent amino-acid identity thresholds are not necessarily conservative for predicting allergenic cross-reactivity. Food and Chemical Toxicology: An International Journal Published for the British Industrial Biological Research Association 81: 141–142.

Hillen, N., and Stevanovic, S. (2006). Contribution of mass spectrometry-based proteomics to immunology. Expert Review in Proteomics 3(6): 653–664.

Jiang, D., Zhu, P., Jiang, H., Ji, J., Sun, X., Gu, W., and Zhang, G. (2015). Fluorescent magnetic bead-based mast cell biosensor for electrochemical detection of allergens in foodstuffs. Biosensors and Bioelectronics 70: 482–490.

Johansson, S. G., Bieber, T., Dahl, R., Friedmann, P. S., Lanier, B. Q., Lockey, R. F., Motala, C., Ortega Martell, J. A., Platts-Mills, T. A., Ring, J., Thien, F., Van Cauwenberge, P., and Williams, H. C. (2004). Revised nomenclature for allergy for global use: Report of the nomenclature review committee of the World Allergy Organization, October 2003. The Journal of Allergy and Clinical Immunology 113(5): 832–836.

Johnson, J., Borres, M. P., Nordvall, L., Lidholm, J., Janson, C., Alving, K., and Malinovschi, A. (2015). Perceived food hypersensitivity relates to poor asthma control and quality of life in young non-atopic asthmatics. PloS One 10(4): e0124675.

Johnson, K. L., Williams, J. G., Maleki, S. J., Hurlburt, B. K., London, R. E., and Mueller, G. A. (2016a). Enhanced approaches for identifying amadori products: application to peanut allergens. Journal of Agricultural and Food Chemistry 64(6): 1406–1413.

Johnson, P. E., Sayers, R. L., Gethings, L. A., Balasundaram, A., Marsh, J. T., Langridge, J. I., and Mills, E. N. (2016b). Quantitative proteomic profiling of peanut allergens in food ingredients used for oral food challenges. Analytical Chemistry 88(11): 5689–5695.

Kagan, R. S. (2003). Food allergy: an overview. Environmental Health Perspectives 111(2): 223–225.

Koppelman, S. J., Bruijnzeel-Koomen, C. A., Hessing, M., and de Jongh, H. H. (1999). Heat-induced conformational changes of Ara h 1, a major peanut allergen, do not affect its allergenic properties. The Journal of Biological Chemistry 274(8): 4770–4777.

Ledesma, A., Barderas, R., Westritschnig, K., Quiralte, J., Pascual, C. Y., Valenta, R., Villalba, M., and Rodriguez, R. (2006). A comparative analysis of the cross-reactivity in the polcalcin family including Syr v 3, a new member from lilac pollen. Allergy 61(4): 477–484.

Leduc, V., Moneret-Vautrin, D. A., Guerin, L., Morisset, M., and Kanny, G. (2003). Anaphylaxis to wheat isolates: immunochemical study of a case proved by means of double-blind, placebo-controlled food challenge. The Journal of Allergy and Clinical Immunology 111(4): 897–899.

Lee, J. Y., and Kim, C. J. (2010). Determination of allergenic egg proteins in food by protein-, mass spectrometry-, and DNA-based methods. Journal of AOAC International 93(2): 462–477.

Leszczynskaa, J., Lackaa, A., and Bryszewskaa, M. (2006). The use of transglutaminase in the reduction of immunoreactivity of wheat flour. Food Agricultural of Immunology 17: 105–113.

Mihajlovic, L., Radosavljevic, J., Nordlund, E., Krstic, M., Bohn, T., Smit, J., Buchert, J., and Cirkovic Velickovic, T. (2016). Peanut protein structure, polyphenol content and immune response to peanut proteins *in vivo* are modulated by laccase. Food and Function 7(5): 2357–2366.

Monaci, L., and van Hengel, A. J. (2008). Development of a method for the quantification of whey allergen traces in mixed-fruit juices based on liquid chromatography with mass spectrometric detection. Journal of Chromatography A 1192(1): 113–120.

Monaci, L., Losito, I., Palmisano, F., and Visconti, A. (2010). Identification of allergenic milk proteins markers in fined white wines by capillary liquid chromatography-electrospray ionization-tandem mass spectrometry. Journal of Chromatography A 1217(26): 4300–4305.

Monaci, L., Losito, I., Palmisano, F., Godula, M., and Visconti, A. (2011). Towards the quantification of residual milk allergens in caseinate-fined white wines using HPLC coupled with single-stage Orbitrap mass spectrometry. Food Additives and Contaminants. Part A, Chemistry, Analysis, Control, Exposure and Risk Assessment 28(10): 1304–1314.

Monaci, L., Pilolli, R., De Angelis, E., Godula, M., and Visconti, A. (2014). Multi-allergen detection in food by micro high-performance liquid chromatography coupled to a dual cell linear ion trap mass spectrometry. Journal of Chromatography A 1358: 136–144.

Monaci, L., De Angelis, E., Bavaro, S. L., and Pilolli, R. (2015). High-resolution Orbitrap-based mass spectrometry for rapid detection of peanuts in nuts. Food Additives and Contaminants. Part A, Chemistry, Analysis, Control, Exposure and Risk Assessment 32(10): 1607–1616.

Mondoulet, L., Paty, E., Drumare, M. F., Ah-Leung, S., Scheinmann, P., Willemot, R. M., Wal, J. M., and Bernard, H. (2005). Influence of thermal processing on the allergenicity of peanut proteins. Journal of Agricultural and Food Chemistry 53(11): 4547–4553.

Nakamura, A., Tanabe, S., Watanabe, J., and Makino, T. (2005). Primary screening of relatively less allergenic wheat varieties. Journal of Nutritional Science and Vitaminology 51(3): 204–206.

Nitride, C., Mamone, G., Picariello, G., Mills, C., Nocerino, R., Berni Canani, R., and Ferranti, P. (2013). Proteomic and immunological characterization of a new food allergen from hazelnut (Corylus avellana). Journal of Proteomics 86: 16–26.

Nowak-Wegrzyn, A., and Fiocchi, A. (2009). Rare, medium, or well done? The effect of heating and food matrix on food protein allergenicity. Current Opinion in Allergy and Clinical Immunology 9(3): 234–237.

Offermann, L. R., Giangrieco, I., Perdue, M. L., Zuzzi, S., Santoro, M., Tamburrini, M., Cosgrove, D. J., Mari, A., Ciardiello, M. A., and Chruszcz, M. (2015). Elusive structural, functional, and immunological features of Act d 5, the green Kiwifruit Kiwellin. Journal of Agricultural and Food Chemistry 63(29): 6567–6576.

Palacin, A., Varela, J., Quirce, S., del Pozo, V., Tordesillas, L., Barranco, P., Fernandez-Nieto, M., Sastre, J., Diaz-Perales, A., and Salcedo, G. (2009). Recombinant lipid transfer protein Tri a 14: a novel heat and proteolytic resistant tool for the diagnosis of baker's asthma. Clinical and Experimental Allergy 39(8): 1267–1276.

Parker, C. H., Khuda, S. E., Pereira, M., Ross, M. M., Fu, T. J., Fan, X., Wu, Y., Williams, K. M., DeVries, J., Pulvermacher, B., Bedford, B., Zhang, X., and Jackson, L. S. (2015). Multi-allergen quantitation and the impact of thermal treatment in industry-processed baked goods by ELISA and liquid chromatography-tandem mass spectrometry. Journal of Agricultural and Food Chemistry 63(49): 10669–10680.

Paschke, A. (2009). Aspects of food processing and its effect on allergen structure. Molecular Nutrition and Food Research 53(8): 959–962.

Picariello, G., Ferranti, P., Fierro, O., Mamone, G., Caira, S., Di Luccia, A., Monica, S., and Addeo, F. (2010). Peptides surviving the simulated gastrointestinal digestion of milk proteins: biological and toxicological implications. Journal of Chromatography B, Analytical Technologies in the Biomedical and Life Sciences 878(3-4): 295–308.

Picariello, G., Mamone, G., Addeo, F., and Ferranti, P. (2011). The frontiers of mass spectrometry-based techniques in food allergenomics. Journal of Chromatography A 1218(42): 7386–7398.

Picariello, G., Mamone, G., Cutignano, A., Fontana, A., Zurlo, L., Addeo, F., and Ferranti, P. (2015). Proteomics, peptidomics, and immunogenic potential of wheat beer (Weissbier). Journal of Agricultural and Food Chemistry 63(13): 3579–3586.

Picariello, G., Ferranti, P., and Addeo, F. (2016). Use of brush border membrane vesicles to simulate the human intestinal digestion. Food Research International.

Plundrich, N. J., Kulis, M., White, B. L., Grace, M. H., Guo, R., Burks, A. W., Davis, J. P., and Lila, M. A. (2014). Novel strategy to create hypoallergenic peanut protein-polyphenol edible matrices for oral immunotherapy. Journal of Agricultural and Food Chemistry 62(29): 7010–7021.

Pomes, A., Chruszcz, M., Gustchina, A., Minor, W., Mueller, G. A., Pedersen, L. C., Wlodawer, A., and Chapman, M. D. (2015). 100 Years later: Celebrating the contributions of x-ray crystallography to allergy and clinical immunology. The Journal of Allergy and Clinical Immunology 136(1): 29–37 e10.

Poms, R. E., Klein, C. L., and Anklam, E. (2004). Methods for allergen analysis in food: a review. Food Additives and Contaminants 21(1): 1–31.

Posada-Ayala, M., Alvarez-Llamas, G., Maroto, A. S., Maes, X., Munoz-Garcia, E., Villalba, M., Rodriguez, R., Perez-Gordo, M., Vivanco, F., Pastor-Vargas, C., and Cuesta-Herranz, J. (2015).

Novel liquid chromatography-mass spectrometry method for sensitive determination of the mustard allergen Sin a 1 in food. Food Chemistry 183: 58–63.

Ramesh, S. (2008). Food allergy overview in children. Clinical Reviews in Allergy and Immunology 34(2): 217–230.

Reuter, A., Luttkopf, D., and Vieths, S. (2009). New frontiers in allergen standardization. Clinical and Experimental Allergy 39(3): 307–309.

Sander, I., Raulf-Heimsoth, M., Duser, M., Flagge, A., Czuppon, A. B., and Baur, X. (1997). Differentiation between cosensitization and cross-reactivity in wheat flour and grass pollen-sensitized subjects. International Archives of Allergy and Immunology 112(4): 378–385.

Sathe, S. K., Teuber, S. S., and Roux, K. H. (2005). Effects of food processing on the stability of food allergens. Biotechnology Advances 23(6): 423–429.

Sathe, S. K., and Sharma, G. M. (2009). Effects of food processing on food allergens. Molecular Nutrition and Food Research 53(8): 970–978.

Schneider, N., Becker, C. M., and Pischetsrieder, M. (2010). Analysis of lysozyme in cheese by immunocapture mass spectrometry. Journal of Chromatography B, Analytical Technologies in the Biomedical and Life Sciences 878(2): 201–206.

Schubert-Ullrich, P., Rudolf, J., Ansari, P., Galler, B., Fuhrer, M., Molinelli, A., and Baumgartner, S. (2009). Commercialized rapid immunoanalytical tests for determination of allergenic food proteins: an overview. Analytical and Bioanalytical Chemistry 395(1): 69–81.

Sealey-Voyksner, J., Zweigenbaum, J., and Voyksner, R. (2016). Discovery of highly conserved unique peanut and tree nut peptides by LC-MS/MS for multi-allergen detection. Food Chemistry 194: 201–211.

Shefcheck, K. J., and Musser, S. M. (2004). Confirmation of the allergenic peanut protein, Ara h 1, in a model food matrix using liquid chromatography/tandem mass spectrometry (LC/MS/MS). Journal of Agricultural and Food Chemistry 52(10): 2785–2790.

Shefcheck, K. J., Callahan, J. H., and Musser, S. M. (2006). Confirmation of peanut protein using peptide markers in dark chocolate using liquid chromatography-tandem mass spectrometry (LC-MS/MS). Journal of Agricultural and Food Chemistry 54(21): 7953–7959.

Sicherer, S. H., and Sampson, H. A. (2006). 9. Food allergy. The Journal of Allergy and Clinical Immunology 117(2 Suppl Mini-Primer): S470–475.

Snegaroff, J., Branlard, G., Bouchez-Mahiout, I., Laudet, B., Tylichova, M., Chardot, T., Pecquet, C., Choudat, D., Raison-Peyron, N., Vigan, M., Kerre, S., and Lauriere, M. (2007). Recombinant proteins and peptides as tools for studying IgE reactivity with low-molecular-weight glutenin subunits in some wheat allergies. Journal of Agricultural and Food Chemistry 55(24): 9837–9845.

Son, D. Y., Scheurer, S., Hoffmann, A., Haustein, D., and Vieths, S. (1999). Pollen-related food allergy: cloning and immunological analysis of isoforms and mutants of Mal d 1, the major apple allergen, and Bet v 1, the major birch pollen allergen. European Journal of Nutrition 38(4): 201–215.

Stasyk, T., and Huber, L. A. (2004). Zooming in: fractionation strategies in proteomics. Proteomics 4(12): 3704–3716.

Steinhart, H., Wigotzki, M., and Zunker, K. (2001). Introducing allergists to food chemistry. Allergy 56 Suppl 67: 9–11.

Suckau, D., Resemann, A., Schuerenberg, M., Hufnagel, P., Franzen, J., and Holle, A. (2003). A novel MALDI LIFT-TOF/TOF mass spectrometer for proteomics. Analytical and Bioanalytical Chemistry 376(7): 952–965.

Tada, Y., Nakase, M., Adachi, T., Nakamura, R., Shimada, H., Takahashi, M., Fujimura, T., and Matsuda, T. (1996). Reduction of 14–16 kDa allergenic proteins in transgenic rice plants by antisense gene. FEBS Letters 391(3): 341–345.

Tanner, G. J., Colgrave, M. L., Blundell, M. J., Goswami, H. P., and Howitt, C. A. (2013). Measuring hordein (gluten) in beer—a comparison of ELISA and mass spectrometry. PloS One 8(2): e56452.

Timperman, A. T., and Aebersold, R. (2000). Peptide electroextraction for direct coupling of in-gel digests with capillary LC-MS/MS for protein identification and sequencing. Analytical Chemistry 72(17): 4115–4121.

Unlu, M., Morgan, M. E., and Minden, J. S. (1997). Difference gel electrophoresis: a single gel method for detecting changes in protein extracts. Electrophoresis 18(11): 2071–2077.

van Hengel, A. J. (2007). Food allergen detection methods and the challenge to protect food-allergic consumers. Analytical and Bioanalytical Chemistry 389(1): 111–118.

Wangorsch, A., Larsson, H., Messmer, M., Garcia-Moral, A., Lauer, I., Wolfheimer, S., Schulke, S., Bartra, J., Vieths, S., Lidholm, J., and Scheurer, S. (2016). Molecular cloning of plane pollen allergen Pla a 3 and its utility as diagnostic marker for peach associated plane pollen allergy. Clinical and Experimental Allergy 46(5): 764–774.

Weber, D., Raymond, P., Ben-Rejeb, S., and Lau, B. (2006). Development of a liquid chromatography-tandem mass spectrometry method using capillary liquid chromatography and nanoelectrospray ionization-quadrupole time-of-flight hybrid mass spectrometer for the detection of milk allergens. Journal of Agricultural and Food Chemistry 54(5): 1604–1610.

Yamanishi, R., Tsuji, H., Bando, N., Yamada, Y., Nadaoka, Y., Huang, T., Nishikawa, K., Emoto, S., and Ogawa, T. (1996). Reduction of the allergenicity of soybean by treatment with proteases. Journal of Nutritional Science and Vitaminology 42(6): 581–587.

Zhang, Q., Noble, K. A., Mao, Y., Young, N. L., Sathe, S. K., Roux, K. H., and Marshall, A. G. (2013). Rapid screening for potential epitopes reactive with a polyclonal antibody by solution-phase H/D exchange monitored by FT-ICR mass spectrometry. Journal of the American Society for Mass Spectrometry 24(7): 1016–1025.

CHAPTER 10

Allergen Quantitation for Food Labeling

Martina Koeberl,[1] *Dean Clarke*[1] and
Andreas L. Lopata[2,*]

Introduction

Food allergies are caused by proteins, termed allergens, which are generally not considered harmful to the human body. Hence, food allergy is a hypersensitive reaction of the human immune system. Currently, sensitization rates to one or more allergen among children are globally 40–50% (Pawankar *et al.*, 2011). Worldwide an estimated 220–250 million people suffer from food allergy (Pawankar *et al.*, 2011). Typical allergic symptoms include mild to severe reactions, such as urticaria, vomiting, rhinitis, asthma and life-threatening anaphylaxis (Ortolani and Pastorello, 2006; Sicherer and Sampson, 2010; Untersmayr and Jensen-Jarolim, 2006). Currently, food allergy is predominately managed through avoidance of the allergen causing an allergic reaction.

Food allergens are proteins that mostly originate from plant or animal sources. Most allergens are water soluble proteins in the range between 3–160 kDa, mostly between 20–70 kDa (Picariello *et al.*, 2011). These proteins can be functional proteins, enzymes or structural proteins (Breiteneder and Mills, 2005a; Jenkins *et al.*, 2007; Radauer *et al.*, 2008). Allergens are very stable, considering chemical or physical treatments, and show a high resistance to pH, denaturing chemicals, heat and degradation by proteases and proteolysis (Breiteneder and Mills, 2005a). Structural elements to enhance the stability

[1] National Measurement Institute, Department of Industry, Innovation and Science, 1/153 Bertie Street, Port Melourne, VIC 3207, Australia.
Email: martina.koeberl@measurement.gov.au; dean.clarke@measurement.gov.au
[2] Molecular Immunology Group, Centre for Biodiscovery and Molecular Development of Therapeutics (BMDT), College of Public Health, Medical and Veterinary Sciences, Pharmacy & Medical Research, James Cook University, 1 Angus Smith Drive, Douglas, QLD 4811, Australia.
* Corresponding author: andreas.lopata@jcu.edu.au

of food allergens are, for example, disulfide bonds and N-glycosylation (Breiteneder and Mills, 2005a). The glycosylation of proteins can increase the ability to become absorbed by respiratory or gastrointestinal mucosa (Breiteneder and Mills, 2005a).

Allergenic proteins with common functions can have common structures. Most allergens, therefore, have highly conserved amino acid sequences, especially if the same protein occurs in different sources, e.g., plant storage proteins or muscle proteins in animals. However, cross-reactivity can occur due to similar amino acid sequences. Therefore, an allergen from one source can cause the same allergic reaction to the protein from a different source. Almost all animal food allergens have homologous proteins in the human proteome. It does seem that proteins are not allergens when they share greater than 62% of amino acid sequence identity with the human homolog protein (Breiteneder, 2008; Pomes, 2008; Sicherer and Sampson, 2010). If the amino acid sequence identity of proteins is less than 54% of the human genome, all proteins can become potential allergens (Breiteneder, 2008). For cross-reactivity between allergens, more than 35–40% amino acid sequence identity is necessary (Breiteneder and Mills, 2005b; Ortolani and Pastorello, 2006). The percentage of the amino acid sequence identity required for cross-reactivity also depends on the structure of the allergen. It was reported, when proteins share the same tertiary structure, the amino acid identity can be as low as 20–30% and still be cross-reactive (Chapman *et al.*, 2001; Pomes, 2008).

To protect allergenic individuals, governments enforce food labeling laws. Accurate and legible labeling is essential information for allergic consumers if they are to comply with their strict avoidance diets. However, different legislations are in place around the world and will be discussed later. Moreover, to enforce legislation the presence of food allergens need to be accurately detected in food samples. Currently, ELISAs are mainly utilized to quantify allergens. ELISAs are based on antibodies as well as the low lateral technique. Another detection method applied for food allergens detection and quantification is based on the presence of DNA. However, the antibody-based methods, as well as the DNA detection methods, have several disadvantages. Therefore recently Mass Spectrometry (MS) techniques have been developed and applied to food allergen analysis. Nonetheless, quantification of allergens using MS is not routinely employed. The different aspects of food allergen detection are explained later.

Analytical difficulties for food allergen detection

Although laws are enacted, the execution and control of declaration laws is almost impossible due to technical difficulties. Food allergens are found in low quantities in diverse and complex matrices, additionally only small amounts of an allergen can trigger the allergic reaction. Moreover, as summarized in Table 10.1, there are various food sources and food allergens, groups are heterogeneous and more than one allergen can be found per food group.

Table 10.1: Allergens are requiring labeling of food products. "The Big 8" food allergens are ordered alphabetically (shaded in purple) and additional allergens are below them as currently required by legislation. "*" represents the numbers of allergenic proteins registered with the International Union of Immunological Societies (IUIS) (http://www.allergen.org). "✔" indicates that the allergen needs to be labeled on every food product. "**" voluntary labeling recommended for 18 other foods.

Source/Allergen	Number of known allergenic proteins*	Codex Alimentarius	Australia/New Zealand	European Union	United States	Canada	China	Hong Kong	Japan**	Korea	Mexico	South Africa
Crustacean/Shellfish	9	✔	✔	✔	✔	✔	✔	✔	✔	✔	✔	✔
Egg	7	✔	✔	✔	✔	✔	✔	✔	✔	✔	✔	✔
Fish	3	✔	✔	✔	✔	✔	✔	✔	–	✔	✔	✔
Milk	8	✔	✔	✔	✔	✔	✔	✔	✔	✔	✔	✔
Soy	7	✔	✔	✔	✔	✔	✔	✔	–	✔	✔	✔
Peanut	17	✔	✔	✔	✔	✔	✔	✔	✔	✔	✔	✔
Tree Nuts	34	✔	✔	✔	✔	✔	✔	✔	–	–	✔	✔
Wheat/Cereals	15	✔	✔	✔	✔	✔	✔	✔	✔	✔	✔	✔
Buckwheat	3	–	–	–	–	–	✔	–	✔	✔	–	–
Celery	6	–	–	✔	–	–	–	–	–	–	–	–
Lupine	1	–	–	✔	–	–	–	–	–	–	–	–
Mollusks/Shellfish	1	–	–	✔	–	✔	✔	–	–	–	–	✔
Mustard	1	–	–	✔	–	✔	–	–	–	–	–	–
Sesame	7	–	✔	✔	–	✔	–	–	–	–	–	–
Sulphur oxide and sulphites		✔	✔	✔	✔	✔	–	✔	–	–	–	–

Therefore the food matrix can be very different and the protocol of food allergen analysis cannot be generalized. Due to all these factors, the analysis of foods allergens is very challenging. Generally, sample preparation includes an extraction step of food matrix to elute the allergen(s). The choice of extraction solvent is dependent on solubility of the allergen. For example, allergens from egg and milk are spread evenly throughout the food product and easily extracted (Goodwin, 2004). Shellfish and fish tissues are uncomplicated to disperse. On the other hand, peanut, tree nuts, sesame and soy contain more oily components and therefore need more attention in allergen extraction (Goodwin, 2004). A complex food matrices to analyze is for example, chocolate, due to their high content of fat, carbohydrates and polyphenols (Goodwin, 2004).

Moreover, food products are often processed during food production. These include chemical and physical treatments, mainly to increase shelf-life.

These processes can significantly alter the physico-chemical and structural properties of allergens, thereby increasing or attenuating their allergenicity (Lepski and Brockmeyer, 2013; Verhoeckx *et al.*, 2015). Moreover, the structure and solubility of an allergen can change. The most important factors that influence the sample preparation of allergen analysis are: (1) Food processing, such as thermal and chemical treatment (Wal, 2003). (2) Oils and fats present in the food matrix, thus can lead to lower solubility of allergens. (3) Carbohydrates can bind to allergens, potentially changing the solubility and structure of the allergen. (4) The Maillard reaction, which occurs when amino acids react with reducing sugars during thermal processing. The Maillard reaction can mainly increase allergenicity, but it was also demonstrated that it can reduce allergenicity (Maleki *et al.*, 2000; Mills *et al.*, 2009; Thomas *et al.*, 2007). (5) Enzymes or chemical denaturation reactions with other food components can lead to structural modifications of allergens aggregation with other food components. (6) Post-translational modification, such as glycosylation and oxidation, can result in changes to the secondary and tertiary structure of an allergen (Thomas *et al.*, 2007).

Overall, many factors are influencing the choice of allergen detection and stability of allergens in complex food matrices. Therefore allergen analysis is complex and challenging. One protocol cannot be applied for all allergens and food sources.

Current methods for food allergen quantification

The major methods for food allergen analysis are based on (1) antibodies 'Enzyme Linked Immunosorbent Assays' (ELISA) and lateral flow or (2) DNA or (3) Mass Spectrometry (MS), as a chemical method, has been recently introduced as alternative method for food allergen analysis, however, is not routinely employed. Illustrated in Fig. 10.1 are the general principals of the three different methods, whereas the first step (Fig. 10.1a) is to extract the allergen from the food matrix. Most allergens are water soluble and therefore for ELISA and MS mainly utilizing aqueous salt solutions for extractions. For DNA extraction and purification organic solvents are used, due to the chemical properties of the DNA. However, due to the fact that food allergens and food matrixes are extremely diverse, it would be beneficial to have different extraction methods for allergens and especially food matrices.

All three food allergen detection methods have advantages and disadvantages and will be explained later. Nevertheless, ELISA is the most commonly employed method for food allergen analysis and quantification. For most of "The Big 8" food allergens ELISA kits and PCR methods are commercial available. The main exceptions are some of the tree nuts, thus only DNA methods are available (Lopata and Lehrer, 2009). For other allergens, which need to be labeled in some countries (Table 10.1) only DNA methods are available, e.g., for mollusks and celery.

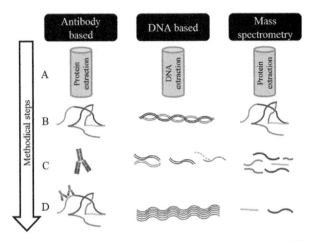

Fig. 10.1: Schematic methodology for food allergen analysis applying three different methods. Letters A–D represent different methodical steps, A shows the extraction; B displays the analyzed product; C summarized the detection method; and D visualizes the detected and quantified product.

Antibody based methods for food allergen quantification—biological method

ELISAs and the lateral flow technique are both based on allergen specific antibodies, applying the same principal (Fig. 10.1). Antibodies are very specific and have a high affinity towards the allergen and can be available as monoclonal or polyclonal antibody, whereas monoclonal antibodies are monospecific and recognize the same epitope of the allergen. Polyclonal antibodies usually recognize more epitopes of one allergen. ELISAs and lateral flow methods are available as competitive or sandwich technique, whereas for the competitive technique the antibodies are covered with other particles and dyes and when the more specific allergens binds with higher affinity to antibodies, the antibodies release the dye. For the sandwich method, the surface is covered with antibodies and if the allergen binds a color change occurs. In terms of applying the antibody based methods for food allergen detection, as shown in Fig. 10.1, the allergen (Fig. 10.1b) becomes extracted from the food matrix, usually using aqueous salt buffers such as Phosphate-Buffered Saline (PBS). The allergen specific antibody (Fig. 10.1c) is applied and binds to the allergen (Fig. 10.1d). In contrast to the lateral flow technique, only ELISA can be used for allergen quantification, as this method uses internal standards for quantification purposes.

The lateral flow technique is therefore mostly used for the fast and rough control of the presence of allergens, e.g., for swapping surfaces. The advantages of lateral flow, summarized in Table 10.2, are the simplicity, practicality, time and the costs. However, lateral flows have poor accuracy results and need to be confirmed by other methods. Moreover, this technique is only a semi-qualitative method for food allergens. Currently they are commercially available for almond, Brazil nut, cashew, coconut, crustacean, egg, hazelnut, macadamia, milk, mustard, pecan nut, peanut, pistachio, sesame, walnuts and wheat (Gluten). It is possible that more, mainly country specific, lateral flows are available for different allergens.

ELISAs are the most common method applied for food allergen analysis and quantification; hence they are available for a range of allergens. The main advantages (Table 10.2) are the selectivity and sensitivity that can be achieved using the allergen specific antibodies. Other advantages are the low detection levels of ELISA, cost effectiveness with respect to machinery and training required for implementation. The Limit Of Quantification (LOQ) for ELISA reported in literature range from 0.3–1.5 ppm and Limit Of Detection (LOD) 0.2–2 ppm, respectively (Monaci and Visconti, 2010). Whereas others found LOD of ELISA kits vary from 1–5 ppm (Chassaigne *et al.*, 2007; Picariello *et al.*, 2011). The LOQ and LOD of allergen analysis are dependent on complexity of allergen and food matrices analyzed.

However, antibody based methods have a range of disadvantages. The major disadvantages of antibodies are that they very often poorly characterized and the real target of the antibody is unknown (Johnson *et al.*, 2014). Moreover,

Table 10.2: Advantages and disadvantages of antibody based methods for food allergen analysis.

ELISA		Lateral flow	
Advantages	**Disadvantages**	**Advantages**	**Disadvantages**
High specificity and affinity for the allergen using antibodies	Target of the antibody very often unknown, antibodies are poorly characterized	High affinity for the allergen using antibodies	Target of the antibody very often unknown, antibodies are poorly characterized
High sensitivity and low detection and quantification limits	Cross-reactivity due to similar allergens		Cross-reactivity due to similar allergens
Available for a range of allergens	Antibody selectivity and specificity can be influenced by food matrix and food processing	Available for a range of allergens	Antibody selectivity and specificity can be influenced by food matrix and food processing
Cost effective	Lack of standards	Very cost effective	Lack of standards
Ease of use	Lack of reference materials	Ease of use	Lack of reference materials
Field portable	Inconsistent allergen targets in different kits	Field portable	Semi-quantitative
Time effective	Uncertainty for results of approx. 20–30%	Time effective	Low accuracy
Simple sample preparation	Conflicting results from different kits for the same allergen	Simple sample preparation	Limited validation data—or International Accreditation
No special training required for laboratory technicians to use it	Limited validation data—or International Accreditation	No special training required to use it	

the food matrix and the food processing, as mentioned later, can influence the allergen and/or the antibody (Lepski and Brockmeyer, 2013; Wal, 2003). Therefore some ELISA kit manufactures advice to add substances to the food extraction protocol, such as fish skin gelatin or skim milk powder, to reduce the effect of different food components, such as oils and fats. Furthermore, cross-reactivity can occur utilizing antibodies, therefore antibody based methods are not suitable to distinguish species (Johnson *et al.*, 2014; Kamath *et al.*, 2013; Kamath *et al.*, 2014; Sakai *et al.*, 2008). Food processing as well as cross-reactivity can lead to false-negative or false-positive results applying antibodies or when using ELISAs to an over and/or underestimation of the food allergen quantified. Furthermore, the quantification of allergens is dependent on the standard used in the commercial available ELISA kit. Unfortunately, standards provided are poorly characterized and therefore generated results using different ELISA kits are not comparable at all (Careri *et al.*, 2008; Rauh, 2012; Shefcheck and Musser, 2004). For example, a comparative study by (Heick *et al.*, 2011a) of two commercially available ELISA kits for soy noted that the detection for spiked flour samples varied by a factor of 10. When they examined hazelnut in spiked processed bread they observed that results between ELISA kits varied by a factor of 3. Quantifying hazelnut in both unprocessed and processed samples using two different ELISA kits resulted in significant differences of up to 40% (Heick *et al.*, 2011a). A similar comparative study of commercial ELISA kits for hazelnut detection by (Cucu *et al.*, 2011) demonstrated that all kits evaluated produced false-positive and false-negative results. In some kits the actual hazelnut protein concentration was 17–49% underestimated and another kit overestimated the concentration by 27%. Johnson *et al.* (2014) performed a multi-laboratory evaluation of egg and milk allergens and demonstrated that all kits underestimated the concentration of egg. Only one kit quantified the milk protein content with acceptable accuracy at 6 and 15 mg/kg. All milk and egg ELISA kits were able to detect the lowest spiked concentration (3 mg/kg); however, LOQ was for egg about 10 mg/kg and for milk 30 mg/kg. This highlights that the current methods would have difficulties to detect allergens in certain types of food consumed in larger quantities.

Although ELISAs are commercially available for many food allergens, most ELISA kits only target a single allergen. Therefore, ELISA are generally not time consuming to perform, however, the time increases when more than one allergen needs to be analyzed. For example, for the analysis of milk allergens, ELISA kits are commercially available to detect casein, β-lactoglobulin and total allergen content (casein and β-lactoglobulin). None of the other known milk allergens including α-lactalbumin, which is also considered as a major allergen in milk, is targeted (Weber *et al.*, 2006).

Overall, ELISA is the most commonly used method for allergen detection and quantification, thus it is highly specific, sensitive and available. Industry and official controls therefore use ELISAs for routine analyzes and screening. However, ELISA is affected by food processing, food matrices and cross-reactivity. Therefore the results of ELISAs are often in dispute due to unexpected component concentrations, lack of validation data for specific food types, conflicting results from different kits and questionable extractability or detection in complex matrices. Cross-reactivity and false negative/positive rates for commercial allergen detection kits are not widely disclosed.

DNA based methods for food allergen quantification—biological method

The DNA method for food allergen analysis used the Polymerase Chain Reaction (PCR) technique and therefore analyzes and quantifies the DNA of the allergen (Fig. 10.1). The DNA becomes extracted from the food matrix (Fig. 10.1a) and then purified (Fig. 10.1b).The extraction is mainly achieved by cell lysis, removal from RNA and proteins, followed by DNA purification which utilizes organic solvents, due to the nature of the DNA. Utilizing specific primers, the DNA or DNA fragments become amplified applying PCR technique (Fig. 10.1c). Therefore the results are based on the numbers of DNA copies (Fig. 10.1d).

The main advantage of the DNA based methods is that it is very specific and sensitive for the allergen as well as for the species (Table 10.3). The presence of one single DNA copy can be sufficient to amplify the DNA with the PCR technique and therefore be easy to detect. Different DNA kits are commercially available, such as for almond, celery, crustaceans, fish, gliadins, hazelnut, lupine, milk mollusks, mustard, peanut, sesame, soy and walnut. It is possible that more, mainly country specific, DNA based methods are available for different allergens. Some of these commercial available kits are approved by the Association of Analytical Communities (AOAC) and therefore are official AOAC methods (Goodwin, 2004). The only AOAC approved method for ELISA is the detection and quantification of gliadins and peanut.

The major disadvantage of DNA based methods is that they do not detect the allergen itself, but the DNA of the allergen. The presence of the DNA does not mean the allergen is actually present in the food sample and vice versa

Table 10.3: Advantages and disadvantages of DNA based methods for food allergen analysis.

DNA Advantages	DNA Disadvantages
High specificity and selectivity for the DNA of the targeted allergen	Not targeting the allergen
	DNA is influenced by food processing
High sensitivity and low detection limits, one DNA copy is potential enough for the detection	Conversion from copy numbers into other units (ppm) is controversial
	Lack of standards materials
Available for a range of allergens	Lack of reference materials
Species identification due to specific primers	Semi-quantitative - quantitative
Simple sample preparation	Special training required for laboratory technicians
	Limited validation data

(Luber *et al.*, 2014). Moreover, due to food processing, the amount and quality of the DNA in the food matrix can vary, and therefore might not be recognized by the applied primers. Furthermore, the DNA detection can be negatively affected by inhibitors such as proteases and polyphenols that can slow or stop the amplification process (Costa *et al.*, 2015). Moreover, the sequence of DNA from the allergen needs to be known, so primers can be designed to amplify the specific DNA from the species and the allergen. The design of primers and the handling of PCR require special training for laboratory technicians. Nevertheless, a large number of allergens are known today and their cDNA sequence has been determined (Müller and Steinhart, 2007). However, sometimes DNA base methods are not suitable for allergen detection, as it was shown by (Lee and Kim, 2010) that DNA could not distinguish between non-allergenic chicken proteins and allergenic egg proteins. Stephen and Vieths (2004) described good DNA to ELISA correlation for the detection of peanut allergen contamination at concentrations greater than 10 ppm in chocolate samples; however, results diverged in concentrations below 10 ppm.

Overall, DNA base methods are commercially available for a range of allergens. Moreover, due to the targeted DNA the method is highly specific and sensitive. However, the actual LOD and LOQ are not certain, thus the conversion of copy numbers to other units needs to be discussed. Moreover the DNA is affected by food processing and food matrices. In summary, DNA base methods only detect the possibility of allergen being present.

Mass spectrometry for food allergen detection and quantification chemical method

There are different mass spectrometry (MS) techniques available, which allows choosing the right application according to the research question and allergen investigated. Moreover, there are two approaches, the bottom-up and top-down strategy, to analyze and identify allergens, whereas the latter is mainly used for a certain type of mass spectrometer, namely Matrix-Assisted Laser Desorption Ionization (MALDI), and more commonly used for the analysis of intact allergens. However, the bottom-up strategy is the most applied technique using Time Of Flight (TOF) or Ion Trap (IT) as mass spectrometer, which is the identification and quantification of peptides derived from the allergen. More information about the bottom-up and top-down strategy are explained by (Monaci, 2009). The general procedure on how to analyze allergens by MS is that the allergen becomes extracted from the food matrix (Fig. 10.1a), using aqueous buffers such as ammonium bicarbonate buffers. The extracted allergen (Fig. 10.1b) then becomes digested (Fig. 10.1c) and the peptides (Fig. 10.1d) become identified. Once the peptides are identified, these peptides can be quantified using TOF, IT and Multiple Reaction Monitoring (MRM). Most commonly digested peptides derived from the allergen become separated via Liquid Chromatography (LC) prior to MS analysis. More details about how to operate MS for allergen detection and quantification, including the steps for allergen method development are explained later.

The advantages of MS techniques are selectivity and specificity (Table 10.4). A peptide becomes identified by exact molecular weight and its amino acid sequence, therefore the chemical and structural information of the peptide is exactly known. With the correctly selected peptide, so-called "Unique signature peptides" (see later) MS can identify and quantify the allergen as well as species-specific allergens (Ortea *et al.*, 2011), and more than one allergen can be quantified in a single analysis (Sancho and Mills, 2010). Moreover, food processing and food matrix have less influence utilizing MS technique compared to antibody or DNA base method (Anđelković *et al.*, 2015; Gomaa and Boye, 2015). Hence, the sensitivity and specificity of an ELISA can depend on the 3-D structure of allergens, whereas MS is based on the structurally independent amino acid sequence (Abdel Rahman *et al.*, 2010; Rauh, 2012). Furthermore, the LOD and LOQ that can be achieved are in a very low concentration range (Heick *et al.*, 2011a; Heick *et al.*, 2011b; Picariello *et al.*, 2011). The MS technique is stable, robust and reproducible. Another main advantage is that the MS analysis requires standards, which are known exactly by their chemical structure, hence results can be compared between methods and laboratories.

The disadvantages of MS techniques are that equipment is very costly (Table 10.4). Moreover, for the development of allergen detection and quantification highly qualified staff is required. Some peptides show poor ionization and therefore not as sensitive for MS detection. High salt content in sample matrix can also influence ionization of analysis; however with additional sample preparation steps the salt content can be reduced. The sample preparation is more time consuming compared to the other food allergen detection methods, as the allergen needs to be digested (see later).

Table 10.4: Advantages and disadvantages of mass spectrometry methods for food allergen analysis.

MS Advantages	MS Disadvantages
High specificity and selectivity for the targeted allergen	High cost of the equipment
High sensitivity and low detection limits	Higher level of expertise and skill required
Stable, robust and reliable method	Output data is complex
Species identification due to signature peptides	Sample preparation is more time-consuming
Food matrix and food processing have less influence on the detection methods	No routinely applicable methods
More than one allergen can be analyzed with one method	Not commercially available
Well characterized standards	
Comparable results and methods	

Using MS for food allergen detection and quantification is a relatively new field; hence, there are currently no commercially available methods, as at present this technique is still in the research and establishing phase. Therefore, this method is currently only applied by research facilities, mainly as confirmation methods for inconclusive ELISA results. Nevertheless, many food allergens have been already analyzed and signature peptides have been identified and quantified, applying different LC/MS systems. A detailed review of the current analyzed food allergens using LC/MS systems is summarized by (Koeberl *et al.*, 2014).

Operating mass spectrometry for allergen analysis

To develop a LC/MS method for allergens analysis a set of methodological steps has to be followed, which includes (1) protein extraction, (2) protein digestion, (3) peptide analysis with LC/MS, (4) peptide identification, (5) selection of unique signature peptides, and (6) quantification of the unique signature peptides using LC/MS, as illustrated in Fig. 10.2. Once the LC/MS method is developed and validated, the allergens can be quantified by (1) protein extraction, (2) protein digestion, and (3) quantification of the unique signature peptides by LC/MS.

　　Digestion of the allergenic protein cleaves large proteins into smaller peptides, thus, potentially matrix interferences and associated interactions

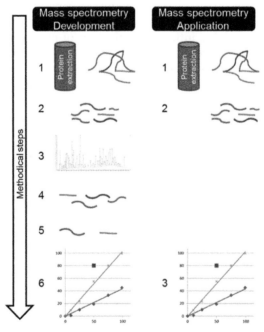

Fig. 10.2: Summary of methical steps for LC/MS development and LC/MS applications for food allergen analysis and quantification.

with other proteins are reduced. These reductions remove complicating factors and make the analysis with LC/MS more reproducible (Shefcheck *et al.*, 2006). Various enzymes are available, with specific cleavage sites. However, the most commonly used enzyme is trypsin, due to the well-known cleavage sites between the amino acid arginine (R) and lysine (K). Trypsin is also preferred, as it occurs naturally in the stomach and therefore is representative *in vivo* cleavage of all proteins.

The digested peptides become analyzed by the LC/MS system. The peptides become ionized, mainly resulting in double charged peptides, and the accurate mass, as well as the retention time, will be monitored (Johnson *et al.*, 2011). Moreover, peptides become fragmented, leading to peptide-specific b-ions and y-ions (Picariello *et al.*, 2011). To ensure the allergen is present "unique signature peptides" need to be identified. A signature peptide is defined as a theoretical tryptic peptide that is exclusively present in one group, but not in any other group. Overall, with the correct selection of the signature peptide, the detection of this peptide ensures the presence of a specific allergen, and additionally a specific allergen originated from a specific species (Heick *et al.*, 2011a; Johnson *et al.*, 2011; Monaci and Visconti, 2009).

Overall, LC/MS techniques have several advantages, especially in the field where antibody and DNA base methods have disadvantages. LC/MS is robust, stable and can easily be automated and standardized, with potential low LOD and LOQ. Another advantage is to have better-defined standards, which makes the comparison of results between methods and laboratories much easier. However, LC/MS is not routinely employed for allergen detection and quantification. Therefore there are no commercial methods available.

Comparison between biological methods and chemical methods for food allergen detection

Several authors have compared detection of ELISA, DNA and MS methods. Weber *et al.* (2006) found that the results of ELISA and MS were comparable when analyzing milk allergens in orange sherbet, lacto-free ice cream, milk powder, oatmeal cereal and cookies extract. On the other hand for milk and soy, especially when products were processed, MS detection was outstanding in comparison to ELISA kits. Heick *et al.* (2011b) found that when analyzing peanut, hazelnut, walnut and almond with ELISA and MS that both methods were capable of detecting the allergens. Lee and Kim (2010) found in their comparison study that DNA is not suitable when analyzing egg allergens, thus, it cannot distinguish between egg and chicken proteins. ELISA was suitable to detect egg allergen in trace amounts whereas MS was not able to detect ovomucoid. Monaci *et al.* (2010) used milk allergen standards and demonstrated a LOD of 1 ppm using LC/TOF. The LOD for spiked wine samples was 5 ppm, thus, LOD and LOQ derived with LC/TOF and LC/IT are comparable with reported ELISA values.

Legislation

The prevalence of food allergies is rising as well as the number of allergens. Consequently, numbers of countries and regulatory bodies have recognized the importance of providing information by enacting laws, regulations or standards for food allergen labeling to protect allergic consumers (Cornelisse-Vermaat *et al.*, 2008; Gendel, 2012).

Ninety percent of all food allergies are caused by eight food groups. These eight groups, often referred to as "The Big 8" food allergies, include egg, fish, milk, peanut, shellfish, soy, tree nuts and wheat. However, every food group contains more than one allergenic protein (Table 10.1) and some food groups are very heterogeneous, e.g., the group of tree nuts. In a botanical taxonomy the group of tree nuts includes various species, nevertheless, the term tree nut was selected to make it more understandable for consumers and are mainly found in the human diet. However, the EU limits the list of tree nuts to eight named species, whereas in Canada nine species are named. The US cites three species of tree nuts as examples, but does not include a complete list of tree nuts (Gendel, 2012). The groups of fish and shellfish (crustacean and mollusks) include numerous species and various allergens, whereas the fish and shellfish have only one major allergen, pavalbumin and tropomyosin respectively (Lopata and Lehrer, 2009; Lopata *et al.*, 2010; Sharp and Lopata, 2014). However, the amount of different species consumed in the human diet and the cross-reactivity between certain species make these two groups very heterogeneous as well.

Food labeling is the primary means of preventing food allergy. Recently many countries have enacted laws to ensure the health of allergic individuals (Table 10.1). The basis for labeling in all countries is provided by the International Codex Alimentarius Commission (a joint committee with delegates from both the Food and Agriculture Organization of the United Nations and the World Health Organization) (Pawankar *et al.*, 2011). Nevertheless, different countries interpret the recommendations given by the Codex Alimentarius differently. As shown in Table 10.1, different countries mandate a different selection of allergens required for food allergy labeling. Already 14 different food groups are required for allergen labeling in the European Union, compared with Japan mandating just six allergens (Cheftel, 2005; Gendel, 2012). However, 18 more allergens are recommended to be voluntarily labeled in Japan, which includes mainly allergens, such as buckwheat or "matsutake" mushrooms, being more common in Japan, compared to other countries (Gendel, 2012; Industry, 2013).

All food products containing one or more allergens listed in Table 10.1 need therefore to be labeled by legislation. However, this is quite challenging for the industry and the food manufactures, as the mandatory labeling changes in different countries. The first line of defense for the allergic individual is the ingredients list, while over complex labels and the lack of labeling in hospitability offers additional challenges. Ingredient list descriptions may not clearly distinguish potential allergenic components. Currently there are 19 different laws, regulations, rules, statements, languages and vocabulary used for food allergen labeling. Six of the labeling regulations (Canada, China, EU, Hong Kong, Mexico, US) contain language that explicitly includes ingredients in the labeling requirement. Another language problem that occurs is that often technical or scientific language is used, which is not understood by consumers. For example, labels are "casein" instead of "milk" or "ovalbumin" instead of "egg". Additional, language can also be too simple using a broad, uninformative term, for example, "textured vegetable protein" instead of "soy" (Gendel, 2012).

Precautionary statements are commonly used on food packaging by the food industry to communicate risk to consumers, especially when potential contamination might occur during the food production. Food allergen labeling as well as precautionary statements are therefore commonly used; however they are quite different and can lead to risky consumer interpretation. Language and allergen statements that are commonly used are for example: "products of", "major food allergen", "may contain", "ingredients that contain protein derived from", "made in a factory that also handles", or "made on the same production line that also processes" (Cheftel, 2005; Gendel, 2012; Van Hengel, 2007).

Overall, the legislation wants to protect allergic consumer by enforcing labeling regulations. However, due to different laws and regulations as well as small amounts that can trigger an allergic reaction the allergic consumer can be confused. The ideal scenario would be to have several food allergen detection methods to be used as important tools in the food manufacturing chain. The ability to confirm the presence or absence of an allergenic protein is valuable information in support of food recalls, food labeling and food production cleaning procedures.

Conclusion

The prevalence of food allergies are increasing worldwide and represent a growing public health concern. Governments protect allergic consumers by regulating the labeling of food products containing potential allergens. However, the number of allergens, as well as the language on food packaging, varies in different countries, possibly leading to confusion for the consumer. Technical methods to detect allergens are either not validated and the limit of detection and quantification is not sensitive enough or just not available. Moreover, there is a lack of well characterized standards or reference materials. Therefore correct or incorrect declarations cannot be verified. The limited range of available commercial allergen detection kits can lead to food recall decisions based on data derived from a single method. More confident decisions are possible when corroborating information is available. Food allergens are highly diverse and complex, therefore detecting and quantifying food allergens remains problematic. To date the most common quantitative methods for allergen analysis is ELISA. However, ELISA methods have several drawbacks. DNA based methods are available, but the DNA based method do not detect the allergen and are therefore not commonly applied. Therefore, the development of new methods for the quantification of food allergens is suggested, which are robust, reliable, comparable, stable, sensitive and easy to standardize. Therefore, allergen detection and quantification using mass spectrometry brings an important advantage over antibody and DNA techniques, especially regarding method reliability and reproducibility. Moreover, well-characterized standards are required for all MS based methods, which can be used as reference materials for Intra- and Inter-laboratory comparison. However, MS is costly and requires trained staff; therefore, it is not routinely employed and currently mainly used as a confirmation method. In conclusion, reliable and reproducible high-throughput detection methods and quantitative determination of allergens are urgently needed for implementing in food industry and control laboratories as a part of quality assurance and quality control during production and distribution, to ensure food safety for allergenic consumers.

Keywords: Food Allergy, Mass Spectrometry, ELISA, DNA, Allergen Detection

References

Abdel Rahman, A. M., Lopata, A. L., O'hehir, R. E., Robinson, J. J., Banoub, J. H., and Helleur, R. J. (2010). Characterization and *de novo* sequencing of snow crab tropomyosin enzymatic peptides by both electrospary ionization and matrix-assisted laser desorption ionization QqToF tandem mass spectrometry. Journal of Mass Spectrometry 45: 372–381.

Anđelković, U., Martinović, T., and Josić, D. (2015). Foodomic investigations of food allergies. Current Opinion in Food Science 4: 92–98.

Breiteneder, H. (2008). Can any protein become an allergen? Revue Française d'Allergologie 48: 135–138.

Breiteneder, H., and Mills, C. E. N. (2005a). Molecular properties of food allergens. Journal of Allergy and Clinical Immunology 115: 14–23.

Breiteneder, H., and Mills, C. E. N. (2005b). Plant food allergens—structural and functional aspects of allergenicity. Biotechnology Advances 23: 395–399.

Careri, M., Elviri, L., Lagos, J. B., Mangia, A., Speroni, F., and Terenghi, M. (2008). Selective and rapid immunomagnetic bead-based sample treatment for the liquid chromatography-electrospray ion-trap mass spectrometry detection of Ara h3/4 peanut protein in foods. Journal of Chromatography A 1206: 89–94.

Chapman, M. D., Smith, A. M., Vailes, L. D., Arruda, L. K., Dhanaraj, V., and Pomes, A. (2001). Recombinant allergens for diagnosis and therapy of allergic disease. Clinical and Experimental Allergy 31: 164–164.

Chassaigne, H., Norgaard, J. V., and Van Hengel, A. J. (2007). Proteomics-based approach to detect and identify major allergens in processed peanuts by capillary LC-Q-TOF (MS/MS). Journal of Agricultural and Food Chemistry 55: 4461–4473.

Cheftel, J. C. (2005). Food and nutrition labelling in the European Union. Food Chemistry 93: 531–550.

Cornelisse-Vermaat, J. R., Pfaff, S., Voordouw, J., Chryssochoidis, G., Theodoridis, G., Woestman, L. *et al.* (2008). The information needs and labelling preferences of food allergic consumers: the views of stakeholders regarding information scenarios. Trends in Food Science & Technology 19: 669–676.

Costa, J., Melo, V. S., Santos, C. G., Oliveira, M. B. P. P., and Mafra, I. (2015). Tracing tree nut allergens in chocolate: A comparison of DNA extraction protocols. Food Chemistry 187: 469–476.

Cucu, T., Platteau, C., Taverniers, I., Devreese, B., De Loose, M., and De Meulenaer, B. (2011). ELISA detection of hazelnut proteins: effect of protein glycation in the presence or absence of wheat proteins. Food Additives & Contaminants. Part A, Chemistry, Analysis, Control, Exposure & Risk Assessment 28: 1–10.

Gendel, S. M. (2012). Comparison of international food allergen labeling regulations. Regulatory Toxicology and Pharmacology 63: 279–285.

Gomaa, A., and Boye, J. (2015). Simultaneous detection of multi-allergens in an incurred food matrix using ELISA, multiplex flow cytometry and liquid chromatography mass spectrometry (LC–MS). Food Chemistry 175: 585–592.

Goodwin, P. R. (2004). Food allergen detection methods: a coordinated approach. Journal of AOAC International 87: 1383–1390.

Heick, J., Fischer, M., and Popping, B. (2011b). First screening method for the simultaneous detection of seven allergens by liquid chromatography mass spectrometry. Journal of Chromatography A 1218: 938–943.

Heick, J., Fischer, M., Kerbach, S., Tamm, U., and Popping, B. (2011a). Application of a liquid chromatography tandem mass spectrometry method for the simultaneous detection of seven allergenic foods in flour and bread and comparison of the method with commercially available ELISA test kits. Journal of AOAC International 94: 1060–1068.

International Organization of the Flavor Industry (2013). Update on Food Allergy Labeling in Japan. Information Letter N°1484.

Jenkins, J. A., Breiteneder, H., and Mills, C. E. N. (2007). Evolutionary distance from human homologs reflects allergenicity of animal food proteins. Journal of Allergy and Clinical Immunology 120: 1399–1405.

Johnson, P. E., Baumgartner, S., Aldick, T., Bessant, C., Giosafatto, V., Heick, J. *et al.* (2011). Current perspectives and recommendations for the development of mass spectrometry methods for the determination of allergens in foods. Journal of AOAC International 94: 1026–1033.

Johnson, P. E., Rigby, N. M., Dainty, J. R., Mackie, A. R., Immer, U. U., Rogers, A. *et al.* (2014). A multi-laboratory evaluation of a clinically-validated incurred quality control material for analysis of allergens in food. Food Chemistry 148: 30–36.

Kamath, S. D., Abdel Rahman, A. M., Komoda, T., and Lopata, A. L. (2013). Impact of heat processing on the detection of the major shellfish allergen tropomyosin in crustaceans and molluscs using specific monoclonal antibodies. Food Chemistry 141: 4031–4039.

Kamath, S. D., Abdel Rahman, A. M., Voskamp, A., Komoda, T., Rolland, J. M., O'hehir, R. E. *et al.* (2014). Effect of heat processing on antibody reactivity to allergen variants and fragments of black tiger prawn: A comprehensive allergenomic approach. Molecular Nutrition & Food Research 58: 1144–1155.

Koeberl, M., Clarke, D., and Lopata, A. L. (2014). Next generation of food allergen quantification using mass spectrometric systems. Journal of Proteome Research 13: 3499–3509.

Lee, J. -Y., and Kim, C. J. (2010). Determination of allergenic egg proteins in food by protein-, mass spectrometry-, and DNA-based methods. Journal of AOAC International 93: 462–477.

Lepski, S., and Brockmeyer, J. (2013). Impact of dietary factors and food processing on food allergy. Molecular Nutrition & Food Research 57: 145–152.

Lopata, A. L., and Lehrer, S. B. (2009). New insights into seafood allergy. Current Opinion in Allergy and Clinical Immunology 9: 270–277.

Lopata, A. L., O'hehir, R. E., and Lehrer, S. B. (2010). Shellfish allergy. Clinical and Experimental Allergy: Journal of the British Society for Allergy and Clinical Immunology 40: 850–858.

Luber, F., Demmel, A., Herbert, D., Hosken, A., Hupfer, C., Huber, I. *et al.* (2014). Comparative assessment of DNA-based approaches for the quantification of food allergens. Food Chemistry 160: 104–111.

Maleki, S. J., Chung, S. Y., Champagne, E. T., and Raufman, J. P. (2000). The effects of roasting on the allergenic properties of peanut proteins. The Journal of Allergy and Clinical Immunology 106: 763–768.

Mills, E. N. C., Sancho, A. I., Rigby, N. M., Jenkins, J. A., and Mackie, A. R. (2009). Impact of food processing on the structural and allergenic properties of food allergens. Molecular Nutrition & Food Research 53: 963–969.

Monaci, L., and Visconti, A. (2009). Mass spectrometry-based proteomics methods for analysis of food allergens. Trac-Trends in Analytical Chemistry 28: 581–591.

Monaci, L., and Visconti, A. (2010). Immunochemical and DNA-based methods in food allergen analysis and quality assurance perspectives. Trends in Food Science & Technology 21: 272–283.

Monaci, L., Losito, I., Palmisano, F., and Visconti, A. (2010). Identification of allergenic milk proteins markers in fined white wines by capillary liquid chromatography-electrospray ionization-tandem mass spectrometry. Journal of Chromatography A 1217: 4300–4305.

Müller, A., and Steinhart, H. (2007). Recent developments in instrumental analysis for food quality. Food Chemistry 101: 1136–1144.

Ortea, I., Canas, B., and Gallardo, J. M. (2011). Selected tandem mass spectrometry ion monitoring for the fast identification of seafood species. Journal of Chromatography A 1218: 4445–4451.

Ortolani, C., and Pastorello, E. A. (2006). Food allergies and food intolerances. Best Practice & Research in Clinical Gastroenterology 20: 467–483.

Pawankar, R., Canonica, G. W., Holgate, S. T., and Lockey, R. F. (2011). WAO White Book on Allergy.

Picariello, G., Mamone, G., Addeo, F., and Ferranti, P. (2011). The frontiers of mass spectrometry-based techniques in food allergenomics. Journal of Chromatography A 1218: 7386–7398.

Pomes, A. (2008). Common structures of allergens. Revue Francaise D Allergologie Et D Immunologie Clinique 48: 139–142.

Radauer, C., Bublin, M., Wagner, S., Mari, A., and Breiteneder, H. (2008). Allergens are distributed into few protein families and possess a restricted number of biochemical functions. Journal of Allergy and Clinical Immunology 121: 847–852.e847.

Rauh, M. (2012). LC-MS/MS for protein and peptide quantification in clinical chemistry. Journal of Chromatography B Analytical Technologies in the Biomedical and Life Sciences 883-884: 59–67.

Sakai, S., Matsuda, R., Adachi, R., Akiyama, H., Maitani, T., Ohno, Y. et al. (2008). Interlaboratory evaluation of two enzyme-linked immunosorbent assay kits for the determination of crustacean protein in processed foods. Journal of AOAC International 91: 123–129.

Sancho, A. I., and Mills, E. N. C. (2010). Proteomic approaches for qualitative and quantitative characterisation of food allergens. Regulatory Toxicology and Pharmacology 58: S42–46.

Sharp, M. F., and Lopata, A. L. (2014). Fish allergy: in review. Clinical Reviews in Allergy & Immunology 46: 258–271.

Shefcheck, K. J., and Musser, S. M. (2004). Confirmation of the allergenic peanut protein, Ara h 1, in a model food matrix using liquid chromatography/tandem mass spectrometry (LC/MS/MS). Journal of Agricultural and Food Chemistry 52: 2785–2790.

Shefcheck, K. J., Callahan, J. H., and Musser, S. M. (2006). Confirmation of peanut protein using peptide markers in dark chocolate using liquid chromatography-tandem mass spectrometry (LC-MS/MS). Journal of Agricultural and Food Chemistry 54: 7953–7959.

Sicherer, S. H., and Sampson, H. A. (2010). Food allergy. The Journal of Allergy and Clinical Immunology 125: S116–125.

Stephan, O., and Vieths, S. (2004). Development of a real-time PCR and a sandwich ELISA for detection of potentially allergenic trace amounts of peanut (Arachis hypogaea) in processed foods. Journal of Agricultural and Food Chemistry 52: 3754–3760.

Thomas, K., Herouet-Guicheney, C., Ladics, G., Bannon, G., Cockburn, A., Crevel, R. et al. (2007). Evaluating the effect of food processing on the potential human allergenicity of novel proteins: international workshop report. Food and Chemical Toxicology 45: 1116–1122.

Untersmayr, E., and Jensen-Jarolim, E. (2006). Mechanisms of type I food allergy. Pharmacology & Therapeutics 112: 787–798.

Van Hengel, A. J. (2007). Food allergen detection methods and the challenge to protect food-allergic consumers. Analytical and Bioanalytical Chemistry 389: 111–118.

Verhoeckx, K. C. M., Vissers, Y. M., Baumert, J. L., Faludi, R., Feys, M., Flanagan, S. et al. (2015). Food processing and allergenicity. Food and Chemical Toxicology 80: 223–240.

Wal, J. M. (2003). Thermal processing and allergenicity of foods. Allergy 58: 727–729.

Weber, D., Raymond, P., Ben-Rejeb, S., and Lau, B. (2006). Development of a liquid chromatography-tandem mass spectrometry method using capillary liquid chromatography and nanoelectrospray ionization-quadrupole time-of-flight hybrid mass spectrometer for the detection of milk allergens. Journal of Agricultural and Food Chemistry 54: 1604–1610.

CHAPTER 11

Shellfish Allergy

Taking the Allergenomics Approach towards Improved Allergen Detection and Diagnostics

Sandip D. Kamath[1,2,3,]* and *Andreas L. Lopata*[1,2,3]

Introduction to Shellfish Allergy

Shellfish is an important source of food and plays a significant role in human nutrition and health. The last decade has witnessed an increase in the worldwide consumption of various seafood products mainly due to changed perceptions of dietary requirements as a result of an increase in awareness of the health benefits of seafood. This in turn has resulted in a growing international trade in shellfish species and products, adding to the popularity and frequency of consumption in many countries (Lopata et al., 2010). However, this increase in the consumption and production has been accompanied by a rise in the incidences of adverse reactions to shellfish in both consumers and seafood processors, respectively.

Shellfish allergy is a long lasting disorder which mostly persists throughout life and is often associated with severe reactions (Lehrer et al., 2003). The allergenic group of shellfish can be broadly classified into crustaceans and mollusks. Of all the various consumed shellfish, prawns are one of the most widely consumed crustacean group and causes the most severe reactions (Lopata and SD, 2016; Matricardi et al., 2016).

[1] Australian Institute of Tropical Health and Medicine, James Cook University, Townsville, QLD, Australia.

[2] Centre for Biodiscovery and Molecular Development of Therapeutics, James Cook University, Townsville, QLD, Australia.

[3] Molecular Allergy Research Laboratory, College of Public Health, Medical and Veterinary Sciences, James Cook University, Townsville, QLD, Australia.

* Corresponding author

Recent population-based studies conducted on food allergy have demonstrated a rise in the prevalence of shellfish allergy. A telephone-based survey conducted in the USA showed 2% of the general population is affected by shellfish allergy (Sicherer *et al.*, 2004). These figures, however, seem to vary according to different geographical regions as shown by a Singapore-based study where 5.3% of children were shown to be affected by this disease (Shek *et al.*, 2010). In Australia, a study conducted by Turner *et al.* demonstrated that 25% of children with definite clinical reaction to seafood were allergic to shrimps (Turner *et al.*, 2011).

A systematic approach to diagnosis requires a careful examination of history linked to an understanding of the clinical manifestations, understanding the epidemiology and immune cause, and incorporation of various test results (Boyce *et al.*, 2010). *In vivo* tests such as Skin Prick Test (SPT) or Oral Food Challenges (OFC) are used to determine a high probability of allergic sensitization (Sicherer and Wood, 2013).

In vitro diagnosis, in contrast, is performed by quantification of allergen-specific IgE antibodies. However, crude preparations of shellfish extracts are mostly used in these tests, which do not represent the exposure to various shellfish species consumed in that region, and may lead to errors in specific diagnosis and identification of the offending species. Understanding the structure and function of these allergens is important not only to the understanding of IgE reactivity in patients and the underlying mechanism but also to the development of sensitive and improved diagnostic platforms. Recent advances in the field of molecular cloning and recombinant technology have enabled the production of purified recombinant allergens that have myriad potential in the field of component-resolved diagnostics and allergen quantification.

Exposure to shellfish allergens can also occur through inhalation leading to occupational allergy and asthma. This is an important aspect of shellfish allergy in terms of occupational health and safety where seafood processing workers are constantly exposed to airborne allergens in bioaerosols generated during the processing activities. It is therefore essential to develop sensitive techniques for the detection and monitoring of these airborne allergens for better management of occupational allergy.

In this chapter, a brief overview will be presented on the classification of shellfish, structural and immunological properties of major and minor shellfish allergens, current advances in diagnostic strategies, novel immunological and chemical methods of allergen detection in food and recent advances in the management of occupational allergy to shellfish.

Classification of Shellfish Species

Several seafood species consumed in different regions of the world are often identified using different common names. Patients may fail to identify the offending source, due to the confusion regarding the use of the various common names for different species of seafood. The most important commonly consumed seafood can generally be classified into chordates (fish), arthropods and mollusks. The two invertebrate phyla of arthropods (crustaceans) and mollusks are generally termed as "shellfish" which are further categorized (Fig. 11.1).

Edible crustaceans can be broadly classified into prawns, crabs and lobsters. Prawns constitute a major part of the consumed and farmed species. Decapods from the Penaeidae family are termed as prawns and those from the Caridae family are called shrimps. Prawns and shrimps thus belong to two different taxonomical classifications with the main anatomical differences being the different overlapping pattern of the segments in the carapace and their brooding methods (Poore, 2004). Mollusca are also a large and diverse group with over 100,000 different species currently identified. Commercially important mollusk species are broadly classified into three categories. Bivalve includes mussel, oyster, clam and scallop; gastropod includes snail, abalone and limpet, and cephalopod includes octopus and squid (Fig. 11.1). Although crustaceans and mollusks, which constitute the majority of the consumed shellfish, are taxonomically different and diverse in nature, clinicians often advise for complete avoidance of both the groups to allergic patients. This is partly due to the cross-reactive nature of some allergenic proteins found in shellfish (Lee *et al.*, 2012). On an evolutionary scale, the consumed shellfish species are closely related to invertebrate species such as house dust mites,

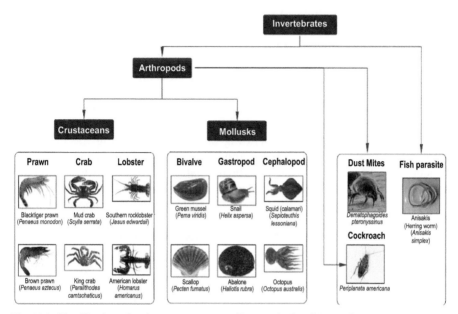

Fig. 11.1: Classification of various crustacean, mollusc, and related invertebrate species.

insects and nematodes. This often leads to immunological and clinical cross-reactivity with these invertebrates in some patients as described in details later in this chapter.

Shellfish allergens

Allergenic proteins are present in different food sources in varying concentrations. More than 1200 allergenic proteins have been identified and sequenced from various sources, and this number is steadily increasing. However, this constitutes only a fraction of the number of proteins that our immune system usually encounters (Traidl-Hoffmann *et al.*, 2009). The most prominent features that might singly or collectively render a protein allergenic are (1) surface features, (2) glycosylation, and (3) protease activity. The elucidation of the primary structure or the amino acid sequence of the allergen helps in predicting the molecular weight, isoelectric point, hydrophobicity and stability using various bioinformatic approaches.

Allergens in shellfish are mainly present in the edible portion of the animal. Over the past 20 years, shellfish allergens, particularly in crustaceans have been identified and sequenced. The first such study was conducted in 1993 by Shanti *et al.* in which the allergens SA-I and SA-II were identified as IgE-binding proteins in *Penaeus indicus* (Indian white shrimp) bearing 86% amino acid identity with Drosophila melanogaster tropomyosin (Shanti *et al.*, 1993). This was later identified to be tropomyosin, the major allergen found in crustaceans and molluscs.

Tropomyosin belongs to a family of highly conserved proteins with multiple isoforms found in muscle and non-muscle tissue of both vertebrate and invertebrate animals (Reese *et al.*, 1999). Tropomyosin exists as a complex with troponin and is involved in muscle contractile function by interacting with actin and myosin (Behrmann *et al.*, 2012; Nevzorov and Levitsky, 2011; Oguchi *et al.*, 2011; Rao *et al.*, 2012). It is present in muscle (skeletal, cardiac and smooth), brain, platelets, fibroblasts, and many other non-muscle cells. In the physiological state, tropomyosin exists as a highly stable α-helical coiled coil homodimeric protein. Depending on alternate splicing mechanisms, different isoforms of tropomyosin are generated, which differ structurally and functionally. These are required for the regulation of contractility in different cell types (Reese *et al.*, 1999). In crustacean species, the fast twitch and the slow twitch isoforms were identified in the tail muscles and the pincer muscles, respectively (Motoyama *et al.*, 2007).

Over the years, several studies have identified tropomyosin to be the major allergen in various shellfish species. According to the Allfam database, tropomyosin is the fourth largest allergen family consisting of 47 tropomyosins identified in various food sources (Radauer *et al.*, 2008).

Other minor allergens have been identified in shellfish such as arginine kinase, myosin light chain and sarcoplasmic calcium binding protein (Abdel

Rahman *et al.*, 2010a; Abdel Rahman *et al.*, 2011; Ayuso *et al.*, 2008; Bauermeister *et al.*, 2011; Chuang *et al.*, 2010; Garcia-Orozco *et al.*, 2007; Giuffrida *et al.*, 2014; Shen *et al.*, 2012). Recent studies have identified novel allergens such as troponin C, triose phosphate isomerase and paramyosin. Allergens such as myosin light chain, sarcoplasmic calcium binding protein, troponin C and paramyosin are involved in muscle contraction and regulation. On the other hand, arginine kinase and triose phosphate isomerase play a role in the metabolic pathways resulting in the ATP production. It is interesting to note that most of the shellfish allergens exist in dimeric or oligomeric states in natural physiological conditions (Fig. 11.2). Recent studies have demonstrated that tropomyosin, myosin light chain and sarcoplasmic calcium binding protein are resistant to heat processing methods whereas arginine kinase and triose phosphate isomerase are heat labile (Abramovitch *et al.*, 2013; Kamath *et al.*, 2013; Kamath *et al.*, 2014a).

Immunological allergen cross-reactivity

One of the important features of major shellfish allergens is the phenomena of IgE antibody cross-reactivity. Tropomyosin is a highly conserved protein among various invertebrate species and demonstrates a high amino acid sequence identity. Because of this, IgE antibodies raised against tropomyosin from a certain species may bind to and trigger an allergic reaction upon exposure to tropomyosin from a different source. This immunological cross-reactivity may be responsible for cross-sensitization and allergic reaction to house dust mites and insects among shellfish allergic patients (Ayuso *et al.*,

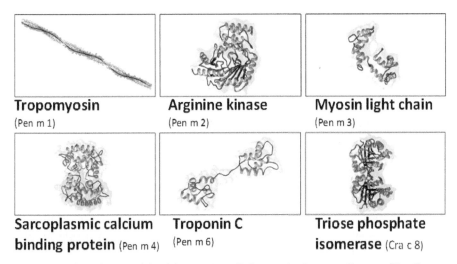

Tropomyosin
(Pen m 1)

Arginine kinase
(Pen m 2)

Myosin light chain
(Pen m 3)

Sarcoplasmic calcium binding protein (Pen m 4)

Troponin C
(Pen m 6)

Triose phosphate isomerase (Cra c 8)

Fig. 11.2: 3D homology models of the top six well-characterized prawn allergens. The allergen names are stated according to the International Union of Immunological Societies (IUIS) Allergen Nomenclature.

2002; Fernandes *et al.*, 2003; Gamez *et al.*, 2014; Purohit *et al.*, 2007). A simple amino acid sequence alignment and comparison of the allergen sequences may be able to predict the level of IgE cross-reactivity. An indepth investigation into the conservation or relevance of specific IgE epitopes among various tropomyosins is essential for understanding the molecular basis of IgE cross-reactivity among various invertebrate species.

Tropomyosin is highly conserved among various crustacean species (prawns, crabs, and lobsters) with amino acid identities reaching 95–100%. Therefore, IgE cross-reactivity is very frequent among crustacean species (Abramovitch *et al.*, 2013; Kamath *et al.*, 2014a; Nakano *et al.*, 2008; Zhang *et al.*, 2006).

Hypersensitivity cross-reaction within mollusk species is often found in allergic individuals. A study in 2006 (Motoyama *et al.*, 2006) determined IgE cross-reactivity of 10 species of cephalopod and found cross-reaction in all species tested. Although immunological and clinical cross-reactivity among crustacean and mollusk species have been documented, these occurrences are not common with the individual often eliciting different clinical symptoms to either group. Nonetheless, complete avoidance of all shellfish species is prescribed. Cross-reactivity has also been shown to play a role in occupational allergy to seafood where a seafood handler elicited asthma and contact urticarial to both shrimps and scallops (Goetz and Whisman, 2000).

Most studies on cross-reactivity have been conducted using tropomyosin as the pan-allergen. Other shellfish allergens may play a role in immunological cross-sensitization. A recent study has shown that allergens other than tropomyosin, such as arginine kinase might also be responsible for seafood-mite cross-reactivity (Gamez *et al.*, 2014; Marinho *et al.*, 2006). Hemocyanin has been demonstrated to play a role in seafood-mite sensitivity as well as being characterized as a cockroach allergen (Giuffrida *et al.*, 2014; Khurana *et al.*, 2014).

Identification and Characterization of Shellfish Allergens

A central aspect of research into food allergy and diagnostics is the identification of novel and putative allergens found in various food and inhalant sources. As diagnostic strategies are increasingly moving from crude extract-based platforms to more purified allergen platform, characterization of allergenic proteins has become an important part of diagnostic research incorporating recent advances in the field of proteomics and bioinformatics. For characterization of allergenic proteins from various crustacean and mollusk species, a general strategy is followed using various immunochemical techniques as summarized in Fig. 11.3. Water soluble total proteins are extracted from the edible portions of the organism, which is used as a starting material. Depending on the heat stability of the allergen, raw or heat-treated crude shellfish extract may be used. Using different techniques such as ion-

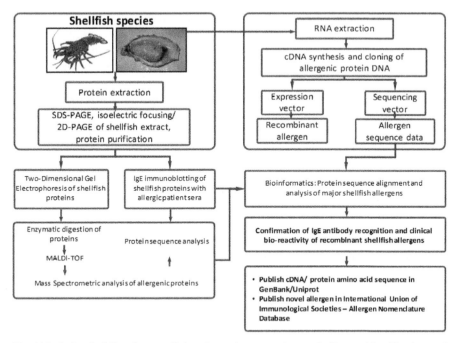

Fig. 11.3: A detailed flowchart outlining the major stages in novel allergen identification and characterization.

exchange chromatography, ammonium sulfate precipitation and sodium dodecyl sulfate-polyacrylamide gel electrophoresis, the natural allergen is isolated or purified from the crude extract. Novel allergens are identified by analyzing their ability to bind to IgE antibodies derived from blood serum of shellfish allergic individuals using 1D or 2D gel electrophoresis and subsequent immunoblotting. According to the International Union of Immunological Societies-allergen nomenclature, a putative protein should be reactive to IgE antibodies from at least five or more allergic individuals to be confirmed as a novel allergen, or more than 50% patient IgE binding to be termed as a major allergen. Identification of the allergenic protein is performed using the mass spectrometric technique. The protein of interest isolated from the SDS-PAGE gel is digested using one of various protease enzymes; trypsin, that is being most commonly used. The generated tryptic peptides are analyzed for their mass to charge ratio using mass spectrometry, and the amino acid sequence is deduced. The protein is identified by analyzing the peptides for homology using different databases (Koeberl *et al.*, 2014a). Alternatively, in the case of very low abundance proteins of interest, it may be difficult to purify the naturally occurring allergen in sufficient quantities for different analytical techniques. In such cases, molecular cloning techniques are employed to generate recombinant allergens as described below.

Recombinant technology has brought tremendous advances to the field of allergen characterization, diagnostics and vaccine development (Ferreira *et al.*, 2014). Many shellfish allergens have been generated and purified as recombinant proteins using *E. coli* expression systems. Currently, black tiger prawn tropomyosin (Pen m 1) is commercially available for Component-Resolved Diagnosis (CRD) for prawn allergy (Thermo Scientific). The advantages of employing recombinant allergens are (a) Large scale production of allergenic proteins (Koeberl *et al.*, 2014b), and (b) Low batch-to-batch variability and validation. Purified recombinant allergens are also being implemented in microarray-based IgE detection platforms.

Diagnosis of shellfish allergy

Diagnostic methods of establishing a true seafood allergy include various *in vivo* and *in vitro* tests to demonstrate the presence of specific IgE antibodies (Lopata and Kamath, 2012; Sastre, 2010). Due to the possible unavailability of the exact species using SPT and blood IgE assays, a detailed clinical history and/or food challenge is performed. Precise evaluation and diagnosis of shellfish allergy using various *in vivo* and *in vitro* tests may result in less restricted dietary requirements.

History

A precise and detailed history is very important to gain information regarding the seafood species under suspicion, nature of the symptoms and the atopic status of the patient. In addition, the identification of the implicated seafood species using specific diagnostic procedures is of importance, where accidental exposure to allergens due to mislabeling is a possibility. A unique or inconsistent history always suggests a non-atopic aetiology, such as contamination with toxins or parasites or intolerance reaction to seafood.

Skin tests

Skin Prick Tests (SPT) are most frequently used *in vivo* allergy testing method. Commercial SPT preparations are available for most shellfish species such as prawns, crabs, lobsters, mussels, oysters, etc. However, many of the species used in these tests are sourced from the northern hemisphere, which are not consumed elsewhere in the world. This often leads to false negative results. In some cases, the source species for allergens is not provided. In addition, much fewer SPT solutions seem to be available for the mollusk group as compared to crustaceans. In certain cases where specific extracts may not be available, skin prick tests or prick to prick tests can be utilized provided their safety and toxin free status are confirmed, and major allergens present.

Blood IgE tests

A precise and reliable *in vitro* assay to quantify the amount of allergen specific IgE antibodies is a valuable tool to support the clinician in confirming or refuting an allergic reaction to seafood, prescribing medication and following up treatment and predicting disease development. Detecting and quantifying IgE antibodies, however, is considerably more complicated than performing many other immunoassays.

There are some complicating factors to be considered:

- The concentration of IgE antibodies in blood is extremely low (0.05% as compared to 75% for the IgG isotype), even in highly sensitized individuals.

- Each allergen source contains a large number of different allergenic components. It is essential for these sources to have enough amounts of the major and minor allergens to be able to detect specific IgE in serum samples.

- The assay must have high enough capacity to bind all IgE antibodies to an allergen in competition with other antibodies with the same specificity from other immunoglobulin classes present in higher concentrations (e.g., IgG).

- To achieve a precise and reproducible test system, total control of the allergen source material is necessary, both in content and in allergenic activity, thus reassuring reproducibility when comparing different patients.

There are several commercial tests available to quantify specific IgE antibodies; however, the most prominent system is the ImmunoCAP (Thermo Scientific), which has been used as a model system to demonstrate the gaps and needs in the context of seafood allergy diagnosis. The ImmunoCAP test (previous known as CAP-RAST) is an *in vitro* diagnostic test to measure the amount of specific IgE antibodies to a given allergen. The accuracy of this assay is dependent on the selection of the correct seafood species and is restricted to the panel of commercially available species.

Due to the vast amount of different shrimp/prawn species worldwide available an ImmunoCAP (f24) including four different species has been developed for increased accuracy in IgE quantification. Many shellfish allergic patients have a concurrent sensitivity to other seafood species, but some patients are truly mono-sensitive to a particular species. In addition, the use of allergens derived from raw or heat treated sources must be considered, as differential allergic responses have been documented (Carnes *et al.*, 2007; Kamath *et al.*, 2014a; Samson *et al.*, 2004). Some of the allergens used in the ImmunoCAP's are derived from heated extracts (e.g., crabs and some prawns), however this information is not provided for most of the crustacean and mollusk allergens. However, a positive history of shellfish allergy and negative

ImmunoCAP result needs further investigation and should be followed up by additional investigations.

Allergen microarray technology

A novel antibody detection system, the allergen microarray has emerged as a promising approach to high-throughput large-scale profiling of allergen interactions for simultaneous monitoring of IgE and IgG antibodies directed against a variety of allergy-eliciting molecules (De Knop *et al.*, 2010; Ferrer *et al.*, 2009; Ott *et al.*, 2008; Wohrl *et al.*, 2006). Some allergens are spotted onto a solid phase (e.g., modified glass slides or nitrocellulose membranes) and subsequently used to bind antibodies from the serum of allergic patients. Detection of allergen-specific antibody binding is accomplished by the addition of specific secondary antibodies that carry an appropriate label for the quantification using fluorescence technology and measured in IU/ml. The major benefit of this technology is its ability to monitor sIgE to several hundred allergen molecules simultaneously using very small volumes (usually 20 µL). The capturing agents are partially purified allergen extracts, highly purified recombinant or natural allergenic components. Importantly, this results in an optimal profiling of the patients IgE response (in one analytical step), identifying major and minor allergens, pan-allergens as well as possible Cross-reactive Carbohydrate Determinants (CCDs).

Double-blind placebo-controlled food challenge (DBPCFC)

The "gold standard" for diagnosis of food allergy is the DBPCFC. Various studies have investigated the minimal shellfish concentrations to elicit clinical reactions. Wu and Williams reported that fatal anaphylaxis occurred after ingestion of three snails (Wu and Williams, 2004). A separate study reported the accumulated amount of as little as 120 mg of dried snail caused a significant decrease in FEV1 (Forced expiration volume) (Pajno *et al.*, 2002). For crustacean Bernstein *et al.* reported that patients in a DBPCFC reacted to 14 gram of shrimp (Bernstein *et al.*, 1982). Similar results were confirmed by Daul *et al.* which reported that the equivalent dose of about four medium-sized shrimps (16 gram) caused reactions in DBPCFC (Daul *et al.*, 1988). However, this technique does not distinguish between allergic (IgE-mediated) and non-allergic hypersensitivity which may involve different antibody types, cellular immune responses and intolerance or toxins. However, performing oral food challenges can improve the quality of life, particularly when the results are favorable (van der Velde *et al.*, 2012).

In summary, various diagnostic tests are used only in support of medical history and epidemiology of the food allergy. While allergists avoid invasive allergy testing, sIgE and total IgE quantification from *in vitro* testing only predicts the severity of clinical symptoms. However, the next generation sIgE quantification involving specific allergen "components" within foods, termed as Component Resolved Diagnosis (CRD) may provide an improved or refined testing platform better able to predict the allergic sensitization in combination with other parameters. Recent advances in PCR-based assays quantification has opened new avenues in allergen-specific IgE quantification which is highly specific and requires as low as 5 uL of serum (derived from a finger prick) (Johnston *et al.*, 2014). This is an added benefit for paediatric allergy testing, where a collection of a sizeable blood volume is a challenge (see Chapter Sophia).

Detection of food allergens

The detection and quantification of allergens are an important responsibility in the food processing industry, where allergenic proteins present in trace amounts may cause accidental exposure and clinical reaction in affected individuals. Allergens may be unintentionally introduced in food products due to sharing of production lines or shared air ventilation. Moreover, certain shellfish products are commonly used as flavoring agents in packed food products thus introducing allergens in trace amounts (Kamath and Lopata, 2014).

To avoid accidental exposure and reaction, food labeling practices and regulations are implemented by specific legislations declaring the allergen contents in the given food product. The basis for labeling in most countries is provided by the International Codex Alimentarius Commission. Different food groups are required for allergen labeling in the European Union as compared to five allergens in Japan (Gendel, 2012). Moreover, the European Commission food labeling law requires crustaceans and mollusks to be declared separately (Becker *et al.*, 2006).

The identification and detection of food allergens remain a challenging issue. Such analysis is complicated by the complex food matrices, the presence of multiple allergens, trace amounts of allergens and partial degradation of allergenic proteins due to processing and shelf life. There is a lack of standardized analytical methods for the detection of shellfish allergens in food including antibody-based methods and mass spectrometric approaches (Koeberl *et al.*, 2014a).

Enzyme linked immunosorbent assay based allergen detection

ELISA based detection kits or lateral flow devices are available for most of the "Big 8" food allergen groups. Previous studies in the past 10 years have attempted to develop analytical methods for the sensitive detection of shellfish allergens. Antibody-based immunoassays have frequently been used for allergen detection because of its ease of use, sensitivity and low assay variability. Monoclonal and polyclonal antibody-based immunoassays have been developed for the detection of the shellfish allergen, tropomyosin (Lopata *et al.*, 2002; Seiki *et al.*, 2007; Werner *et al.*, 2007; Zhang *et al.*, 2014). An important factor in the development of ELISA based detection is to validate the effect of the food matrix, and food protein extraction buffer; both of which can negatively affect the limit of quantitation. Monoclonal antibody-based assays tend to show high specificity but low sensitivity. However, polyclonal antibody-based methods are highly sensitive, but may not be able to distinguish between crustacean, mollusk or other invertebrate allergens. However, most of these assays differ in their sensitivity and specificity to various shellfish species. One important factor to be considered is the effect of heat processing on allergen detection. In addition to protein denaturation and degradation, heat processing has been demonstrated to affect antibody binding (Kamath *et al.*, 2013; Kamath *et al.*, 2014a). ELISA-based methods have been used not only for detection of shellfish allergens in food products but also to quantify airborne crab allergen tropomyosin, which has been demonstrated to cause occupational asthma and allergy (Kamath *et al.*, 2014b).

Polymerase chain reaction (PCR) based detection methods

Various PCR-based allergen detection methods have been designed and validated. A study in 2011 by Taguchi *et al.* used the PCR technique for the detection of shrimp and crab genomic DNA as a means of detecting trace amounts of allergenic content (Taguchi *et al.*, 2011). In another study, a PCR-based method and DNA extraction procedure was developed and validated to detect the fish parasite Anisakis simplex proteins, which are known to cross-react to shellfish allergen-specific IgE and cause adverse reactions (Lopez and Pardo, 2010). Multi-analyte detection methods have also been demonstrated for the fish allergen parvalbumin, capable of detecting parvalbumin from several fish species using the multi-analyte (xMAP) technology (Hildebrandt, 2010). A PCR-based biosensor chip was developed, capable of detecting eight different food allergen sources including shrimp (Wang *et al.*, 2011). Shrimp derived components were detected using 16S rRNA genes and real-time fluorescent PCR technology (Cao *et al.*, 2011). A recent study has demonstrated PCR assay coupled with capillary electrophoresis for the simultaneous detection of 10 food allergens (Cheng *et al.*, 2016). An essential factor however for PCR-based methods is intra-assay variability and repeatability in different laboratories, which must be accordingly tested and validated before being used as a commercial test kit.

Mass Spectrometric-based Detection Methods

Recent advances in the use of next-generation mass spectrometric approaches provide an opportunity to improve the sensitivity of analytical methods for allergen detection and overcome the drawbacks of ELISA based assays such as matrix interference and intra-assay variations. Moreover, multiple allergens may be detected in a broad concentration range (up to five magnitudes). The major advantage of mass spectrometric based allergen detection methods is the extremely high sensitivity, reproducibility and robust validation of detection protocols. Recent studies have focused on the characterization of specific or unique regions of allergenic proteins called signature peptides. These peptides are increasingly being used for the detection and quantification of allergens from different food sources using mass spectrometric approaches. New advances in the mass spectrometric analysis of proteins have enabled the complete sequencing of proteins using enzymatic digestion methods and identification of the generated peptides mass, called *de novo* sequencing (Abdel Rahman *et al.*, 2010b). Mass spectrometric analysis of allergens requires a set of methodological steps involving protein digestion for generation of peptides, elucidation of these peptides for their sequence data and analysis using bioinformatic tools and protein databases. Most commonly, databases such as SEQUEST and Mascot are utilized for this purpose. The generated peptides are identified based on their mass-to-charge ratio and the allergen is finally identified by matching the derived amino acid sequence to known proteins. Digestion of the allergenic protein in question is commonly performed before MS analysis. For generating of allergen-specific peptides, various enzymes were tested such as trypsin, Glu-C V8 and AspN. Recent studies have developed a liquid chromatography-tandem mass spectrometry method for the detection and quantification of crustacean tropomyosin and arginine kinase (Abdel Rahman *et al.*, 2012; Nagai *et al.*, 2015).

Occupational Exposure to Shellfish Allergens

Occupational allergy and asthma are serious health concerns, affecting seafood-processing workers. According to the Food and Agricultural Organisation (FAO), over 45 million people are involved in the fishery and aquaculture industry (Jeebhay and Lopata, 2012; Lopata and Jeebhay, 2013). The increase in consumption and subsequent increase in fishing and harvesting activities in the last three decades have been associated with exposure to allergenic seafood proteins, allergic disease and asthma. Workers in this industry are exposed to seafood, involved in the manual or automated processing of crabs, prawns, mussels or fish (Jeebhay and Cartier, 2010).

The aetiology and development of allergic diseases are due to the interactions between genetic, environmental and host factors which give rise to different allergic disease phenotypes. Occupational allergy to seafood can manifest as both upper and lower respiratory symptoms, as well as urticaria and protein contact dermatitis. Rhinitis and conjunctivitis may also occur which may precede chest symptoms. The prevalence of occupational asthma in seafood processing workers is between 2 and 36% (Jeebhay and Cartier, 2010; Jeebhay *et al.*, 2008; Lopata and Lehrer, 2009). About 7% of the workers with ingestion-related allergy develop asthma symptoms associated with inhalational allergen exposure (Jeebhay *et al.*, 2005; Jeebhay *et al.*, 2008).

Conversely, there are rare cases of workers with occupational asthma who subsequently developed ingestion-related allergic symptoms to the same seafood species (Jeebhay *et al.*, 2001).

Exposure and inhalation of seafood allergens depend on the generation of bioaerosols during the manual or automated processing activities in the factories. While automated processes reduce direct contact with the seafood, it may also lead to increased bioaerosol production. In some cases, processing of the seafood is performed on board the shipping vessel which is characterized by confined spaces and inadequate ventilation systems (Bonlokke *et al.*, 2012). The generated bioaerosols contain muscle, exoskeleton and visceral contents as well as various allergenic proteins.

Various shellfish species are of considerable commercial importance, particularly king crab, snow crab and black tiger prawn which are processed on a large scale. Several studies have been conducted analyzing the airborne exposure of crustacean allergens in various processing activities (Abdel Rahman *et al.*, 2012; Bonlokke *et al.*, 2012; Cartier *et al.*, 1986; Gill *et al.*, 2009; Howse *et al.*, 2006; Malo *et al.*, 1997; Scharer *et al.*, 2002). A recent study by Abdel Rahman *et al.* has demonstrated the presence of major shrimp allergens in the bioaerosols generated in a processing facility particularly in the butchering section (Abdel Rahman *et al.*, 2013). Processing procedures can vary from filleting, freezing, drying, cooking and high-pressure techniques (Thomassen *et al.*, 2016). Specific activities that are known to cause excessive bioaerosol generation are butchering, meat grinding, degutting, boiling, degilling and cleaning of processing lines or storage tanks with high-pressure water hoses. In addition, there has been recent evidence that high-temperature and high-pressure processing may affect the nature, dose and allergenicity of food.

Recent studies have developed advanced methods for monitoring and quantifying airborne shellfish allergens for better management of occupational exposure. Abdel Rahman *et al.* have developed and validated mass spectrometric-based detection and quantification platforms for the detection of crab (Abdel Rahman *et al.*, 2012; Abdel Rahman *et al.*, 2011; Abdel Rahman *et al.*, 2010b; Abdel Rahman *et al.*, 2010c) and prawn (Abdel Rahman *et al.*, 2010a; Abdel Rahman *et al.*, 2013) allergens, tropomyosin and arginine kinase. Previous studies have employed IgE antibodies sources from shellfish allergic patients for the detection of airborne shellfish allergens. However, a recent study by Kamath *et al.* has demonstrated the use of a highly sensitive ELISA-based assay, using tropomyosin-specific polyclonal antibodies, for the detection and quantification of crab allergen tropomyosin in the breathing zones of workers in Norwegian crab processing factories (Kamath *et al.*, 2014b). Better characterization of the allergen repertoire in commonly consumed shellfish species, along with the development of standardized approaches to identify and quantify allergens, is of utmost importance for improved management of occupational allergies.

Summary

A central aspect of food allergy research is the characterization of major and minor allergens in different shellfish species. This is a daunting task, given the diversity and availability of various shellfish species consumed across the world. For this reason, it is not possible to have a single standard diagnostic test or allergen detection method for all species. However, recent advances in allergen characterization with the advent of proteomic and transcriptomic approaches have accelerated the process of identifying novel and putative allergenic proteins from shellfish. Although current diagnostic methods for shellfish allergy are based on whole shellfish extract, current research is gradually moving towards component resolved diagnosis for faster, accurate and sensitive diagnosis, resulting in decreased incidences of false-negative test results. This has led to a prime focus on single allergen characterization using natural or recombinant allergens. This approach is also paving the way for the development of novel immunotherapeutic research for food allergy; something which is in its nascent stage as compared to therapeutics for inhalant and aero-allergens.

Detection of food allergens plays a crucial role in food labeling regulations, allergen content in processed food, food contamination as well as monitoring of airborne allergens which pose a risk to occupational health and safety. Recent advances in the field of immunological- and chemical-based technologies have resulted in the developed of ultra-sensitive, accurate and efficient allergen detection platforms. Future research on method development should focus on the characterization of various shellfish species to incorporate the diversity of allergenic proteins in crustaceans, mollusks as well as other invertebrates.

Keywords: Food allergy, Allergen, Prawn, Tropomyosin, Crustacean, Mollusc, Arginine kinase, Sarcoplasmic calcium binding protein, Skin prick test, Food challenge, Recombinant proteins, Shellfish, Diagnosis

References

Abdel Rahman, A. M., Kamath, S., Lopata, A. L., and Helleur, R. J. (2010a). Analysis of the allergenic proteins in black tiger prawn (*Penaeus monodon*) and characterization of the major allergen tropomyosin using mass spectrometry. Rapid Communications in Mass Spectrometry 24(16): 2462–2470.

Abdel Rahman, A. M., Lopata, A. L., O'Hehir, R. E., Robinson, J. J., Banoub, J. H., and Helleur, R. J. (2010b). Characterization and *de novo* sequencing of snow crab tropomyosin enzymatic peptides by both electrospray ionization and matrix-assisted laser desorption ionization QqToF tandem mass spectrometry. Journal of Mass Spectrometry 45(4): 372–381.

Abdel Rahman, A. M., Lopata, A. L., Randell, E. W., and Helleur, R. J. (2010c). Absolute quantification method and validation of airborne snow crab allergen tropomyosin using tandem mass spectrometry. Analytica Chimica Acta 681(1-2): 49–55.

Abdel Rahman, A. M., Kamath, S. D., Lopata, A. L., Robinson, J. J., and Helleur, R. J. (2011). Biomolecular characterization of allergenic proteins in snow crab (*Chionoecetes opilio*) and *de novo* sequencing of the second allergen arginine kinase using tandem mass spectrometry. Journal of Proteomics 74(2): 231–241.

Abdel Rahman, A. M., Gagne, S., and Helleur, R. J. (2012). Simultaneous determination of two major snow crab aeroallergens in processing plants by use of isotopic dilution tandem mass spectrometry. Analytical and Bioanalytical Chemistry 403(3): 821–831.

Abdel Rahman, A. M., Kamath, S. D., Gagne, S., Lopata, A. L., and Helleur, R. (2013). Comprehensive proteomics approach in characterizing and quantifying allergenic proteins from northern shrimp: toward better occupational asthma prevention. Journal of Proteome Research 12(2): 647–656.

Abramovitch, J. B., Kamath, S., Varese, N., Zubrinich, C., Lopata, A. L., O'Hehir, R. E., and Rolland, J. M. (2013). IgE Reactivity of blue swimmer crab *Portunus pelagicus* tropomyosin, Por p 1, and other allergens; cross-reactivity with black tiger prawn and effects of heating. PLoS ONE 8(6): e67487.

Ayuso, R., Reese, G., Leong-Kee, S., Plante, M., and Lehrer, S. B. (2002). Molecular basis of arthropod cross-reactivity: IgE-binding cross-reactive epitopes of shrimp, house dust mite and cockroach tropomyosins. International Archives of Allergy and Applied Immunology 129(1): 38–48.

Ayuso, R., Grishina, G., Bardina, L., Carrillo, T., Blanco, C., Ibanez, M. D., Sampson, H. A., and Beyer, K. (2008). Myosin light chain is a novel shrimp allergen, Lit v 3. Journal of Allergy and Clinical Immunology 122(4): 795–802.

Bauermeister, K., Wangorsch, A., Garoffo, L. P., Reuter, A., Conti, A., Taylor, S. L., Lidholm, J., Dewitt, A. M., Enrique, E., Vieths, S., Holzhauser, T., Ballmer-Weber, B., and Reese, G. (2011). Generation of a comprehensive panel of crustacean allergens from the North Sea Shrimp Crangon crangon. Molecular Immunology 48(15-16): 1983–1992.

Becker, W., Branca, F., Brasseur, D., Bresson, J., Flynn, A., Jackson, A., Lagiou, P., Løvik, M., Mingrone, G., Moseley, B., Palou, A., Przyrembel, H., Salminen, S., Strobel, S., Berg, H., and Loveren, H. (2006). Opinion of the scientific panel on dietetic products, nutrition and allergies (NDA) related to the evaluation of molluscs for labelling purposes. The EFSA Journal (Vol. 327, pp. 1–25). European Food Safety Authority.

Behrmann, E., Muller, M., Penczek, P. A., Mannherz, H. G., Manstein, D. J., and Raunser, S. (2012). Structure of the rigor actin-tropomyosin-myosin complex. Cell 150(2): 327–338.

Bernstein, M., Day, J. H., and Welsh, A. (1982). Double-blind food challenge in the diagnosis of food sensitivity in the adult. The Journal of Allergy and Clinical Immunology 70(3): 205–210.

Bonlokke, J. H., Gautrin, D., Sigsgaard, T., Lehrer, S. B., Maghni, K., and Cartier, A. (2012). Snow crab allergy and asthma among Greenlandic workers—a pilot study. International Journal of Circumpolar Health 71.

Boyce, J. A., Assa'ad, A., Burks, A. W., Jones, S. M., Sampson, H. A., Wood, R. A., Plaut, M., Cooper, S. F., Fenton, M. J., Arshad, S. H., Bahna, S. L., Beck, L. A., Byrd-Bredbenner, C., Camargo, C. A., Jr., Eichenfield, L., Furuta, G. T., Hanifin, J. M., Jones, C., Kraft, M., Levy, B. D., Lieberman, P., Luccioli, S., McCall, K. M., Schneider, L. C., Simon, R. A., Simons, F. E., Teach, S. J., Yawn, B. P., and Schwaninger, J. M. (2010). Guidelines for the diagnosis and management of food allergy in the United States: report of the NIAID-sponsored expert panel. The Journal of Allergy and Clinical Immunology 126(6 Suppl): S1–58.

Cao, J., Yu, B., Ma, L., Zheng, Q., Zhao, X., and Xu, J. (2011). Detection of shrimp-derived components in food by real-time fluorescent PCR. Journal of Food Proteomics 74(10): 1776–1781.

Carnes, J., Ferrer, A., Huertas, A. J., Andreu, C., Larramendi, C. H., and Fernandez-Caldas, E. (2007). The use of raw or boiled crustacean extracts for the diagnosis of seafood allergic individuals. Annals of Allergy Asthma & Immunology 98(4): 349–354.

Cartier, A., Malo, J. L., Ghezzo, H., McCants, M., and Lehrer, S. B. (1986). IgE sensitization in snow crab-processing workers. The Journal of Allergy and Clinical Immunology 78(2): 344–348.

Cheng, F., Wu, J., Zhang, J., Pan, A., Quan, S., Zhang, D., Kim, H., Li, X., Zhou, S., and Yang, L. (2016). Development and inter-laboratory transfer of a decaplex polymerase chain reaction assay combined with capillary electrophoresis for the simultaneous detection of ten food allergens. Food Chemistry 199: 799–808.

Chuang, J. G., Su, S. N., Chiang, B. L., Lee, H. J., and Chow, L. P. (2010). Proteome mining for novel IgE-binding proteins from the German cockroach (*Blattella germanica*) and allergen profiling of patients. Proteomics 10(21): 3854–3867.

Daul, C. B., Morgan, J. E., Hughes, J., and Lehrer, S. B. (1988). Provocation-challenge studies in shrimp-sensitive individuals. The Journal of Allergy and Clinical Immunology 81(6): 1180–1186.

De Knop, K. J., Bridts, C. H., Verweij, M. M., Hagendorens, M. M., De Clerck, L. S., Stevens, W. J., and Ebo, D. G. (2010). Component-resolved allergy diagnosis by microarray: potential, pitfalls, and prospects. Advances in Clinical Chemistry 50: 87–101.

Fernandes, J., Reshef, A., Patton, L., Ayuso, R., Reese, G., and Lehrer, S. B. (2003). Immunoglobulin E antibody reactivity to the major shrimp allergen, tropomyosin, in unexposed Orthodox Jews. Clinical and Experimental Allergy 33(7): 956–961.

Ferreira, F., Wolf, M., and Wallner, M. (2014). Molecular approach to allergy diagnosis and therapy. Yonsei Medical Journal 55(4): 839–852.

Ferrer, M., Sanz, M. L., Sastre, J., Bartra, J., del Cuvillo, A., Montoro, J., Jauregui, I., Davila, I., Mullol, J., and Valero, A. (2009). Molecular diagnosis in allergology: application of the microarray technique. Journal of Investigational Allergology and Clinical Immunology 19 Suppl 1: 19–24.

Gamez, C., Zafra, M. P., Boquete, M., Sanz, V., Mazzeo, C., Ibanez, M. D., Sanchez-Garcia, S., Sastre, J., and Del Pozo, V. (2014). New shrimp IgE-binding proteins involved in mite-seafood cross-reactivity. Mol Nutr Food Res. 2014 Sep; 58(9): 1915–25. doi: 10.1002/mnfr.201400122.

Garcia-Orozco, K. D., Aispuro-Hernandez, E., Yepiz-Plascencia, G., Calderon-de-la-Barca, A. M., and Sotelo-Mundo, R. R. (2007). Molecular characterization of arginine kinase, an allergen from the shrimp litopenaeus vannamei. International Archives of Allergy and Immunology 144(1): 23–28.

Gendel, S. M. (2012). Comparison of international food allergen labeling regulations. Regulatory Toxicology and Pharmacology 63(2): 279–285.

Gill, B. V., Rice, T. R., Cartier, A., Gautrin, D., Neis, B., Horth-Susin, L., Jong, M., Swanson, M., and Lehrer, S. B. (2009). Identification of crab proteins that elicit IgE reactivity in snow crab-processing workers. The Journal of Allergy and Clinical Immunology 124(5): 1055–1061.

Giuffrida, M. G., Villalta, D., Mistrello, G., Amato, S., and Asero, R. (2014). Shrimp allergy beyond Tropomyosin in Italy: clinical relevance of Arginine Kinase, Sarcoplasmic calcium binding protein and Hemocyanin. European Annals of Allergy and Clinical Immunology 46(5): 172–177.

Goetz, D. W., and Whisman, B. A. (2000). Occupational asthma in a seafood restaurant worker: cross-reactivity of shrimp and scallops. Annals of Allergy Asthma & Immunology 85(6): 461–466.

Hildebrandt, S. (2010). Multiplexed identification of different fish species by detection of parvalbumin, a common fish allergen gene: a DNA application of multi-analyte profiling (xMAP) technology. Analytical and Bioanalytical Chemistry 397(5): 1787–1796.

Howse, D., Gautrin, D., Neis, B., Cartier, A., Horth-Susin, L., Jong, M., and Swanson, M. C. (2006). Gender and snow crab occupational asthma in Newfoundland and Labrador, Canada. Environmental Research 101(2): 163–174.

Jeebhay, M. F., Robins, T. G., Lehrer, S. B., and Lopata, A. L. (2001). Occupational seafood allergy: a review. Occupational Environmental Medicine 58(9): 553–562.

Jeebhay, M. F., Robins, T. G., Seixas, N., Baatjies, R., George, D. A., Rusford, E., Lehrer, S. B., and Lopata, A. L. (2005). Environmental exposure characterization of fish processing workers. Annals Occupational Hygiene 49(5): 423–437.

Jeebhay, M. F., Robins, T. G., Miller, M. E., Bateman, E., Smuts, M., Baatjies, R., and Lopata, A. L. (2008). Occupational allergy and asthma among salt water fish processing workers. American Journal of Industrial Medicine 51(12): 899–910.

Jeebhay, M. F., and Cartier, A. (2010). Seafood workers and respiratory disease: an update. Current Opinion in Allergy and Clinical Immunology 10(2): 104–113.

Jeebhay, M. F., and Lopata, A. L. (2012). Occupational allergies in seafood-processing workers. Advances Food Nutrition Research 66: 47–73.

Johnston, E. B., Kamath, S. D., Lopata, A. L., and Schaeffer, P. M. (2014). Tus-Ter-lock immuno-PCR assays for the sensitive detection of tropomyosin-specific IgE antibodies. Bioanalysis 6(4): 465–476.

Kamath, S. D., Abdel Rahman, A. M., Komoda, T., and Lopata, A. L. (2013). Impact of heat processing on the detection of the major shellfish allergen tropomyosin in crustaceans and molluscs using specific monoclonal antibodies. Food Chemistry 141(4): 4031–4039.

Kamath, S. D., and Lopata, A. L. (2014). Sensitivity to Shellfish: An Overview of Food Allergy to Crustaceans and Molluscs. New York: Nova Publishers.

Kamath, S. D., Rahman, A. M., Voskamp, A., Komoda, T., Rolland, J. M., O'Hehir, R. E., and Lopata, A. L. (2014a). Effect of heat processing on antibody reactivity to allergen variants and fragments of black tiger prawn: A comprehensive allergenomic approach. Molecular Nutrition and Food Research 58(5): 1144–1155.

Kamath, S. D., Thomassen, M. R., Saptarshi, S. R., Nguyen, H. M., Aasmoe, L., Bang, B. E., and Lopata, A. L. (2014b). Molecular and immunological approaches in quantifying the air-borne food allergen tropomyosin in crab processing facilities. International Journal of Hygiene and Environmental Health 217(7): 740–750.

Khurana, T., Collison, M., Chew, F. T., and Slater, J. E. (2014). Bla g 3: a novel allergen of German cockroach identified using cockroach-specific avian single-chain variable fragment antibody. Annals of Allergy Asthma and Immunology 112(2): 140–145.e141.

Koeberl, M., Clarke, D., and Lopata, A. L. (2014a). Next generation of food allergen quantification using mass spectrometric systems. Journal of Proteome Research 13(8): 3499–3509.

Koeberl, M., Kamath, S. D., Saptarshi, S. R., Smout, M. J., Rolland, J. M., O'Hehir, R. E., and Lopata, A. L. (2014b). Auto-induction for high yield expression of recombinant novel isoallergen tropomyosin from King prawn (Melicertus latisulcatus) for improved diagnostics and immunotherapeutics. Journal of Immunology Methods 415: 6–16.

Lee, A. J., Gerez, I., Shek, L. P. C., and Lee, B. W. (2012). Shellfish allergy—an Asia-Pacific perspective. Asian Pacific Journal of Allergy Immunology 30(1): 3–10.

Lehrer, S. B., Ayuso, R., and Reese, G. (2003). Seafood allergy and allergens: a review. Marine Biotechnology 5(4): 339–348.

Lopata, A. L., Luijx, T., Fenemore, B., Sweijd, N. A., and Cook, P. A. (2002). Development of a monoclonal antibody detection assay for species-specific identification of abalone. Marine Biotechnology 4(5): 454–462.

Lopata, A. L., and Lehrer, S. B. (2009). New insights into seafood allergy. Current Opinion in Allergy and Clinical Immunology 9(3): 270–277.

Lopata, A. L., O'Hehir, R. E., and Lehrer, S. B. (2010). Shellfish allergy. Clinical and Experimental Allergy 40(6): 850–858.

Lopata, A. L., and Kamath, S. (2012). Shellfish allergy diagnosis—gaps and needs. Current Allergy & Clinical Immunology 25(2): 60–66.

Lopata, A. L., and Jeebhay, M. F. (2013). Airborne seafood allergens as a cause of occupational allergy and asthma. Current Allergy and Asthma Reports 13(3): 288–297.

Lopata, A. L., and Kamath, S.D. (2016). Allergy to crustacean and mollusks (shellfish). pp. 173–183. In: Kleine-Tebbe, J. Matricardi, P. M., Hoffmann H. J., Valenta R., and Ollert M. (eds.). EAACI Molecular Allergology User's Guide. Published by the European Academy of Allergy and Clinical Immunology.

Lopez, I., and Pardo, M. A. (2010). Evaluation of a real-time polymerase chain reaction (PCR) assay for detection of anisakis simplex parasite as a food-borne allergen source in seafood products. Journal of Agricultural and Food Chemistry 58(3): 1469–1477.

Malo, J. L., Chretien, P., McCants, M., and Lehrer, S. (1997). Detection of snow-crab antigens by air sampling of a snow-crab production plant. Clinical and Experimental Allergy 27(1): 75–78.

Marinho, S., Morais-Almeida, M., Gaspar, A., Santa-Marta, C., Pires, G., Postigo, I., Guisantes, J., Martinez, J., and Rosado-Pinto, J. (2006). Barnacle allergy: allergen characterization and cross-reactivity with mites. Journal of Investigational Allergology and Clinical Immunology 16(2): 117–122.

Matricardi, P. M., Kleine-Tebbe, J., Hoffmann, H. J., Valenta, R., Hilger, C., Hofmaier, S. et al. (2016). EAACI molecular allergology user's guide. Pediatric of Allergy Immunology 27(Suppl 23): 1–236.

Motoyama, K., Ishizaki, S., Nagashima, Y., and Shiomi, K. (2006). Cephalopod tropomyosins: identification as major allergens and molecular cloning. Food Chemistry Toxicology 44(12): 1997–2002.

Motoyama, K., Suma, Y., Ishizaki, S., Nagashima, Y., and Shiomi, K. (2007). Molecular cloning of tropomyosins identified as allergens in six species of crustaceans. Journal of Agricultural and Food Chemistry 55(3): 985–991.

Nagai, H., Minatani, T., and Goto, K. (2015). Development of a method for crustacean allergens using liquid chromatography/tandem mass spectrometry. Journal of AOAC International 98(5): 1355–1365.

Nakano, S., Yoshinuma, T., and Yamada, T. (2008). Reactivity of shrimp allergy-related IgE antibodies to krill tropomyosin. International Archives of Allergy and Immunology 145(3): 175–181.

Nevzorov, I. A., and Levitsky, D. I. (2011). Tropomyosin: Double helix from the protein world. Biochem.-Moscow 76(13): 1507–1527.

Oguchi, Y., Ishizuka, J., Hitchcock-DeGregori, S. E., Ishiwata, S., and Kawai, M. (2011). The Role of Tropomyosin Domains in Cooperative Activation of the Actin-Myosin Interaction. Journal of Molecular Biology 414(5): 667–680.

Ott, H., Baron, J. M., Heise, R., Ocklenburg, C., Stanzel, S., Merk, H. F., Niggemann, B., and Beyer, K. (2008). Clinical usefulness of microarray-based IgE detection in children with suspected food allergy. Allergy 63(11): 1521–1528.

Pajno, G. B., La Grutta, S., Barberio, G., Canonica, G. W., and Passalacqua, G. (2002). Harmful effect of immunotherapy in children with combined snail and mite allergy. The Journal of Allergy and Clinical Immunology 109(4): 627–629.

Poore, G. (2004). Marine Decapod Crustacea of Southern Australia: A Guide to Identification. Melbourne.

Purohit, A., Shao, J., Degreef, J. M., van Leeuwen, A., van Ree, R., Pauli, G., and de Blay, F. (2007). Role of tropomyosin as a cross-reacting allergen in sensitization to cockroach in patients from Martinique (French Caribbean island) with a respiratory allergy to mite and a food allergy to crab and shrimp. European Annals of Allergy and Clinical Immunology 39(3): 85–88.

Radauer, C., Bublin, M., Wagner, S., Mari, A., and Breiteneder, H. (2008). Allergens are distributed into few protein families and possess a restricted number of biochemical functions. The Journal of Allergy and Clinical Immunology 121(4): 847–852 e847.

Rao, J. N., Rivera-Santiago, R., Li, X. E., Lehman, W., and Dominguez, R. (2012). Structural analysis of smooth muscle tropomyosin alpha and beta Isoforms. Journal of Biological Chemistry 287(5): 3165–3174.

Reese, G., Ayuso, R., and Lehrer, S. B. (1999). Tropomyosin: an invertebrate pan–allergen. International Archives of Allergy and Immunology 119(4): 247–258.

Samson, K. T., Chen, F. H., Miura, K., Odajima, Y., Iikura, Y., Naval Rivas, M., Minoguchi, K., and Adachi, M. (2004). IgE binding to raw and boiled shrimp proteins in atopic and nonatopic patients with adverse reactions to shrimp. International Archives of Allergy and Immunology 133(3): 225–232.

Sastre, J. (2010). Molecular diagnosis in allergy. Clinical and Experimental Allergy 40(10): 1442–1460.

Scharer, L., Hafner, J., Wuthrich, B., and Bucher, C. (2002). Occupational protein contact dermatitis from shrimps. A new presentation of the crustacean-mite syndrome. Contact Dermatitis 46(3): 181–182.

Seiki, K., Oda, H., Yoshioka, H., Sakai, S., Urisu, A., Akiyama, H., and Ohno, Y. (2007). A reliable and sensitive immunoassay for the determination of crustacean protein in processed foods. Journal of Agricultural and Food Chemistry 55(23): 9345–9350.

Shanti, K. N., Martin, B. M., Nagpal, S., Metcalfe, D. D., and Rao, P. V. S. (1993). Identification of tropomyosin as the major shrimp allergen and characterization of its IgE-binding epitopes. Journal of Immunology 151(10): 5354–5363.

Shek, L. P. C., Cabrera-Morales, E. A., Soh, S. E., Gerez, I., Ng, P. Z., Yi, F. C., Ma, S., and Lee, B. W. (2010). A population-based questionnaire survey on the prevalence of peanut, tree nut, and shellfish allergy in 2 Asian populations. The Journal of Allergy and Clinical Immunology 126(2): 324–U350.

Shen, H. W., Cao, M. J., Cai, Q. F., Ruan, M. M., Mao, H. Y., Su, W. J., and Liu, G. M. (2012). Purification, cloning, and immunological characterization of arginine kinase, a novel allergen of *Octopus fangsiao*. Journal of Agricultural and Food Chemistry 60(9): 2190–2199.

Sicherer, S. H., Munoz-Furlong, A., and Sampson, H. A. (2004). Prevalence of seafood allergy in the United States determined by a random telephone survey. The Journal of Allergy and Clinical Immunology 114(1): 159–165.

Sicherer, S. H., and Wood, R. A. (2013). Advances in diagnosing peanut allergy. The Journal of Allergy and Clinical Immunology: In Practice 1(1): 1–13.

Taguchi, H., Watanabe, S., Temmei, Y., Hirao, T., Akiyama, H., Sakai, S., Adachi, R., Sakata, K., Urisu, A., and Teshima, R. (2011). Differential detection of shrimp and crab for food labeling using polymerase chain reaction. Journal of Agricultural and Food Chemistry 59(8): 3510–3519.

Thomassen, M. R., Kamath, S. D., Lopata, A. L., Madsen, A. M., Eduard, W., Bang, B. E., and Aasmoe, L. (2016). Occupational Exposure to Bioaerosols in Norwegian Crab Processing Plants. Annals of Occupational Hygiene. 2016 Aug;60(7): 781–94. doi: 10.1093/annhyg/mew030. Epub 2016 May 28.

Traidl-Hoffmann, C., Jakob, T., and Behrendt, H. (2009). Determinants of allergenicity. The Journal of Allergy and Clinical Immunology 123(3): 558–566.

Turner, P., Ng, I., Kemp, A., and Campbell, D. (2011). Seafood allergy in children: a descriptive study. Annals of Allergy Asthma and Immunology 106(6): 494–501.

van der Velde, J. L., Flokstra-de Blok, B. M., de Groot, H., Oude-Elberink, J. N., Kerkhof, M., Duiverman, E. J., and Dubois, A. E. (2012). Food allergy-related quality of life after double-blind, placebo-controlled food challenges in adults, adolescents, and children. The Journal of Allergy and Clinical Immunology 130(5): 1136–1143 e1132.

Wang, W., Han, J. X., Wu, Y. J., Yuan, F., Chen, Y., and Ge, Y. Q. (2011). Simultaneous detection of eight food allergens using optical thin-film biosensor chips. Journal of Agricultural and Food Chemistry 59(13): 6889–6894.

Werner, M. T., Faeste, C. K., and Egaas, E. (2007). Quantitative sandwich ELISA for the determination of tropomyosin from crustaceans in foods. Journal of Agricultural and Food Chemistry 55(20): 8025–8032.

Wohrl, S., Vigl, K., Zehetmayer, S., Hiller, R., Jarisch, R., Prinz, M., Stingl, G., and Kopp, T. (2006). The performance of a component-based allergen-microarray in clinical practice. Allergy 61(5): 633–639.

Wu, A. Y., and Williams, G. A. (2004). Clinical characteristics and pattern of skin test reactivities in shellfish allergy patients in Hong Kong. Allergy & Asthma Proceedings 25(4): 237–242.

Zhang, H., Lu, Y., Ushio, H., and Shiomi, K. (2014). Development of sandwich ELISA for detection and quantification of invertebrate major allergen tropomyosin by a monoclonal antibody. Food Chemistry 150(0): 151–157.

Zhang, Y., Matsuo, H., and Morita, E. (2006). Cross-reactivity among shrimp, crab and scallops in a patient with a seafood allergy. Journal of Dermatology 33(3): 174–177.

CHAPTER 12

Bioinformatics Approaches to Identifying the Cross-Reactive Allergenic Risk of Novel Food Proteins

Ping Song,* Rod A. Herman and *Siva Kumpatla*

Introduction

The use of bioinformatics to investigate the evolutionary and functional relationship between proteins based on Amino Acid (AA) sequence is well established. The AA sequence of a protein largely dictates its folding conformation and physicochemical properties. The more similar two proteins are in AA sequence; the more likely they are to share similar evolutionary origins and physicochemical properties. The majority of allergies are mediated by the binding of immunoglobulin E (IgE) antibodies to specific sites (epitopes) on allergenic proteins. These epitopes have specific physicochemical properties recognized by these IgE antibodies. Therefore, it is expected that proteins sharing more similar AA sequences are more likely to cross-react with the same IgE antibodies and thus be cross-reactive allergens.

Food allergens are almost always proteins, but most food proteins are not allergens (Bannon, 2004). Evaluation of allergic potential is essential whenever novel proteins are brought into contact with humans, either through food, cosmetics or other modes of contact. Bioinformatics approaches for assessing the cross-reactive allergenic risk for novel proteins have been investigated in the scientific literature. The main application has been to assess novel food proteins (either new to the food supply or newly characterized). Much of the research in this area has been driven by regulatory requirements aimed at the

Dow AgroSciences LLC, Zionsville Road, Indianapolis, IN 46268, USA.
* Corresponding author: psong@dow.com

safety assessment of novel proteins introduced into food crops by modern methods of biotechnology (transgenesis). Here we review this research and its applications towards identifying the allergenic potential of novel food proteins. This chapter expands upon and updates an earlier publication (Song, 2015).

Government Regulations Relating to Bioinformatics Assessment of Allergen Cross-Reactive Risk

Food allergy is a growing public health concern, especially in developed countries. For example, as many as 5% of children and 3–4% of adults in westernized countries have food allergies (Branum and Lukacs, 2008; Gupta *et al.*, 2011; Liu *et al.*, 2011; Sicherer and Sampson, 2010; Sicherer, 2011). Notably, the prevalence appears to be rising. Although the diversity of the human diet is great, there are just a few foods that account for the majority of food allergies (Sampson, 2004; Sicherer and Sampson, 2010). There is a risk that humans could be exposed to new allergens or cross-reactive allergens when they are introduced and consumed. Most of the food allergies are mediated by antigen-specific IgE antibodies. One allergen can be cross-reactive with the IgE antibodies of another allergen, resulting in patients who are initially sensitized to one allergen subsequently reacting to another protein with a similar protein sequence or structure (Vieths *et al.*, 2002). In the majority of commercialized genetically modified food crops, a novel protein that is not naturally present in that host food crop is expressed from the inserted transgene. The newly expressed protein could be encoded by a gene derived from a known or unknown allergenic source. Alternatively, a novel open reading frame that could encode a novel protein might be created in the junction regions of a transgene insert after insertion of an exogenous DNA sequence into the host genome. Theoretically, these novel proteins carry the potential to be cross-reactive allergens. Therefore, an allergenicity assessment is necessary when a transgene is introduced into a food crop to express a novel protein. It is noteworthy that the same risk also occurs in the introduction of new food such as fuzzy kiwifruit and traditional food crop breeding programs that make use of natural or induced mutation, or crosses with wild crop relatives (interspecies hybridization), but lack of knowledge of what changes have occurred hampers a bioinformatics analysis of allergenic risk for traditionally bred crops (Herman and Ladics, 2014).

Since the first launch of transgenic food crops, allergenicity has been one of the most frequently voiced concerns about the safety of food derived from biotechnology. For the sake of human food safety and public health, international organizations including the United Nations Food and Agriculture Organization (FAO) and World Health Organization (WHO) and their joint Codex Alimentarius (Latin for "food of code") Commission have issued guidelines on evaluation of allergenicity of foods derived from biotechnology. Through a Joint Expert Consultation on Foods Derived from Biotechnology, FAO/WHO have published recommendations to strengthen the process used to protect consumers from the risk that some Genetically Modified Organisms (GMOs) could pose for a small percentage of people with food allergies. The FAO/WHO Consultation proposed an extensive methodology to evaluate the allergenicity of foods derived from sources with known allergenicity, as well as from sources with no known allergenicity. The methodology includes an initial comparison of the similarity of the protein's AA sequences with those of known allergens using bioinformatics tools followed by, when necessary, more in-depth investigation using various other scientific testing techniques including serum screening, etc. (FAO/WHO, 2001). The Codex Alimentarius Commission establishes international standards, guidelines or other recommendations known as Codex Alimentarius through deliberations among representatives of Codex Alimentarius Members which includes 165 countries. Reflecting growing concern about the safety and nutritional aspects of foods derived from biotechnology, Codex Alimentarius Commission decided in 1999 to undertake "the consideration of standards, guidelines or other recommendations for foods derived from biotechnology or traits introduced into foods by biotechnology." Since then, Codex Alimentarius Commission has held several sessions on this topic and the guidelines regarding allergenicity risk assessment of food derived from biotechnology (CODEX, 2009). Following these guidelines, regulatory agencies such as European Food Safety Authority (EFSA) have published risk assessment guidelines specific to evaluation of potential allergenicity for newly expressed proteins (EFSA, 2010, 2011). Evaluation of sequence similarity between the newly expressed proteins and known allergens using bioinformatics tools has become one of the components in all these guidelines and government regulations across countries.

Over the past decade, a weight-of-evidence approach, which encompasses a variety of investigations, has been developed and widely adopted, although a decision tree approach was recommended in the FAO/WHO guideline (FAO/WHO, 2001; Astwood *et al.*, 2003; Metcalf *et al.*, 1996; CODEX, 2009). Bioinformatics assessment for potential protein allergenicity is a part of this approach. This approach has been consistently reviewed and improved on ever since the launch of the first transgenic food crops. According to the current guideline, comparison of the newly expressed proteins with known allergens for AA sequence similarity should be conducted using > 35% identity over 80 amino acids (> 35%/80aa+) as criteria to judge if the newly expressed protein has potential to be a cross-reactive allergen. In some cases, not only the newly expressed protein(s) is subject to comparison with known allergens, but also all the reading frames from a stop to stop codon in all six *in silico* reading-frame translations in the whole transgenic insert as well as the region across the border junctions must be evaluated (EFSA, 2011).

Bioinformatics Research on Prediction of Allergen Cross-Reactivity

The biological function of a protein is largely controlled by the AA sequence that determines the tertiary structure of the protein. Allergenic proteins generally contain linear or conformational epitopes recognized by specific IgE antibodies (Pomès, 2010; Ladics *et al.*, 2014). By using specific databases containing the primary sequences or identified linear/conformational epitopes of known allergens, the potential allergenicity of a given protein can be assessed based on sequence/structure similarity with known allergens or structure similarity with known epitopes. With the rapid advances in bioinformatics methodology, many protein sequence similarity search or structure prediction tools, ranging from simple short segment (epitope) match to sophisticated 3-D structure modeling and comparisons, along with various databases designed for those search tools, have been tested over decades for prediction of potential allergenicity of a given protein (Song, 2015).

Allergen databases

To facilitate a bioinformatics investigation of potential cross-reactive allergenicity of protein, one needs to know the AA sequence of previously identified allergens. While massive protein databases such as the NCBI (National Center for Biotechnology Information) non-redundant protein-sequence database (http://www.ncbi.nlm.nih.gov/protein) contain known allergens, a dedicated allergen database is preferred because the statistical measurement (E-value) of most popular search algorithms such as BLAST (Altschul *et al.*, 1990, 1997) and FASTA (Person and Lipman, 1988) are associated with database size (smaller databases have more statistical power to detect structural and functional relationships). When searching for very distant relationships, one should always use the smallest database that is likely to contain the homolog of interest (Pearson, 1999). Thus, a dedicated allergen database is desirable for implementing bioinformatics methods to assess the potential allergenicity of a novel protein present in a transgenic food crop or new food source. For this reason, a number of allergen-sequence databases have been created (Table 12.1) since the regulatory frame work on GMOs was formulated (Song, 2015).

Currently, there are more than 13 publically available allergen databases that focus on allergen sequence/structure along with various bioinformatics tools for prediction of protein allergenicity (Table 12.1; Gendel, 2006, 2009; Mari *et al.*, 2006, 2009). Biological/biomedical information is also included in some of the allergen sequence databases along with various bioinformatics tools that allow users to search their protein sequences against the hosted database to evaluate the potential allergenicity of their proteins. Assessment of potential

Table 12.1: Publicly accessible allergen database sites with search tools.

Database Name	Website	Type	Sequence similarity search tools
Allergenonline	http://www.allergenonline.org/	Biomedical information/ Sequence	1. Sliding window FASTA search for > 35% /80aa+ with default setting 2. Whole sequence FASTA search with default setting 3. Search for contiguous 8-mer match
Allergome (Mari *et al.*, 2006, 2009)	http://www.allergome.org/	Biomedical information/ Sequence	1. BLASTp search with Expect value set to 100 2. FASTA search with default setting 3. SSEARCH search with default setting 4. Two databases for search: Allergome and Uniprot (User can define minimum and maximum identity in BLASTp search and minimum and maximum similarity in FASTA search)
Allergen Database for Food Safety	http://allergen.nihs.go.jp/ADFS/	Biomedical information/ Sequence	1. BLASTp for sequence identity with default setting of search parameters 2. BLASTp search for short mer matches with Expectation set at 2000, PAM30 Matrix, and Gap Cost of Existence: 7 and Extension: 2
AlgPred (Saha and Raghava, 2006)	http://www.imtech.res.in/raghava/algpred/	Sequence	1. Mapping of IgE epitopes and PID 2. MEME/MAST motif 3. SVM module based on amino acid composition 4. SVM module based on dipeptide composition 5. Blast search on allergen representative peptides (ARPs) 6. Hybrid Approach (SVMc+IgEepitope+ARPs BLAST+MAST)
AllerMatch (Fiers *et al.*, 2004)	http://www.allermatch.org/index.html	Sequence	1. Sliding window FASTA search for > 35%/80aa+ 2. Whole sequence FASTA search 3. Search for contiguous short mer (defined by user) match
APPEL (Cui *et al.*, 2007)	http://jing.cz3.nus.edu.sg/cgi-bin/APPEL	Sequence	Prediction through sequence-derived protein structure and physicochemical properties

Table 12.1 contd. ...

... Table 12.1 contd.

Database Name	Website	Type	Sequence similarity search tools
SDAP (Structural Database of Allergenic Proteins) (Ivanciuc *et al.*, 2003; Schein *et al.*, 2006)	http://fermi.utmb.edu/SDAP/index.html	Sequence	1. Sliding window FASTA search for > 35%/80aa+ 2. Whole sequence FASTA search 3. Search for contiguous short mer (defined by user; default is 6) match 4. Pepetidie match with known allergen 5. Peptide similarity based on the five dimensional descriptors E1-E5 of amino acids properties derived from a pool of 237 physicochemical properties
AllerHunter	http://tiger.dbs.nus.edu.sg/AllerHunter/running.html	Sequence	1. Sliding window search for > 35%/80 aa+ 2. Cross-reactivity prediction using SVM (vector support machine)
Allerginia	http://allergenia.gzhmu.edu.cn	Sequence	1. Sliding window search for > 35%/80aa+ using BLASTp or FASTA 2. Cross-reactivity prediction using SVM (vector support machine) based on allergen family featured peptides (SORTALLER)
proAP	http://gmobl.sjtu.edu.cn/proAP/main.html	Sequence	1. Sliding window search for > 35% /80aa+ using BLASTp 2. Sliding window search for contiguous short mer (defined by user) match 3. Motif-based method 4. SVM-AAC method
Allerdictor (Dang and Lawrence, 2014)	http://allerdictor.vbi.vt.edu	Sequence	Sequence-based allergen prediction tool that models protein sequences as text documents and employs support vector machine in text classification for allergen prediction
AllerTop (Dimitrov *et al.*, 2013a)	http://www.pharmfac.net/allertop	Sequence	Uses a model based on amino acid z-descriptors, ACC protein transformation and *k* nearest neighbors (*k*NN) clustering to classify protein
AllergenFP (Dimitrov *et al.*, 2013b)	http://ddg-pharmfac.net/AllergenFP/	Sequence	Uses binary descriptor fingerprints generated by *E*-descriptors, auto-cross covariance (ACC) transformation, and Tanimoto coefficient similarity calculation to classify protein.

allergenicity of transgenic proteins continues to be part of the requirements for regulatory approval of transgenic crops. Bioinformatics analysis to identify cross-reactive allergenic risk is a part of the weight-of-evidence evaluation system. Due to the regulatory requirement to assess the cross-reactive allergenic risk of novel proteins expressed in Genetically Modified (GM) crops, a database has been created specifically for this purpose (http://www.allergenonline. org/). This database is curated by the Food Allergy Research and Resource Program (FARRP) group at the University of Nebraska. Because aero-allergens and food allergens are sometimes known to cross-react (pollen-food allergy), the database contains both types of protein allergen sequences. One of the features of this database is the implementation of an expert peer review process using established criteria. As such, this database is widely used in regulatory assessment for potential protein allergenicity of transgenic proteins in food crops (Randhawa *et al.*, 2011; Verma *et al.*, 2012; Zou *et al.*, 2013).

Linear epitope identification and prediction

Linear epitopes are present in many known allergens. To identify potential shared linear epitopes, a straightforward approach is to search for matches of short segments of contiguous amino acids between a candidate sequence and known allergens. This is typically done by parsing a query sequence into all overlapping fragments of a given length (sliding window approach) and comparing each of them with allergens in a database (or a collection of known Ig Epitopes) for an exact match. Regarding the minimum length used for such matches, the FAO/WHO (2001) guideline suggests matches as short as six contiguous amino acids based on the hypothetical epitope size for IgE epitope binding. However, many studies indicated that a simple search of short contiguous AA matches with an allergen sequence might not be appropriate because not all short AA sequences represent allergenic epitopes, resulting in extremely high numbers of false-positive matches. For example, incremental increases in length of short-mer searches showed no significant improvement in allergen detection (Wong *et al.*, 2014), but for match sizes from 6–8, the specificity improved from 23 to 95%. One approach to reducing false-positive matches was to profile any short-mer (6 AA) protein sequence matches to identify hydrophilic sites because of their tendency to be a part of antibody-binding epitopes (Hopp and Woods, 1981; Kleter and Peijnenburg, 2003). In spite of further evaluation after identification of short-mer matches, it has been concluded that the use of less than eight-AA window sizes is prone to high rates of false positives and were of no predictive value (Stadler and Stadler, 2003; Silvanovich *et al.*, 2006). Through recognition of high false-positive potential, Codex Alimentarius guideline (2009) recommends that "the size of the contiguous amino acid search should be based on a scientifically justified rationale in order to minimize the potential for false negative or false positive results". Furthermore, the use of any short segment of AA sequence match for predicting the allergenic potential of proteins has also been debated (Goodman *et al.*, 2008; Cressman and Ladics, 2009; Herman *et al.*, 2009). Consequently, the use of less than an eight-AA sliding window match is no longer used due to the high probability of random alignments. Through acknowledgment of the extremely high false positive rate and limited scientific value to the risk assessment of potential allergenicity, EFSA (2010, 2011) discontinued support for the short peptide match search for assessment of potential protein allergenicity.

It is commonly known that an allergenic protein must contain at least two IgE binding epitopes to secure the cross-linking to IgE on mast cells and basophils. Other approaches using specific epitope database and bioinformatics algorithm have been explored. Although a comprehensive and extensive public epitope database is not currently available, it has been reported that about 150 linear IgE-binding epitopes have been determined (Bannon and Ogawa, 2006) in known allergens. The use of structural and physicochemical properties of the known epitopes to predict the potential linear epitope of a given protein has been investigated. Methods based on the physicochemical properties were first deployed in the SDAP (Structural Database of Allergenic Proteins) along with tools associated with epitope prediction (Ivanciuc *et al.*, 2003a, 2003b, 2009a, 2009b, 2009c). Based on the physicochemical properties, the PD (Property Distance) similarity index is calculated between a query sequence and each sequence from all the epitopes in the SDAP database, thus generating a list of similar sequences identified in allergenic proteins. The similarity between a known epitope and the query sequence decreases with the increment of PD values, and a threshold value between 7.5 and 9 is recommended to determine peptides with similar properties. However, this method is limited by the availability of known epitopes within known allergens.

Searching Allergen-Specific Motifs

Motifs in a group of functional proteins also referred to as super secondary structures, are small substructures that are structurally similar. Distinctive motifs can be identified within the overall protein structure. Given that protein motifs commonly exist within protein families or groups of proteins that are functionally related, it is logical to expect that cross-reactive allergens share common motifs. By grouping known allergens into Pfam families followed by motif extraction or multiple sequence alignment of allergenic protein sequences, a set of motifs were used to predict cross-reactive allergens (Ivanciuc *et al.*, 2009a). Tools for discovering motifs in a group of related protein sequences such as MEME (Multiple Em for Motif Elicitation) and PSI-BLAST (Position-specific iterative BLAST) have also been tested to identify motifs/profiles in known allergens (Bailey *et al.*, 1994, 1998). An allergenic motif database was created by MEME and used for identifying cross-reactive allergens using MAST (Motif Alignment and Search Tool) (Saha and Raghava,

2006). In one evaluation of the effect of *E*-value using a MAST approach, it was found that the specificity and sensitivity changed slightly when the cut-off E-value was below 0.1, but the specificity decreased from 96.97% at E-value of 0.1 to 66.67 at E-value of 1.0 (Wong *et al.*, 2014). Considering accuracy, iteration motif elicitation with a MAST *E*-value of 0.5 was recommended. In another publication, a PSI (Position-Specific Iterated)-BLAST was used to search a set of training allergen sequences, followed by filtering and optimization to create allergen profiles or PSSMs (Position Specific Score Matrices) (Lim *et al.*, 2008). By RPS-BLAST (reverse PSI-BLAST, Marchler-Bauer *et al.*, 2002) of the allergen profiles or PSSMs, the potential allergenicity of a query protein could be predicted when using an *E*-value of 10^{-9} as a threshold. This method resulted in a significant improvement in accuracy and specificity with similar sensitivity when compared with the method proposed by FAO/WHO guideline (Lim *et al.*, 2008). One disadvantage of motif based prediction is that the motif database has to be re-constructed once new or cross-reactive allergens are identified.

Due to the fact that motifs do not always exist in all allergens, a combination of sequence similarity searches and motif identification was also evaluated. In one approach, a query protein was first scanned for the matches with the motifs extracted from known allergens. In the case where a negative result was generated from motif scanning, the query protein was compared with the known allergen sequences in which no motifs were identified using local alignment tools such as FASTA or BLASTp (Stadler *et al.*, 2003). In another approach, known allergens were first clustered into different sequence groups by multiple sequence alignment using the ClustalW (Thompson *et al.*, 1994) program and PAM scoring matrix. Then the motifs from each sequence group were extracted using a wavelet analysis, followed by generation of an HMM (Hidden Markov Model) profile for each motif (Li *et al.*, 2004; Riaz *et al.*, 2005). The allergens from the sequence group in which no motifs were detected were grouped as a separate allergen database. For protein allergenicity prediction, a query protein was first compared with all the profiles of identified motifs using the HMMER (a software package used by Pfam for building and search profile HMMs) program. Similar to the aforementioned approach, a BLASTp search against the no-motif allergen database was performed if no matching profile was detected in the first step. This approach also showed improved sensitivity and precision when compared with the methods outlined in the FAO/WHO (2001) guideline.

Machine Learning Models

In addition to regular bioinformatics tools such as sequence alignment and motif identification, more sophisticated algorithms derived from computerized learning or machine learning systems, such as Support Vector Machines (SVM), have been introduced to predict protein allergenicity. SVM are statistical learning methods originally developed based on structural risk minimization principles (Cortes and Vapnik, 1995; Vapnik, 1995; Joachims, 1999). For protein allergenicity prediction, the SVM methods generally employ a kernel function to project input vectors consisting of allergens and non-allergens into a high-dimensional feature space and then selecting a hyperplane within the space that maximizes the separation of the allergens and non-allergens (Muh et al., 2009). In an initial study, a computerized learning system combining pattern extraction through sequence alignment by FASTA with the k-Nearest-Neighbor (kNN) classification algorithm was used to classify protein sequences associated with allergenicity and non-allergenicity (Zorzet et al., 2002). Afterwards, a more comprehensive performance comparison using a larger number of allergens and non-allergens along with three different classification algorithms concluded that the linear Gaussian classifier was the most useful among the three tested supervised machine learning algorithms, followed by the quadratic Gaussian and kNN classifiers (Soeria-Atmadja et al., 2004).

Several modified SVM-based methods were developed and investigated. Using one method, an allergenicity detector was created by sequence alignment using a FASTA search of a set of designated or validated allergens and non-allergens, followed by an external cross-validation procedure (Soeria-Atmadja et al., 2005). Using another method, an allergenicity detector was generated using the following procedure: (1) Filtered Length-adjusted Allergen Peptides (FLAPs) were created to serve as a database; (2) a query protein and a training set of allergens and non-allergens were aligned to the sequences in the database to extract feature vectors used to create a detector (Soeria-Atmadja et al., 2006). Other modified SVM-based methods to predict protein allergenicity or cross-reactive allergens included an SVM detector constructed from sequence-derived structural and physicochemical properties of allergens and non-allergens (Cui et al., 2007) and an SVM-pairwise system (Muh et al., 2009). Recently, another modified SVM approach using allergen family featured peptides to create a detector was reported (Zhang et al., 2012). Performance evaluation of a SVM-based method (Saha and Raghava, 2006) indicated an accuracy of 91.70% with respective sensitivity and specificity of 92.82 and 90.59% (Wong et al., 2014). Compared with the FAO/WHO methods, SVM-based methods usually displayed a significant improvement in specificity while maintaining similar sensitivity. Similar to motif-based approach, the SVM needs to be re-built after the discovery of new or cross-reactive allergens. However, one performance comparison study including various allergenicity prediction methods indicated that the motif identification based on position-specific scoring metrics outperformed SVM-based methods in specificity and sensitivity (Lim et al., 2009).

Text classification techniques were recently used to predict protein allergenicity (Dang and Lawrence, 2014). This combined method models the overlapping k-length peptides (k-mer) from each allergen and non-allergens in a given dataset as text documents (sequence representations) and applies a text classification algorithm NB (Naive Bayes) or SVM to the k-mer sequence representation for allergen prediction. For the three datasets tested, the combined method performed better than BLAST and MEM (Maximal Exact Match) with higher precision while maintaining the same sensitivity. This method identified < 1% of the ~ 540,000 proteins in the Swiss-Prot database as allergens.

Use of Tertiary Structure

The biological function of a protein typically depends on its tertiary structure. The tertiary structure of a folded protein is complex and dependent on the position of each AA in the protein, the local 3-dimensional structure, as well as the global 3-dimensional structure. Understanding the 3-dimensional structures of allergens provides knowledge for the development of advanced bioinformatics tools that will more accurately predict protein allergenicity. Conformational epitopes are estimated to represent for 90% of all B-cell epitopes (Van Regenmortel *et al.*, 1996). They are spatially clustered, and surface-exposed arrangements of AA residues and mapping of these epitopes requires the availability of structural models. Currently, more than a hundred entries of non-redundant allergen tertiary structures have been deposited in the protein data bank (PDB, http://www.rcsb.org/pdb/home/home.do). Based on the domains identified in the Pfam database, the 3-D structures of known allergens were classified into 19 families (Radauer *et al.*, 2006, 2008; Dall'Antonia *et al.*, 2014).

Molecular modeling combined with B-cell and T-cell epitope mapping tools based on hydrophilicity, chain flexibility/mobility, solvent accessibility, polarity, exposed surface and turns, was reported to identify epitopes and their sequences. After identification of high sequence identity and similarity with a known 3-D structure protein, the tertiary structure of Cur I 3, a major allergen of *Curvalarialunata*, was generated by sequencing homology modeling, and its epitopes were mapped using this structure and T-B-cell and T-cell epitope identification tools (Sharma *et al.*, 2009). Most of the published structure-based prediction methods of conformational epitopes focus on the prediction of antigenicity in the proteins without computational tools specifically developed for prediction of allergenicity (Furmonaviciene *et al.*, 2005; Guarnei *et al.*, 2005; Guarnei *et al.*, 2006). Recently, one tool named SPADE (Surface comparison-based prediction of allergenic discontinuous epitopes, Dall'Antonia *et al.*, 2011) was specifically developed for conformational epitope prediction. The SPADE method uses the quantitative analysis of geometric and physicochemical surface parameters, and the subsequent correlation between surface similarity scores and immunologic data, to extract key features including Cα superposition RMSD (Root Mean Standard Deviation), overall surface similarity, and IgE CR (%) (Cross-Reactivity) from a given protein. This method successfully predicted the IgE-reactive surface portions of two hypoallergenic Bet v 1 isoforms when at least two structural models and IgE reactivity data were available, which was consistent with the result from IgE epitope-mapping studies (Dall'Antonia *et al.*, 2011, 2014).

Local Sequence Alignment using Sequence Identity as a Criterion

Sequence alignment profiles are generally used to infer higher-order structure or function (i.e., secondary and tertiary structures) of proteins because higher-order structure and function largely depend on the arrangement of amino acids. The most widely used pair wise protein sequence comparison methods are local sequence alignment tools such as FASTA (Pearson and Lipman, 1988) and BLAST (Altschul *et al.*, 1990, 1997). For protein allergenicity assessment based on local sequence alignment results, implementation of scientifically justified criteria is essential to facilitate the sequence similarity search and ensure the biological relevance of sequence alignments while maintaining scientifically justified sensitivity and specificity. Evaluation of potential cross-reactivity between a newly expressed protein in a Genetically Modified (GM) food crop and known allergens based on sequence identity generated by local alignment was developed 14 years ago and documented by FAO/WHO/Codex Alimentarius (FAO/WHO, 2001; CODEX, 2009). The FAO/WHO/Codex Alimentarius method specified a threshold of > 35% amino-acid identity over a stretch of 80 amino acids (> 35%/80aa+) for a given alignment between a query protein and known allergens. The original intention was to have a conservative approach that is able to detect known cross-reactive allergens across even the most disparate AA sequences. While the FAO/WHO method recommends that a FASTA or BLAST search be conducted in an 80-mer sliding-window fashion, there is no defined approach in the Codex Alimentarius guideline. Due to the authority and influence of FAO/WHO/Codex Alimentarius, a local sequence alignment with known allergens combined with a criterion of > 35%/80aa+ is currently the most commonly used method of the regulatory assessment of transgenic proteins for potential allergenicity.

In the sliding window search for > 35%/80aa+, a query sequence (> 80 AA) is first parsed into sequentially overlapping stretches of 80 AA long, followed by searching each stretch against an allergen database using FASTA or BLASTp and identifying the alignments with > 35% identity over 80 amino acids or more (due to AA gaps existed in the alignments) regardless of *E*-value associated with the alignments. Over the years, many studies have been conducted to evaluate the performance of the sliding window search for > 35%/80aa+ using local sequence alignment tools such as FASTA. It is widely acknowledged that the sliding window search for > 35%/80aa+ displays a very low specificity in spite of high sensitivity. As such, the sliding window search for > 35%/80aa+ generates many false positives when used for evaluation of novel protein for potential allergenicity (Cressman and Ladics, 2009; Guarneri, 2010; Ladics *et al.*, 2007; Stadler and Stadler, 2003; Silvanovich *et al.*, 2009). One study indicated when the identity threshold was increased from 25 to 70%; the specificity was improved from 20.33 to 99.39% with a slight drop in sensitivity (Wong *et al.*, 2014). Because of its high false-positive rate, a conventional FASTA (using the whole sequence as a query) but still with a criterion of > 35%/80aa+ was proposed to improve the poor specificity of the sliding window method (Cressman and Ladics, 2009; Silvanovich *et al.*, 2009). In retrospect, this high false-positive rate is not surprising because the sliding-window search for > 35%/80aa+ does not take account of the statistical power such as reflected by *E*-values of the local alignment algorithms (e.g., FASTA) available for differentiating true protein relationships from biologically insignificant relationships.

In addition to its high positive rate, the FAO/WHO/Codex Alimentarius threshold of > 35%/80aa+, either achieved by sliding-window or conventional FASTA search, fails to address the following scenarios: (1) when a query sequence has a much higher identity with a known allergen (e.g., 90%) within an alignment of less than 80 amino acids with a known allergen; (2) when a query sequence is shorter than 29 amino acids (29/80 = 35%), which is often the case when evaluating non-intended reading frames generated by transgene insert in a GM event; (3) the effect of variable *E*-value settings when running a local alignment search (e.g., FASTA or BLASTp) on the number of returned alignments containing > 35%/80aa+. In the latter case, for example, the same query protein could sometimes have greater numbers of > 35%/80aa+ alignments with known allergens in a database when a FASTA search was run with an *E*-value set to 100 instead of the default setting of 10. To address the scenarios of > 35% identity over less than 80 amino acids, EFSA specifically requires a conversion to an identity over 80 amino acids (EFSA, 2011). More recent work also raised a question about the ability of the FAO/WHO/Codex Alimentarius criterion (> 35%/80aa+) to detect sequences with very high similarity but low identity (Herman *et al.*, 2015).

To avoid false positive hits, a statistical measurement needs to be taken into account when using local alignment algorithm to evaluate the quality of a given alignment. Two investigations indicated that a combination of a conventional FASTA search of the whole protein sequence with a biologically meaningful *E*-value is superior to the 80-mer sliding window search for > 35%/80aa+ (Ladics *et al.*, 2007; Cressman and Ladics, 2009). The *E*-value or expectation calculated by the local sequence alignment tools is the number of times one would expect to see a score equal to or greater than that is expected by chance alone in a search of a given database (Pearson, 1999). A threshold *E*-value of 3.9 E-07 is sufficiently conservative to identify allergen sequence homology in the Bet v allergen family containing homologous protein sequences associated with known biological cross-reactivity (Silvanovich *et al.*, 2009). Another study indicated that a BLAST search of a full-length protein sequence using an *E*-value of 0.1 as a cut-off achieved the correct recognition of all known allergens with 100% sensitivity and a reduced false positive rate (Guarneri, 2010). However, the *E*-value of a given local sequence alignment changes with the size (number of entries and the number of total amino acids) in the database, as noted in the publication on the FASTA search algorithm (Pearson, 1999): "Because *E* increases linearly with the number of database entries, a similarity found in a search of a bacterial genome with 1000–5000 entries will be 50 to 2500 fold more significant than an alignment with exactly the same score found in the OWL redundant protein database (250,000 entries, Bleasby, 1994). Thus, when searching for very distant relationships, one should always use the smallest database that is likely to contain the homolog of interest". Since a well-managed allergen database is updated periodically (addition of newly discovered allergen sequences, removal of allergens without scientific evidence, or sequence information updates), simply using a fixed E-value as a threshold in assessment of proteins for potential allergenicity may not be appropriate because the degree of significance will change as the size of the database changes.

One way to minimize the effect of database size is through temporarily fixing the database size (number of sequences) at some arbitrary value (-Z) and specifying the statistical calculation (-z) in the options of FASTA algorithm (Andre Silvanovich, pers. comm.). Recently, a novel approach to one-to-one local alignment using FASTA combined with an E-value threshold has been explored to address some of the shortfalls of other approaches involving local sequence alignment (Song *et al.*, 2014). In a one-to-one approach, the E-value of a given alignment between a query protein and a known allergen (in this case, each single allergen in a given database serves as a database and aligned with a query respectively) is fixed according to $E = Dmn2^{-b}$ (D = number of entries in the database; m and n are the number of amino acids from the two sequences involved in an alignment; b = the bit score of the alignment). In contrast to > 35%/80aa+ criterion, irrespective of whether it is derived from 80-mer sliding window or conventional search, the 1:1 FASTA approach eliminates the technical issues resulting from short query sequences (≤ 29 aa) with high identity to known allergens, high identity over less than 80 AA stretches, and different E-value settings when conducting a search. The one-to-one FASTA search displayed sensitivity equivalent to the whole sequence FASTA for > 35%/80aa+ with improved specificity when using an E-value of 1.0 E-9 as a threshold. A further study, using groups of known cross-reactive peanut allergens, indicated the sensitivity of this approach is superior to the conventional FASTA search and equivalent to 80-mer sliding window FASTA search for > 35%/80aa+ recommended by WHO/FAO (Song *et al.*, 2015).

Other sequence based prediction tools

For a cross-reaction to take place between a protein and a known allergen, it is likely that in excess of 50–70% sequence identity over a significant span of the target protein and an allergen is needed (Alberse, 2000). Review of sequence identities among allergenic and non-allergenic homologs of pollen allergens found that at least 50% sequence identity across the length of the protein sequence is the prerequisite for allergenic cross-reactivity between a protein of interest and a known allergen (Radauer and Breitender, 2006). Sliding-window searches for identity over 80 aa+ also indicated that the best accuracy was achieved when the criterion was set to 55% (Wong *et al.*, 2014).

Using the Needleman-Wunsch global alignment algorithm (Needleman and Wunsch, 1970), it was found that ≥ 30% overall identity between a query protein and a known allergen could be used as a threshold for potential cross-reactivity (Song *et al.*, 2014). One weakness of the global alignment is the bias when global alignments are computed between a short query sequence and a known allergen with a much longer length. Thus, direct use of a global alignment tool combined with sequence identity to compare a short query sequence (e.g., a partial protein sequence) with a known allergen might fail to identify cross-reactive allergens that carry significant sequence homology with known allergens.

Instead of using the whole allergen sequences in an allergen database for a sequence alignment search, a modified approach is to use a collection of 24-mer peptides extracted from known allergens and non-allergens as a database. A method of Automated Selection of Allergen-Representative Peptides (ASARP) was used to compile a collection of short Allergen-Representative Peptides (ARPs) (Björklund *et al.*, 2005). In the ASARP, all the peptides with a pre-defined length from two peptide repositories, one from true allergens and the other from proteins without any connection with allergy were first extracted. Next, a similarity score for each peptide extracted from known allergens is computed based on its alignment with each peptide extracted from the non-allergen repository, followed by merging these individual similarity scores into one or several global similarity scores. A set of ARPs were created based on the global similarity scores of each allergen peptide. For protein allergenicity prediction using DASARP (Detection based on ASARP), a query protein is parsed into sequentially overlapping peptides with the same length as the ARPs, followed by extraction of the highest scores and statistical analysis after generation of similarity scores by comparing each peptide with all ARPs using un-gapped alignments. Proteins with a score above the statistic detection threshold are implicated as potential allergens. It was found that the highest detection rates were consistently obtained with a peptide length of 24 amino acids after testing different peptide lengths ranging from 6 to 35 amino acids. DASARP outperformed the simple sliding window search for short-mer matches and yielded results comparable with that using the local alignment for > 35%/80aa+ (FAO/WHO method). When taking account of the E-values of alignments in the test of this method, it was observed that the E-value of 0.001 provided a reasonably high sensitivity of 83.58% with a low false-positive rate of 2.14% (Saha and Raghava, 2006).

Allergenicity prediction using descriptor fingerprints was tested and developed (Dimitrov *et al.*, 2013a, 2013b). In this method, protein sequences of allergens and non-allergens were represented by E-descriptors (Venkatarajan and Braun, 2001) and autocross covariance (ACC) transformation, followed by generation of binary descriptor fingerprints and a Tanimoto coefficient similarity calculation. However, in the leave-one-out cross-validation, the specificity and sensitivity were both less than 90% using this approach.

Future Perspectives

The increasing desire to seek healthy and diversified food sources or ingredients could lead to more novel food, i.e., novel proteins to be brought into the human diet. During the course of introduction of novel proteins for human consumption through food, cosmetics or other modes of contacts, there is a risk for humans to be exposed to new allergens or across-reactive allergens. While new allergens and cross-reactive allergens can be identified after the occurrence of allergenic incidences or clinical cases, a preventive and desirable way is to analyze all the proteins in a food source for their potential allergenicity by means of bioinformatics. Whole genome sequencing by Next-Generation Sequencing (NGS) technology makes such an approach possible. Up to date, genomes from more than 20 food/fruit/vegetable crops, including maize (*Zea mays*), soybean (*Glycine max*), rice (*Orizya sativa* ssp. Japonica and sativa), wheat (*Triticumaestivum*), barley (*Hordeumvulgare*), potato (*Solanum tuberosum*), sorghum (*Sorghum bicolor*), Chinese cabbage (*Brassica rapa*), tomato (*Solanumlycopersicum*), adzuki bean (*Vignaangularis*), banana (*Musaacuminata*), pepper (*Capsicum annuum*), etc. have been sequenced (https://en.wikipedia. org/wiki/List_of_sequenced_plant_genomes). Many genome sequences of animals and fishes have also been published (https://en.wikipedia.org/ wiki/List_of_sequenced_animal_genomes). With the dramatic advance of NGS technology and the decreasing cost of whole genome sequencing, more and more genomes from food/fruit/vegetable crops, fruit trees, animals and fishes will be sequenced. Literally, all the genes that encode proteins in the whole genome of a given food source, plant, animal or fish, etc., can be identified and annotated using modern bioinformatics algorithms. Thus, the potential of an allergenicity risk for a novel food could be evaluated as long as its genome sequence is available. These identified proteins, including the hypothetical ones, can be analyzed using bioinformatics tools for their potential allergenicity to human. The combination of whole genome sequencing and bioinformatics tools for prediction of potential protein allergenicity will add significant value for public health by helping prevent at-risk individuals from being exposed to new allergens or cross-reactive allergens.

Since the publication of the FAO/WHO/Codex Alimentarius guidelines on protein allergenicity assessment for products derived from modern biotechnology, various bioinformatics methods, including motif identification using a collection of known motifs in allergens, SVM-based machine-learning models to detect allergens, IgE epitope identification using physicochemical properties of known allergens, 3-D structure modeling and prediction, and combinations of these approaches, etc., have been evaluated for their application in the prediction of protein allergenicity. The FAO/WHO/Codex Alimentarius suggested criterion of > 35%/80aa+ has become the benchmark used in the regulatory assessment of transgenic protein safety in spite of its drawbacks (Thomas et al., 2007; Ladics, 2008). To overcome the drawbacks caused by a simple search for > 35%/80aa+, a statistical measurement such as *E*-value should be used to determine the biological relevance of sequence alignments between a query protein and allergens. While the current and new bioinformatics methods for prediction of protein allergenicity can be further explored and developed, the 1:1 FASTA with a biologically relevant *E*-value is currently recommended as supplementary to the FAO/WHO method/ criterion due to its simplicity and improved sensitivity and specificity over other approaches. However, one should always keep in mind that protein allergenicity assessment using bioinformatics applications does not confirm allergenicity per se, but instead, it identifies the potential of protein to be allergenic or cross-reactive and guides the design of further allergenicity assessment experiments such as serum screening.

Keywords: Allergenicity, bioinformatics, regulation, alignment, protein, similarity, prediction, database, epitope, allergen, sequences

References

Aalberse, R. C. (2000). Structural biology of allergens. The Journal of Allergy and Clinical Immunology 106: 228–238.

Altschul, S. F., Gish, W., Miller, W., Myers, E. W., and Lipman, D. J. (1990). A basic local alignment search tool. Journal of Molecular Biology 215: 403–410.

Altschul, S. F., Madden, T. L., Schaffer, A. A., Zhang, J., Zhang, Z., Miller, W. *et al.* (1997). Gapped BLAST and PSI-BLAST: a new generation of protein database search programs. Nucleic Acids Research 25: 3389–3402.

Astwood, J. D., Bannon, G. A., Dobertand, R. L., and Fuchs, R. L. (2003). Food biotechnology and genetic engineering. pp. 51–70. *In*: D.D. Metcalfe, H.A. Sampson and R.A. Simon (eds.). Food Allergy, 3rd ed. Blackwell Scientific Inc., Boston, MA, USA.

Bailey, T. L., and Elkan, C. (1994). Fitting a mixture model by expectation maximization to discover motifs in biopolymers. pp. 28–36. *In*: Proceedings of the Second International Conference on the Intelligent Systems for Molecular Biology. AAAI Press. Menlo Park, CA, USA.

Bailey, T. L., and Gribskov, M. (1998). Combining evidence using *P*-values: application to sequence homology searches. Bioinformatics 14: 48–54.

Bannon, G. A. (2004). What makes a food protein an allergen? Current Allergy and Asthma Reports 4: 43–46.

Bannon, G., and Ogawa, T. (2006). Evaluation of available IgE-binding epitope data and its utility in bioinformatics. Molecular Nutrition & Food Research 50: 638–644.

Björklund, Å. K., Soeria-Atmadja, D., Zorzet, A., Hammerling, U., and Gustadsson, M. B. (2005). Supervised identification of allergen-representative peptides for *in silico* detection of potentially allergenic proteins. Bioinformatics 21: 39–50.

Branum, A., and Lukacs, S. (2008). Food allergy among U.S. children: Trends in prevalence and hospitalizations. National Center for Health Statistics Data Brief 2008. (http://www.cdc.gov/nchs/data/databriefs/db10.htm)

Codex Alimentarius Commission. (2009). Assessment of possible allergenicity. pp. 20–23. *In*: Foods Derived from Modern Biotechnology. World Health Organization, Food and Agricultural Organization of the United Nations. Rome, Italy.

Cortes, C., and Vapnik, V. (1995). Support-vector networks. Machine Learning 20: 273–297.

Cressman, R. F., and Ladics, G. S. (2009). Further evaluation of the utility of "sliding window" FASTA in predicting cross-reactivity with allergenic proteins. Regulatory Toxicology and Pharmacology 54: 20–25.

Cui, J., Han, L. Y., Lin, H., Ung, C. Y., Tang, Z. Q., Zheng, C. J., Cao, Z. W., and Chen, Y. Z. (2007). Computer prediction of allergen proteins from sequence-derived protein structural and physicochemical properties. Journal of Molecular Immunology 44: 514–520.

Dall'Antonia, F., Gieras, A., Devanaboyina, S. C., Valenta, R., and Keller, W. (2011). Prediction of IgE-binding epitopes by means of allergen surface comparison and correlation to cross-reactivity. Journal of Allergy and Clinical Immunology 28: 872–879.

Dall'Antonia, F., Pavkov-Keller, T., Znager, K., and Keller, W. (2014). Structure of allergens and structure based epitope predictions. Methods 66: 3–21.

Dang, H. X., and Lawrence, C. B. (2014). Allerdictor: fast allergen prediction using text classification techniques. Bioinformatics 30: 1120–1128.

Dimitrov, I., Naneva, L., Doytchinova, I., and Bangov, I. (2013a). Allergen FP: allergenicity prediction by descriptor fingerprints. Bioinformatics 30: 846–851.

Dimitrov, I., Flower, D. R., and Doytchinova, I. (2013b). AllerTOP—a server for *in silico* prediction of allergens. BMC Bioinformatics 14(Suppl 6): S4.

EFSA. (2010). EFSA Panel on GMOs: Scientific opinion on the assessment of allergenicity of GM plants and microorganisms and derived food and feed. EFSA Journal 8: 1168.

EFSA. (2011). Guidance for risk assessment of food and feed from genetically modified plants. EFSA Journal 9: 2150.

FAO/WHO. (2001). Evaluation of allergenicity of genetically modified foods. pp. 22–25. *In*: Report of a Joint FAO/WHO Expert Consulation on Allergenicity of Foods Derived from Biotechnology, FAO/WHO. Rome, Italy.

Fiers, M. W., Kleter, G. A., Nijland, H., Peijnenburg, A. A., Nap, J. P., and van Ham, R. C. (2004). Allermatch, a web tool for the prediction of potential allergenicity according to current FAO/WHO Codex Alimentarius guideline. BMC Bioinformatics 5: 133.

Furmonaviciene, R., Sutton, B. J., Glaser, F., Laughton, C. A., Jones, N., Sewell, H. F. *et al.* (2005). An attempt to define allergen-specific molecular surface features: a bioinformatics approach. Bioinformatics 21: 4201–4204.

Gendel, S. M., and Jenkins, J. A. (2006). Allergen sequence database. Molecular Nutrition and Food Research 50: 633–637.

Gendel, S. M. (2009). Allergen Databases and allergen semantics. Regulatory Toxicology and Pharmacology 54: S7–S10.

Goodman, R. E., Vieth, S., Sampson, H. A., Hill, D., Ebisawa, M., Taylor, S. L., and Van, R. R. (2008). Allergenicity assessment of genetically modified crops—what makes sense? Nature Biotechnology 296: 73–81.

Guarneri, F., Guarneri, C., and Benvenga, S. (2005). Identification of potentially cross-reactive peanut-lupine proteins by computer-assisted search for amino acid sequence homology. International Archives of Allergy and Immunology 138: 273–277.

Guarneri, F., Guarneri, C., Guarneri, B., and Benvenga, S. (2006). *In silico* identification of potential new latex allergens. Clinical and Experimental Allergy 36: 916–919.

Guarneri, F. (2010). *In silico* allergen identification: proposal for a revision of FAO/WHO guideline. Atti della Accademia Peloritana dei Pericolanti - Classe di Scienze Fisiche, Matematiche e Naturali 88: C1A1002006.

Gupta, R. S., Springston, M. R., Warrier, B. S., Rajesh, K., Pongracic, J., and Holl, J. L. (2011). The prevalence, severity, and distribution of childhood food allergy in the United States. Journal of Pediatric 128: e9–e17.

Herman, R. A., Song, P., and Thirumalaiswamy, A. S. (2009). Value of eight-amino-acid matches in predicting the allergenicity status of proteins: an empirical bioinformatics investigation. Clinical and Molecular Allergy 7: 9 [DOI:10.1186/1476-7961-7-9].

Herman, R. A., and Ladics, G. S. (2014). Endogenous allergen upregulation: Transgenic vs. traditionally bred crops. Food and Chemical Toxicology 49: 2667–2669.

Herman, R. A., Song, P., and Kumpatla, S. (2015). Percent amino-acid identity thresholds are not necessarily conservative for predicting allergenic cross-reactivity. Food and Chemical Toxicology 81: 141–142.

Hopp, T. P., and Woods, K. R. (1981). Prediction of protein antigenic determinants from amino acid sequences. Proceedings of the National Academy of Sciences USA 78: 3824–3828.

Ivanciuc, O., Catherine, H. S., and Braun, W. (2003). SDAP: database and computational tools for allergenic proteins. Nucleic Acids Research 31: 359–362.

Ivanciuc, O., Mathura, V., Midoro-Horiuti, T., Braun, W., Goldblum, R. M., and Schen, C. H. (2003). Detecting potential IgE sites on food proteins using a sequence and structure database, SADP-food. Journal of Agricultural and Food Chemistry 51: 4830–4837.

Ivanciuc, O., Garcia, T., Torres, M., Schen, C. H., and Braun, W. (2009). Characteristic motifs for families of allergenic proteins. Molecular Immunology 46: 559–568.

Ivanciuc, O., Schen, C. H., Gacia, T., Oezguen, N., Negi, S. S., and Braun, W. (2009). Structural analysis of linear and conformational epitopes of allergens. Regulatory Toxicology and Pharmacology 54: 511–519.

Ivanciuc, O., Gacia, T., Torres, M., Schen, C. H., Xie, L., Hillman, G., R. M. *et al.* (2009). The property distance index PD predicts peptides that cross-react with IgE antibodies. Molecular Immunology 46: 873–883.

Joachims, T. (1999). Making large-scale SVM learning practical. pp. 169–184. *In*: B. Schölkopf, C.J.C. Burges and A.J. Smola (eds.). Advances in Kernel Methods Support Vector Learning. MIT Press, Cambridge, MA USA and London.

Kleter, G. A., and Peijnenburg, Ad A. C. M. (2003). Presence of potential allergy-related linear epitopes in novel proteins from conventional crops and the implication for the safety assessment of these crops with respect to the current testing of genetically modified crops. Plant Biotechnology Journal 1: 371–380.

Ladics, G. S., Bannon, G. A., Silvanovich, A., and Cressman, R. R. (2007). Comparison of conventional FASTA identity searches with the 80 amino acid sliding window FASTA search for the elucidation of potential identities to known allergens. Molecular Nutrition and Food Research 51: 985–998.

Ladics, G. S. (2008). Current CODEX guidelines for assessment of potential protein allergenicity. Food and Chemical Toxicology 46: S22–S23.

Ladics, S. G., Fry, J., Goodman, R., Herouet-Guicheney, C., Hoffmann-Sommergruber, K., Madsen, C. B. *et al.* (2014). Allergic sensitization: screening methods. Clinical and Translational Allergy 4: 13–18.

Li, K. B., Issac, P., and Krishnan, A. (2004). Predicting allergenic proteins using wavelet transform. Bioinformatics 20: 2572–2578.

Lim, S. J., Tong, J. C., Chew, F. T., and Tammi, M. (2008). The value of position-specific scoring metrics for assessment of protein allergenicity. BMC Bioinformatics 9: S21 [DOI: 10.1186/1471-2105-9-S12-S21].

Liu, A. H., Jaramillo, R., Sicherer, S. H., Wood, R. A., Bock, A. B., Burks, A. W. *et al.* (2010). National prevalence and risk factors for food allergy and relationships to asthma: Results from the National Health and Nutrition Examination Survey 2005–2006. The Journal of Allergy and Clinical Immunology 126: 798–806.

Marchler-Bauer, A., Panchenko, A. R., Shoemaker, B. A., Thiessen, P., Geer, L. Y., and Bryant, S. H. (2002). CDD: a database of conserved domain alignments with links to domain three-dimensional structure. Nucleic Acids Research 30: 281–3.

Mari, A., Scal, E., Palazzo, P., Ridolfi, S., Zennaro, D., and Carabella, G. (2006). Bioinformatics applied to allergy: Allergen database, from collecting sequence information to data integration. The Allergome platform as a model. Cellular Immunology 244: 97–100.

Mari, A., Rasi, C., and Palazzo, P. (2009). Allergen databases: current status and perspectives. Current Allergy and Asthma Reports 9: 376–383.

Metcalfe, D. D., Astwood, J. D., Townsend, R., Sampson, H. A., Taylor, S. L., and Fuchs, R. L. (1996). Assessment of the allergenic potential of foods derived from genetically engineered crop plants. Critical Reviews in Food Science and Nutrition 36: S165–S186.

Muh, H. C., Tong, J. C., and Tammi, M. T. (2009). AllerHunter: A SVM-poairwise system for assessment of allergenicity and allergic cross-reactivity in proteins. PloS One 4: e5861.

Needleman, S. B., and Wunsch, C. D. (1970). A general method applicable to the search for similarities in the amino acid sequence of two proteins. Journal of Molecular Biology 48: 443–453.

Pearson, W. R., and Lipman, D. J. (1988). Improved tools for biological sequence comparison. Proc. Natl. Acad. Sci. USA 85: 2444–2448.

Pearson, W. R. (1999). Flexible Sequence similarity searching with the FASTA3 program package. Methods in Molecular Biology 132: 185–219.

Pomés, A. (2010). Relevant B cell epitopes in allergic disease. International Archives of Allergy and Immunology 152: 1–11.

Radauer, C., and Breiteneder, H. (2006). Pollen allergens are restricted to few protein families and show distinct patterns of species distribution. The Journal of Allergy and Clinical Immunology 117: 141–147.

Randhawa, G. J., Singh, M., and Grover, M. (2011). Bioinformatic analysis for allergenicity assessment of *Bacillus thuringiensis* Cryproteins expressed in insect-resistant food crops. Food and Chemical Toxicology 49: 356–362.

Riaz, T., Hor, H. L., Krishnan, A., Tang, F., and Li, K. B. (2005). Web Allergen: a web server for predicting allergenic proteins. Bioinformatics 21: 2570–2671.

Saha, S., and Raghava, G. P. S. (2006). AlgPred: prediction of allergenic proteins and mapping of IgE epitopes. Nucleic Acids Research 34: W202–W209.

Sampson, H. A. (2004). Update on food allergy. The Journal of Allergy and Clinical Immunology 113: 805–809.

Sharma, V., Singh, B. P., Gaur, S. N., Pasha, S., and Arora, N. (2009). Bioinformatics and immunologic investigation on B and T cell epitopes of *Cur l 3*, a major allergen of *Curvularialunata*. Journal of Proteome Research 8: 2650–2655.

Sicherer, S. H., and Sampson, H. A. (2010). Food allergy. Journal of Allergy and Clinical Immunology 125: S116–S125.

Sicherer, S. H. (2011). Epidemiology of food allergy. Journal of Allergy and Clinical Immunology 127: 594–602.

Silvanovich, A., Nemeth, M. A., Song, P., Herman, R., Tagliani, L., and Bannon, G. (2006). The value of short amino acid sequence matches for prediction of protein allergenicity. Toxicological Sciences 90: 252–258.

Soeria-Atmadja, D., Zorzet, A., Gustafsson, M. G., and Hammerling, U. (2004). Statistical evaluation of local alignment features predicting allergenicity using supervised classification algorithms. International Archives of Allergy and Immunology 133: 101–112.

Soeria-Atmadja, D., Wallman, M., Björklund, Å. K., Isaksson, A., Hammerling, U., and Gustadsson, M. G. (2005). External cross-validation for unbiased evaluation of protein family detectors: application to allergens. Proteins: Structure, Function, and Bioinformatics 61: 918–925.

Soeria-Atmadja, D., Lundell, T., Gustadsson, M. G., and Hammerling, U. (2006). Computational detection of allergenic proteins attains a new level of accuracy with *in silico* variable-length peptide extraction and machine learning. Nucleic Acids Research 13: 3779–3793.

Song, P., Herman, R. A., and Kumpatla, S. (2014). Evaluation of global sequence comparison and 1:1 FASTA local alignment in regulatory allergenicity assessment of transgenic proteins in food crops. Food Chemistry Toxicology 71: 142–148.

Song, P. (2015). Bioinformatics application in regulatory assessment for potential allergenicity of transgenic proteins in food crops. pp. 397–411. *In*: R.R. Watson and V.R. Reedy (eds.). Genetically Modified Organisms in Food, Production, Safety, Regulation and Public Health. Academic Press. Waltham, MA, USA.

Song, P., Herman, R. A., and Kumpatla, S. (2015). 1:1 FASTA update: Using the power of E-values in FASTA to detect potential allergen cross-reactivity. Toxicology Reports 2: 1145–1148.

Stadler, M. B., and Stadler, B. M. (2003). Allergenicity prediction by protein sequence. FASEB Journal 17: 1141–1143.

Thomas, K., Herouet-Guicheney, C., Ladics, G., McClain, S., MacIntosh, S., Privalle, L., and Woolhiser, M. (2008). Current and future methods for evaluating the allergenic potential of proteins: International workshops report 23–25 October 2007. Food and Chemical Toxicology 46: 3219–3225.

Thompson, J. D., Higgins, D. G., and Gibson, T. J. (1994). CLUSTAL W: improving the sensitivity of progressive multiple sequence alignment through sequence weighting, position-specific gap penalties and weight matrix choice. Nuclear Acids Research 22: 4673–4680.

Van Regenmortel, M. H. V. (1999). Mapping epitope structure and activity: from one-dimensional prediction to four-dimensional description of antigenic specificity. Methods 9: 465–472.

Vapnik, V., Golowich, S. E., and Smola, A. (1995). Support vector method for function approximation, regression estimation and signal processing. pp. 281–287. *In*: M.C. Mozer,

M.I. Jordan and T. Petsche (eds.). Advances in Neural Information Processing Systems 9: Proceedings of the 1996 Conference. MIT Press, Cambridge, MA, USA.

Venkatarajan, M. S., and Braun, W. (2001). New quantitative descriptors of amino acids based on multidimensional scaling of a large number of physical-chemical properties. J. Mol. Model 7: 445–453.

Verma, A. K., Misra, A., Subash, S., Das, M., and Dwivedi, P. D. (2011). Computational allergenicity prediction of transgenic proteins expressed in genetically modified crops. Immunopharmacology and Immunotoxicology 33: 410–422.

Vieths, S., Scheurer, S., and Ballmar-Weber, B. (2002). Current understanding of cross-reactivity of food allergens and pollen. Annals of the New York Academy of Sciences 964: 47–68.

Wang, J., Yu, Y., Zhao, Y., Zhang, D., and Li, J. (2014). Evaluation and integration of existing methods for computational prediction of allergens. BMC Bioinformatics 14 (Suppl 4): S1.

Zhang, L., Huang, Y., Zou, Z., He, Y., Chen, X., and Tao, A. (2012). SORTALLER: predicting allergens using substantially optimized algorithm on allergen family featured peptides. Bioinformatics 28: 2178–2179.

Zorzet, A., Gustafsson, M. G., and Hammerling, U. (2002). Prediction of food protein allergenicity: a bio-informatic learning systems approach. *In Silico* Biology 2: 525–534.

Zou, Z., He, Y., Ruan, L., Sun, B., Chen, H., Chen, D. *et al.* (2012). A bioinformatics evaluation of potential allergenicity of 85 candidate genes in transgenic organisms. Chinese Science Bulletin 57: 1824–1832.

CHAPTER 13

The Pollen-Food Syndrome
A Molecular Perspective

Claudia Asam, Lorenz Aglas, Sara Huber, Fátima Ferreira and *Anargyros Roulias**

Introduction

The allergy towards various foods is a global health issue, and the prevalence in both developed and developing countries is still rising. Approximately 3% of the population is affected by IgE-associated food allergies (Valenta *et al.*, 2015). The 287 food allergens so far identified and acknowledged by the WHO/IUIS nomenclature sub-committee (www.allergen.org) can be classified into two groups depending on the sensitization process that initiates allergic diseases. Class I food allergens are the elicitors of classical food allergies where it is thought that the primary sensitization takes place in the gastrointestinal tract directed against these rather stable food allergens. In contrast, allergies against class II food allergens are pollen-related and primary sensitization is considered to be induced from inhaled aeroallergens such as pollen allergens. The cross-reaction is based on the binding of an IgE antibody, primarily produced against an aeroallergen, to homologous structures on a—not necessarily botanically related—food allergen (Egger *et al.*, 2006). Notably, the reactions against the concerned food allergens can occur already after the first ingestion of this food, as the sensitization can have already happened against another allergen (Kelso *et al.*, 1998). The prevalence for pollen-food allergies can show rather large variations according to the geographic area and the methodology used to diagnose the allergy. It is estimated that 60% of food allergies in older children

Department of Molecular Biology, University of Salzburg, Hellbrunnerstrasse 34, 5020 Salzburg, Austria.
Emails: Claudia.Asam@sbg.ac.at; Lorenz.Aglas@sbg.ac.at; Sara.Huber@sbg.ac.at; Fatima.Ferreira@sbg.ac.at
* Corresponding author: Anargyros.Roulias@sbg.ac.at

and adults are associated with cross-reactions to inhalant allergies (Werfel *et al.*, 2015). Therefore, it should be kept in mind that the increasing numbers of pollen allergic patients will certainly be followed by increasing numbers of patients suffering from pollen-food syndromes. The onset of the symptoms usually starts minutes after ingestion of the food. Most frequent occurrences include local reactions restricted to the oral mucosa; however, also rare systemic reactions like anaphylaxis can be induced. Usually, the symptoms gradually resolve themselves after minutes to hours (Sampson, 1999). With regards to the source of food allergens, 90% of the class I food allergens can be clustered into the "big 8", while a view on class II food allergens shows quite a heterologous picture and clustering them in protein families is more reasonable (www.fda.gov). Within this chapter, we will focus on class II food allergens involved in pollen-food syndromes and give a comprehensive overview on the main concerned protein families.

Historical Background

In the early 1940s, the observation that there is a link between seasonal allergies and hypersensitivity reactions towards food was stated several times (Tuft and Blumstein, 1942). A scientist in 1948 observed that patients allergic to pollen from catkin-bearing trees developed compromising reactions in the mouth after eating hazelnuts, and similar symptoms after eating raw apples (Kelso, 2000). Now we know that he described the cross-reactivity between allergens belonging to the pathogenesis-related protein family 10 (PR-10) from Fagales tree pollen (especially birch) and a variety of nuts, fresh fruits, and vegetables. In 1987 Amlot *et al.* defined in a study with 80 highly atopic patients the term "oral allergy syndrome". It was characterized by oral mucosal symptoms that occasionally spread to the body, triggered by the exposure to food and the thereby IgE-induced release of mediators. It often correlated with positive skin prick tests to food allergens. However, no detailed description of the food allergens was made, and no concomitant allergies of the patients towards inhaled allergens were mentioned (Amlot *et al.*, 1987). One year later Ortolani *et al.* reported on 262 birch pollinosis patients showing symptoms similar to the oral cavity restricted symptoms, as described by Amlot *et al.* after eating fruits and vegetables. By naming these findings including OAS they correlated the term with localized oral symptoms of pollen allergic patients after ingesting fruits and vegetables (Kondo and Urisu, 2009; Ortolani *et al.*, 1988). Since then some confusion and controversy about the term OAS existed as some scientists and authors used the term under different definitions, i.e., Liccardi *et al.* described oral symptoms towards egg allergens also as OAS, which would rather belong to classical food allergies, setting off a discussion with Kelso (Kelso, 1995; Liccardi and D'Amato, 1994). To avoid further confusions, the terms "pollen-food syndrome" (PFS) or "pollen-food allergy syndrome" (PFAS) seemed like a proper improvement; more descriptive and specific. This way, describing cross-reactive allergic reactions to plant-derived food allergens that were primarily induced by sensitization towards aeroallergens would be less confusing. The advantage of this new terminology was also the inclusion of less common systemic reactions towards some pollen-related food allergens, since the OAS was, by definition, restricted to the oral cavity (Lessof, 1996).

As previously mentioned, clustering the PFS-eliciting group 2 food allergens into protein families is less heterologous than bundling them by source. Next the relevant protein families and their allergens will be discussed in more detail.

Molecular Background of Allergens Involved in the Pollen-Food Syndrome

Allergic reactions to one food allergen can be triggered by various aeroallergen sources, as different sensitizing protein families can be involved in the sensitization process and these different protein families could have a homolog in the concerned food. This is the case for apple, which could cross-react with the profilin or the PR-10 protein from birch, as well as the non-specific Lipid Transfer Protein (nsLTP) from the grass. This example shows the necessity of knowledge about the composition of the allergenic source on a molecular level (Andersen *et al.*, 2011). This necessity is also highlighted in the case of peach allergy where allergens from three different protein families are involved, more than one sensitization route has been observed, and even severe symptoms can be elicited (Price *et al.*, 2015).

Pathogenesis-Related Protein Family 10 (PR-10)

Properties and function of PR-10 proteins

To protect themselves against ubiquitous infections, plants have developed several mechanisms. One of these mechanisms is the pathogen- and stress-driven induction of gene-expression of so-called Pathogen-Related (PR) proteins participating in general defense. Currently, PR proteins are divided into 17 classes, while many common food and aeroallergens belonging to PR proteins are clustered in the PR-10 family. The first identified PR-10 protein was found in parsley, followed by several common allergens (Sinha *et al.*, 2014). The PR-10 proteins are encoded by a diverse multigene family, sharing a small size of around 160 amino acids and a similar molecular mass of around 17 kDa. They exhibit a similar secondary structure and appear usually intracellular and cytosolic. Three α-helices embedded in an antiparallel β-sheet consisting of 7 β-strands constitute their 3D fold with an amphiphilic Y-shaped intrinsic cavity traversing their core. This pocket-like structure is solvent-accessible via, in most cases, two to three openings on the surface. This unique structural feature may be the key for unraveling the biological function of PR-10 proteins (Fernandes *et al.*, 2013). In a detailed crystallographical analysis of the major birch pollen allergen Bet v 1 together with a wide spectrum of ligands, it was reported that the binding pocket of Bet v 1 comprises a promiscuous ligand-complex binding site. Moreover, depending on different isoforms and the presence of other ligands, varying binding modes of Bet v 1 could be found (Kofler *et al.*, 2012). Recently the glycosylated flavonol quercetin-3-O-sophoroside (Q3OS) was found to be a physiological ligand of Bet v 1 (Seutter von Loetzen *et al.*, 2014). However, the precise function of several PR-10 proteins still remains elusive. A sub-class of PR-10 proteins exhibits a group of food and pollen proteins with allergenic characteristics.

Sensitizing PR-10 molecules

Belonging to the botanical order of Fagales, birch (*Betula verrucosa*) and the related tree species alder (*Alnus glutinosa*), hornbeam (*Carpinus betulus*), hop-hornbeam (*Ostrya carpinifolia*), hazelnut (*Corylus avellana*), beech (*Fagus sylvatica*), chestnut (*Castanea sativa*) and oak (*Quercus alba*) represent the main elicitors of early seasonal rhinitis in the temperate climate zone of the northern hemisphere (D'Amato *et al.*, 1998). Fagales trees can be found nearly all around the globe while almost all species prefer a temperate climate, especially in northern America and Europe (Asam *et al.*, 2015). The major allergens from Fagales trees are Aln g 1, Bet v 1, Car b 1, Cas s 1, Cor a 1, Fag s 1, Ost c 1 and Que a 1 with Bet v 1 being generally acknowledged as the main sensitizer and marker allergen of this family. However, inhibition experiments revealed that, beside birch, several other Fagales species might have the potential to (co-)sensitize susceptible individuals (Hauser *et al.*, 2011). A high percentage of Fagales allergic patients develop oral reactions against a variety of fresh fruits, nuts and vegetables.

Cross-Reactive Foods

Fruits from the orders Rosales (e.g., apple, cherry, strawberry), Solanales (tomato) and Ericales (kiwi), vegetables from the order Apiales (carrot, celery) as well as nuts from Fagales (hazelnut) and pulses from Fabales (mung bean, soy, peanut) are implicated in cross-reactivities towards IgE antibodies initially produced against Fagales pollen allergens (Table 13.1). Several studies showed that, due to the weak resistance against heat and pepsin digestion of PR-10 proteins, patients could tolerate these foods after cooking (Andersen *et al.*, 2011).

Clinical Manifestations

Among birch pollen allergic patients more than 90% are sensitized to the major birch pollen allergen Bet v 1. Approximately 70% of birch pollen

Table 13.1: Molecule based pollen-food association.
o, +, x: suggested, but not proven, allergens from the PR10, Profilin and nsLTP family, respectively, at the end of the table.
a-i: letter code indicating proven cross-reactivities between PFS sensitizers and associated plant foods.
All proteins listed are based on WHO/IUIS nomenclature subcommittee acknowledged entries.

Protein Family	PFS sensitizer Source Molecule		Association Food Molecule		Symptoms	Evidence strength factor	References
PR10°	European white birch *Betula verrucosa*	Bet v 1[a]					
			Apple *Malus domestica*	Mal d 1[a]	OAS	Inhibition IB	(Chang et al., 2005; Ebner et al., 1991; Mauro et al., 2011; Sinha et al., 2014; Vanek-Krebitz et al., 1995)
			Carrot *Daucus carota*	Dau c 1[a]	Oral and/or systemic	Inhibition IB	(Bollen et al., 2007; Hoffmann-Sommergruber et al., 1999)
			Celery *Apium graveolens*	Api g 1[a]	Oral and/or systemic	Inhibition IB	(Bollen et al., 2007; Breiteneder et al., 1995; Luttkopf et al., 2000)
			Gold kiwi *Actinidia chinensis*	Act c 8[a]	Oral and/or systemic	Inhibition IB, Inhibition ELISA	(Lucas et al., 2004; Oberhuber et al., 2008)
			Hazelnut *Corylus avellana*	Cor a 1.04[a]	OAS	Microarray	(De Knop et al., 2011)
			Kiwi *Actinidia deliciosa*	Act d 8[a]	Oral and/or systemic	Inhibition IB, Inhibition ELISA	(Lucas et al., 2004; Oberhuber et al., 2008)
			Mung bean *Vigna radiata*	Vig r 1[a]	OAS	Inhibition IB	(Mittag et al., 2005)
			Peach *Prunus persica*	Pru p 1[a]	OAS	Inhibition IB	(Gaier et al., 2008; Gamboa et al., 2007; Pastorello et al., 1994)
			Peanut *Arachis hypogaea*	Ara h 8[a]	OAS	RAST inhibition assay	(Hurlburt et al., 2013; Mittag et al., 2004)
			Pear *Pyrus communis*	Pyr c 1[a]	OAS	Inhibition IB	(Karamloo et al., 2001)

	Food source	Allergen	Oral or systemic (sometimes severe)	Method	References
	Soybean *Glycine max*	Gly m 4[a]	OAS	Histamine release assay, Inhibition IB	(Berkner et al., 2009; Julka et al., 2012)
	Strawberry *Fragaria ananassa*	Fra a 1[a]	OAS	Inhibition IB, Basophil degranulation assay	(Karlsson et al., 2004)
	Sweet cherry *Prunus avium*	Pru av 1[a]	OAS	Inhibition IB, Histamine release assay	(Neudecker et al., 2001; Scheurer et al., 1997; Scheurer et al., 1999)
	Tomato *Solanum lycopersicum*	Sola l 4[a]	OAS	Inhibition ELISA, Inhibition IB	(Wangorsch et al., 2015)
Profilin+	Apple *Malus domestica*	Mal d 4[b]	OAS	IB, ImmunoCAP	(Cudowska et al., 2005; Rossi et al., 1996)
European white birch *Betula verrucosa* — Bet v 2[b]	Banana *Musa acuminata*	Mus a 1[b]	OAS (systemic reactions possible)	Inhibition IB, EAST inhibition	(Reindl et al., 2002)
Bermuda grass *Cynodon dactylon* — Cyn d 12[c]	Carrot *Daucus Carota*	Dau c 4[b,d]	OAS	Inhibition IB	(Ballmer-Weber et al., 2001)
Mugwort *Artemisia vulgaris* — Art v 4[d]	Celery *Apium graveolens*	Api g 4[b,d]	OAS	Inhibition IB, Histamine release assay	(Luttkopf et al., 2000; Niederberger et al., 1998; Pauli et al., 1988; Scheurer et al., 2000; Scheurer et al., 2001; Vallier et al., 1988)
Olive *Olea europea* — Ole e 2[e]	Kiwi fruit *Actinidia deliciosa*	Act d 9[b,f]	OAS	Inhibition IB	(Pastorello et al., 1996)
Timothy *Phleum pratense* — Phl p 12[f]					

Table 13.1 contd. ....

... Table 13.1 contd.

Protein Family	PFS sensitizer Source Molecule	Association Food Molecule	Symptoms	Evidence strength factor	References
		Litchi *Litchi chinensis* Lit c 1[b]	OAS, U	Inhibition IB, Inhibition ELISA	(Song et al., 2007)
		Muskmelon *Cucumis melo* Cuc m 2[b,c,f]	OAS	Inhibition ELISA	(Sankian et al., 2005; Tordesillas et al., 2010)
		Peach *Prunus persica* Pru p 4[b,e]	OAS, U	IB	(Rodriguez-Perez et al., 2003; van Ree et al., 1995; Vieths et al., 2002)
		Peanut *Arachis hypogaea* Ara h 5[b,f]	OAS	Microarray assay	(Bublin and Breiteneder, 2014; Cabanos et al., 2010)
		Pear *Pyrus communis* Pyr c 4[b]	OAS	Inhibition IB, Histamine release assay	(Scheurer et al., 2001)
		Pineapple *Ananas comosus* Ana c 1[b]	OAS	Inhibition IB, EAST inhibition	(Reindl et al., 2002)
		Soybean *Glycine max* Gly m 3[b]	OAS	EAST inhibition	(Rihs et al., 1999)
		Sweet cherry *Prunus avium* Pru av 4[b]	OAS	Inhibition IB, Histamine release assay	(Scheurer et al., 2001)
		Sweet orange *Citrus sinensis* Cit s 2[b]	OAS (systemic reactions possible)	Histamine release assay	(Crespo et al., 2006; Lopez-Torrejon et al., 2005; Sloane and Sheffer, 2001)
		Tomato *Solanum lycopersicum* Sola l 1[b]	OAS (systemic reactions possible)	Inhibition ELISA	(Foetisch et al., 2001; Westphal et al., 2004)

nsLTPs[x]					
London plane tree *Platanus acerifolia*		Pla a 3[g]			
Mugwort *Artemisia vulgaris*		Art v 3[h]			
Olive *Olea europea*		Ole e 7[i]			
	Apple *Malus domestica*	Mal d 3[h]	A, U	ELISA inhibition assay	(Diaz-Perales *et al.*, 2000; Gomez *et al.*, 2014)
	Cabbage *Brassica oleracea*	Bra o 3[h]	A, OAS, U	CAP-inhibition assay	(Palacin *et al.*, 2006)
	Celery *Apium graveolens*	Api g 2[h]	A, OAS, ANG	SPHIAa	(Gadermaier *et al.*, 2011)
	Chestnut *Castanea sativa*	Cas s 8[h]	A, OAS, U, ANG	ELISA inhibition assay	(Diaz-Perales *et al.*, 2000; Sanchez-Monge *et al.*, 2006)
	Hazelnut *Corylus avellana*	Cor a 8[h]	A, U, ANG, V, B	Inhibition assay	(Flinterman *et al.*, 2008; Le *et al.*, 2013b)
	Gold Kiwi *Actinidia chinensis*	Act c 10[h]	OAS	microarray SPHIAa	(Bernardi *et al.*, 2011; Le *et al.*, 2013a)
	Kiwi *Actinidia deliciosa*	Act d 10[h]	OAS	SPHIAa	(Bernardi *et al.*, 2011; Le *et al.*, 2013a)
	Lettuce *Lactuca sativa*	Lac s 1[g,h]	A	Inhibition IB	(Bascones *et al.*, 2009; Hartz *et al.*, 2007; San Miguel-Moncin *et al.*, 2003)
	Mulberry *Morus nigra*	Mor n 3[h]	A, OAS, U	SPHIAa	(Ciardiello *et al.*, 2010)
	Peach *Prunus persica*	Pru p 3[g,h]	A, OAS	ELISA inhibition assay	(Diaz-Perales *et al.*, 2000; Gadermaier *et al.*, 2009; Lauer *et al.*, 2007; Lombardero *et al.*, 2004; Sanchez-Lopez *et al.*, 2012; Pascal *et al.*, 2014; Uasuf *et al.*, 2015)

Table 13.1 contd....

...Table 13.1 contd.

Protein Family	PFS sensitizer Source Molecule	Association Food Molecule	Symptoms	Evidence strength factor	References
		Peanut *Arachis hypogaea*	Ara h 9[h]	A, OAS, U, ANG	SPT, ImmunoCap	(Garcia-Blanca et al., 2015)
		Pomegranate *Punica granatum*	Pun g 1[bi]	A, U, ANG, V, B	Inhibition IB	(Almeida et al., 2015)
		Wheat *Triticum aestivum*	Tri a 14[h]	A	SPT, specific IgE ELISA	(Palacin et al., 2010)

°Alder (*Alnus glutinosa*) Aln g 1; Hornbeam (*Carpinus betulus*) Car b 1; Chestnut (*Castanea sativa*) Cas s 1; Hazel (*Corylus avellana*) Cor a 1.01; European beech (*Fagus sylvatica*) Fag s 1; White oak (*Quercus alba*) Que a 1; European hop-hornbeam (*Ostrya carpinfolia*) Ost c 1 (Hauser et al., 2011; Kos et al., 1993; Niederberger et al., 1998).

⁺Annual mercury (*Mercurialis annua*) Mer a 1; Barley (*Hordeum vulgare*) Hor v 12; Burning bush (*Kochia scoparia*) Koc s 2; English plantain (*Plantago lanceolata*) Pla l 2, Hazel (*Corylus avellana*) Cor a 2; Lambsquarters (*Chenopodium album*) Che a 2; Mesquite (*Prosopis juliflora*) Pro j 2; Needle bush (*Acacia farnesiana*) Aca f 2; Para rubber tree (latex) (*Hevea brasiliensis*) Hev b 8; Pellitory-of-the-Wall (*Parietaria Judaica*) Par j 3; Redroot pigweed (*Amaranthus retroflexus*) Ama r 2; Rice (*Oryza sativa*) Ory s 12; Russian thistle (*Salsola kali*) Sal k 4; Saffron crocus (*Crocus sativus*) Cro s 2; Short ragweed (*Ambrosia artemisiifolia*) Amb a 8; Wheat (*Triticum aestivum*) Tri a 12.

ˣOriental plane (*Platanus orientalis*) Pla or 3; Short ragweed (*Ambrosia artemisiifolia*) Amb a 6; Pellitory-of-the-wall (*Parietaria judaica*) Par j 1, Par j 2; Pellitory (*Parietaria officinalis*) Par o 1.

*Oral allergy syndrome (**OAS**); anaphylaxis (**A**); urticaria (**U**); angioedema (**ANG**); vomiting (**V**); and bronchoconstriction (**B**); Immunoblot (**IB**); Basophil activation test (**BAT**); Skin prick test (**SPT**); Single point highest inhibition-achievable assay (**SPHIAa**); Enzymeallergosorbent test (**EAST**); Enzyme-linked immunosorbent assay (**ELISA**).

allergic individuals develop birch pollen-related food allergies due to cross-reactivity. As already mentioned, Bet v 1 seems to be the only established major sensitizer causing birch-pollen related food allergies and is the most relevant allergen associated with clinical reactions (Geroldinger-Simic *et al.*, 2011). Symptoms after ingestion of raw fruits and vegetables typically manifest at the site of allergen exposure, as contact urticaria of the oral mucosa (OAS). Allergic reactions to PR-10 proteins occur immediately after food intake and last for about 30 minutes until they dissipate. Clinical reactions include itching, tingling or oedema of the lips and tongue as well as hoarseness and irritation of the throat. Sometimes patients also experience itching of the ears. However, a few PR-10-related antigens, particularly Api g 1 (from celery) and Gly m 4 (from soybean) are reported to cause systemic and severe IgE-mediated reactions such as asthma, precordial burning and even anaphylactic shock (Ballmer-Weber *et al.*, 2000; Kleine-Tebbe *et al.*, 2002; Yamamoto *et al.*, 2015). Anaphylactic reactions such as swollen tongue, angioedema, urticaria, rhinoconjunctivitis and/or hypotension are reported to occur within 15–30 minutes after consumption.

The reason why the symptoms caused by PR-10 proteins (and/or profilins) tend to be rather mild, is that these molecules are very sensitive to heat and proteolytic degradation. Thus, the process of ingestion and digestion destroys their conformational IgE epitopes leading to the loss of their IgE-binding capacity. Api g 1 and Gly m 1, however, are denaturation- and heat-resistant exceptions allowing them to cause symptoms even after cooking (Ana M. Gimenez-Arnau, 2014).

Profilins

Function and properties of profilins

Profilins are a family of small, 12–15 kDa, highly conserved proteins expressed in all eukaryotic cells and some viruses (Santos and Van Ree, 2011). The first profilin was identified in 1977 by Carlsson *et al.* (Carlsson *et al.*, 1977) as a low-molecular-weight, actin-associated, profilamentous protein complex involved in monomeric actin storage and polymerization. Since then, a large amount of literature has provided insight on the association of profilins with essential cell processes as cell proliferation, differentiation, growth, motility and cytokinesis (Krishnan and Moens, 2009). In plant cells, profilins bind actin as well as two other kinds of ligands, like poly-L-proline and phosphoinositides. Due to their ligand-binding ability, profilins are multifunctional molecules with an established role in plasma membrane-actin cytoskeleton interactions, signal transduction, organelle location and vesicle trafficking (Sun *et al.*, 2013). However, the exact molecular mechanisms implicating profilin in all the aforementioned functions remains mostly to be discovered (Krishnan and Moens, 2009).

Within the plantae kingdom, profilins are highly conserved proteins with sequence identities never below 75%, even between members from distantly related organisms. Due to this conservation of amino acid sequence, profilins possess highly similar structures and, as already discussed, biological functions (Hauser, 2008). Many profilins have already been studied in detail and the elucidation of their three-dimensional structures has revealed a well-conserved structural core mainly consisting of anti-parallel β-sheets surrounded by α-helices (Xue and Robinson, 2013). The conserved structure of profilins, combined with the fact that they are vital components of essential cellular processes and thus, ubiquitously spread among all organisms, constitutes them as very important proteins in the context of allergy. Profilins are designated as panallergens contributing to a large number of cross-reactivity cases between aeroallergens and food allergens (Hauser *et al.*, 2010).

The first allergenic profilin to be identified and characterized was Bet v 2 from birch pollen (Valenta *et al.*, 1991). Following that, profilins were found and classified as allergens in grass and weed pollen as well as in plant foods (Santos and Van Ree, 2011). Since then, the list of identified allergenic profilins in other pollen sources and plant foods is growing ever longer (Table 13.1).

Profilins as Panallergens

Due to the attributes of profilins described above (conserved structures and ubiquitous distribution), profilin sensitization could lead to allergic reactions to a multitude of pollen and plant food sources triggered by profilin-specific IgE (Asero *et al.*, 2008). Thus, sensitization to profilins is considered a high-risk allergy factor and, in the context of the pollen-food syndrome, the potential cause of a great portion of allergic reactions to plant-foods.

Unlike PR-10s, there is more than one protein confirmed to act as a sensitizer in the profilin protein family. The most significant profilin-specific IgE inducers are Phl p 12 and Bet v 2 from grass and birch pollen, respectively, while the sensitizing potency between the two depends on their geographical distribution (Asero *et al.*, 2015; Santos and Van Ree, 2011). Mugwort profilin Art v 4 has also been shown to lead to cross-reactions with plant-food profilins (Wopfner *et al.*, 2002). Profilins in ragweed and olive pollen have also been implicated in the pollen-food syndrome, but no studies confirming them as primary sensitizers have been performed (Werfel *et al.*, 2015).

Sensitization to pollen profilins is connected to a large number of cross-reactions to plant-foods, with *Rosaceae* fruits and nuts, *Apiaceae* fruits and vegetables as well as melons, bananas, kiwis, oranges, tomatoes and peanuts being the most common cases (Table 13.1). However, the role of profilins as elicitors of clinical symptoms is still controversial because sensitization and immunological cross-reactivity are not always directly linked with clinical manifestations (Santos and Van Ree, 2011).

Clinical Manifestations

Despite their panallergen properties and their involvement in a multitude of cases, profilins elicit (Asero, 2003) symptoms rather similar to PR-10 OAS with mild reactions involving the lips, tongue and throat. Additionally, itching of the ears can also occur in some cases. The progression of symptoms elicited by profilins also resembles PR-10 PFS with an almost immediate onset and a maximum duration of half an hour. Nonetheless, rare profilin-mediated systemic reactions to zucchini and anaphylactic reactions to lychi fruit have also been documented (Fah *et al.*, 1995; Reindl *et al.*, 2000). Allergic reactions to Act d 8 from kiwi is also capable of causing severe reactions, particularly in young children (Lucas *et al.*, 2004).

Non-specific Lipid Transfer Proteins (nsLTPs)

Function and properties of nsLTPs

Plant non-specific lipid transfer proteins are small, basic proteins with a wide distribution throughout higher plants. Although a number of different classification systems have been proposed, nsLTPs are mainly categorized according to their molecular weight into the 9 kDa nsLTP1 and the 7 kDa nsLTP2 subfamilies (Liu *et al.*, 2015). Along with seed storage proteins and inhibitors of α-amylase and trypsin, nsLTPs belong to the large protein superfamily of prolamines (Egger *et al.*, 2010). Although nsLTPs were originally discovered and named for their *in vitro* ability to bind and transfer lipids between membranes, such a role *in vivo* has been ruled out. The actual biological function of nsLTPs remains unclear and is still under debate. Nevertheless, several lines of evidence reveal the involvement of nsLTPs in various important plant cytology, growth, development and defense mechanisms (Liu *et al.*, 2015). In fact, their role in plant defense has been conclusively proven, designating them as the 14th member of the pathogenesis-related protein class (PR-14) (Salcedo *et al.*, 2007).

Despite their differences in amino acid sequence, nsLTPs share similar tertiary structures with the characteristic backbone formed by an eight-cysteine motif (C-Xn-C-Xn-CC-Xn-CXC-Xn-C-Xn-C) and stabilized by four disulfide bonds linking the cysteine residues. Determination of several plant nsLTP 3D structures by either X-ray crystallography or nuclear magnetic resonance spectroscopy reveals a typical fold consisting of a α-helical compact domain comprised of four α-helices, connected by short loops, and a non-structured C-terminal tail. The main feature of the nsLTP fold is a large internal tunnel-like cavity along the axis of the molecule which can accommodate a wide variety of lipid types and displays a high plasticity and flexibility upon binding (Liu *et al.*, 2015). This robust protein structure is further stabilized by a multitude of intramolecular H-bonds providing nsLTPs with their characteristic high thermal stability and proteolytic resistance (Scheurer *et al.*, 2004; Gaier *et al.*, 2008).

A great portion of nsLTPs represents major plant food and pollen allergens, especially in the Mediterranean area. Allergenic nsLTPs have been identified in many fruits (predominately *Rosaceae* spp.), vegetables, nuts as well as in pollens (Table 13.1).

The Sensitizer Debate

Unlike PR-10 proteins and profilins, the sensitization route of nsLTPs is not completely clear and is rather complicated. nsLTPs are mainly considered to be a class I or "true" food allergens capable of causing allergies without the involvement of pollen nsLTPs (Zuidmeer and van Ree, 2007). Pru p 3, the nsLTP from peach, is the most clinically relevant member of this protein family and plays a central role in the allergic sensitization to nsLTPs (Egger *et al.*, 2010). In the context of the pollen-food syndrome, the pollen nsLTPs Art v 3 from mugwort and Pla a 3 from the plane tree have been shown to cross-react with Pru p 3 (Garcia-Selles *et al.*, 2002) (Lauer *et al.*, 2007). However, which of them acts as the primary sensitizer is still unclear.

Depending on the study population and the occurring epidemiological factors, clinical association between nsLTPs from pollen and plant foods can be explained by primary sensitization to either a food (classic food allergy) or pollen (pollen-food syndrome) allergen (Zuidmeer and van Ree, 2007). A recent study suggested an additional nsLTP sensitization pathway involving the development of respiratory symptoms (food-pollinosis syndrome) due to Pru p 3 sensitization and cross-reactivity with Art v 3 (Sanchez-Lopez *et al.*, 2014) highlighting the complexity of the nsLTP pollen-food syndrome.

Clinical Manifestations

In contrast to proteins of the PR-10 and the profilin family, nsLTPs are heat-stable molecules that possess a high degree of resistance to proteolytic digestion by the gastrointestinal tract. In allergic patients, these proteolysis-resistant allergens are eliciting severe systemic reactions such as urticaria, angioedema, dyspnea and anaphylaxis. Cofactors like Non-Steroidal Anti-Inflammatory Drugs (NSAIDs) and physical exercises have been shown to favor the development of systemic reactions towards nsLTPs (Pascal *et al.*, 2012; Salcedo *et al.*, 2007).

The manifestation of severe systemic clinical symptoms induced by nsLTPs is largely associated with a certain geographical region. In principal, most reported cases of nsLTP-induced systemic reactions are distributed in the Mediterranean area (Italy and Spain), whereas in central and northern Europe it has hardly been observed (Pastorello and Robino, 2004; Reuter *et al.*, 2006; Zuidmeer and van Ree, 2007).

Beside severe systemic symptoms, allergic reactions to nsLTPs can also manifest also as (local) mild symptoms, as described for profilin and PR-10 proteins. At this point it should be mentioned that patients sensitized to nsLTPs, who possess a co-sensitization to profilin or PR-10 proteins or both, are less likely to develop severe reactions (Gamboa *et al.*, 2007; Pastorello *et al.*, 2011; Scala *et al.*, 2015).

Conclusion

The pollen-food syndrome is a molecularly and clinically fascinating condition with ever-growing significance for patients and clinicians. A great portion of food allergies is associated with cross-reactions to plant foods in adults with pre-existing pollen allergies. PFS mostly manifests itself as a local and mild reaction that does not pose a real threat to the patient. However, there can be cases where the symptoms are severe and systemic. Furthermore, the implication of multiple proteins from different antigenically distinct families in the reactions against a single allergenic source is not a rare occurrence. Differences in geography and dietary habits, leading to individual differences in the exposure to pollen and plant food allergens, must also be taken into account.

Despite the fact that for almost 80 years the field of allergy has been tackling the PFS with increasing intensity, there are many of its aspects that remain unclear. With the exception of birch PFS and the PR-10 protein family members' established role in the majority of the cases, there is much left to be elucidated. In the case of profilins, although their relevance as panallergens in the process of multiple pollen sensitization has already been demonstrated, their clinical significance is still rather controversial. Given their panallergen attributes, profilins are implicated in practically every PFS case but no clear link between profilin sensitization and clinical manifestations has been established. Regarding nsLTPs, the specific geographical distribution of their sources and distinct molecule properties render them the most complicated proteins involved in the pollen-food syndrome. nsLTPs cause the most severe reactions with the highest frequency and their role in causing PFS seems to be outweighed by their involvement in classical food allergies. Only a very limited amount of studies have focused on the association of nsLTPs in PFS, making this a highly debatable subject.

So far 15 PR-10s, 20 profilins and 16 nsLTPs identified in pollen and plant foods have been associated with pollen-food cross-reactivities. In Table 13.1 we summarize all allergens from these protein families and display the confirmed cross-reactions between pollen and food allergens.

Pollen-food syndrome is a very important allergy and should not be underestimated in clinical practice. Moreover, there is a certain need for basic and clinical studies that will investigate the pathomechanism of PFS in depth allowing for better understanding of the disease.

Acknowledgements

Lorenz Aglas and Fatima Ferreira were supported by the European Union 7th Framework program (FP7-HEALTH-2013-INNOVATION-1). Lorenz Aglas was also supported by the Austrian Science Funds (FWF) project 23417. Sara Huber was supported by the FWF project 26125. Claudia Asam and Anargyros Roulias were supported by FWF project 27589. All authors acknowledge the University of Salzburg´s priority program "Allergy-Cancer-BioNano Research Centre" for supporting this work.

Keywords: Pollen-food syndrome, PR-10, profilin, nsLTP, cross-reactive IgE, pollen allergen sensitization, plant food allergy, IgE antibody

References

Almeida, E. M., Bartolome, B., Faria, E. G., Sousa, N. G., and Luis, A. S. (2015). Pomegranate anaphylaxis due to cross-reactivity with Peach LTP (Pru p 3). Allergology and Immunopathology (Madrid) 43(1): 104–106.

Amlot, P. L., Kemeny, D. M., Zachary, C., Parkes, P., and Lessof, M. H. (1987). Oral allergy syndrome (OAS): symptoms of IgE-mediated hypersensitivity to foods. Clinical Allergy 17(1): 33–42.

Ana, M., and Gimenez-Arnau, H. I. M. (2014). Contact Urticaria Syndrome. CRC Press.

Andersen, M. B., Hall, S., and Dragsted, L. O. (2011). Identification of european allergy patterns to the allergen families PR-10, LTP, and profilin from Rosaceae fruits. Clinical Reviews in Allergy and Immunology 41(1): 4–19.

Asam, C., Hofer, H., Wolf, M., Aglas, L., and Wallner, M. (2015). Tree pollen allergens-an update from a molecular perspective. Allergy 70(10): 1201–1211.

Asero, R. (2003). How long does the effect of birch pollen injection SIT on apple allergy last? Allergy 58(5): 435–438.

Asero, R., Monsalve, R., and Barber, D. (2008). Profilin sensitization detected in the office by skin prick test: a study of prevalence and clinical relevance of profilin as a plant food allergen. Clinical and Experimental Allergy: Journal of the British Society for Allergy and Clinical Immunology 38(6): 1033–1037.

Asero, R., Tripodi, S., Dondi, A., Di Rienzo Businco, A., Sfika, I., Bianchi, A., Candelotti, P., Caffarelli, C., Povesi Dascola, C., Ricci, G., Calamelli, E., Maiello, N., Miraglia Del Giudice, M., Frediani, T., Frediani, S., Macri, F., Moretti, M., Dello Iacono, I., Patria, M. F., Varin, E., Peroni, D., Comberiati, P., Chini, L., Moschese, V., Lucarelli, S., Bernardini, R., Pingitore, G., Pelosi, U., Tosca, M., Cirisano, A., Faggian, D., Plebani, M., Verga, C., and Matricardi, P. M. (2015). Prevalence and clinical relevance of IgE sensitization to profilin in childhood: A multicenter study. International Archives of Allergy and Immunology 168(1): 25–31.

Ballmer-Weber, B. K., Vieths, S., Luttkopf, D., Heuschmann, P., and Wuthrich, B. (2000). Celery allergy confirmed by double-blind, placebo-controlled food challenge: a clinical study in 32 subjects with a history of adverse reactions to celery root. The Journal of Allergy and Clinical Immunology 106(2): 373–378.

Ballmer-Weber, B. K., Wuthrich, B., Wangorsch, A., Fotisch, K., Altmann, F., and Vieths, S. (2001). Carrot allergy: double-blinded, placebo-controlled food challenge and identification of allergens. The Journal of Allergy and Clinical Immunology 108(2): 301–307.

Bascones, O., Rodriguez-Perez, R., Juste, S., Moneo, I., and Caballero, M. L. (2009). Lettuce-induced anaphylaxis. Identification of the allergen involved. Journal of Investigational Allergology and Clinical Immunology 19(2): 154–157.

Berkner, H., Neudecker, P., Mittag, D., Ballmer-Weber, B. K., Schweimer, K., Vieths, S., and Rosch, P. (2009). Cross-reactivity of pollen and food allergens: soybean Gly m 4 is a member of the Bet v 1 superfamily and closely resembles yellow lupine proteins. Bioscience Reports 29(3): 183–192.

Bernardi, M. L., Giangrieco, I., Camardella, L., Ferrara, R., Palazzo, P., Panico, M. R., Crescenzo, R., Carratore, V., Zennaro, D., Liso, M., Santoro, M., Zuzzi, S., Tamburrini, M., Ciardiello, M. A., and Mari, A. (2011). Allergenic lipid transfer proteins from plant-derived foods do not immunologically and clinically behave homogeneously: the kiwifruit LTP as a model. PLoS One 6(11): e27856.

Bollen, M. A., Garcia, A., Cordewener, J. H., Wichers, H. J., Helsper, J. P., Savelkoul, H. F., and van Boekel, M. A. (2007). Purification and characterization of natural Bet v 1 from birch pollen and related allergens from carrot and celery. Molecular Nutrition & Food Research 51(12): 1527–1536.

Breiteneder, H., Hoffmann-Sommergruber, K., O'Riordain, G., Susani, M., Ahorn, H., Ebner, C., Kraft, D., and Scheiner, O. (1995). Molecular characterization of Api g 1, the major allergen of celery (Apium graveolens), and its immunological and structural relationships to a group of 17-kDa tree pollen allergens. European Journal of Biochemistry/FEBS 233(2): 484–489.

Bublin, M., and Breiteneder, H. (2014). Cross-reactivity of peanut allergens. Current Allergy and Asthma Reports 14(4): 426.

Cabanos, C., Tandang-Silvas, M. R., Odijk, V., Brostedt, P., Tanaka, A., Utsumi, S., and Maruyama, N. (2010). Expression, purification, cross-reactivity and homology modeling of peanut profilin. Protein Expression and Purification 73(1): 36–45.

Carlsson, L., Nystrom, L. E., Sundkvist, I., Markey, F., and Lindberg, U. (1977). Actin polymerizability is influenced by profilin, a low molecular weight protein in non-muscle cells. Journal of Molecular Biology 115(3): 465–483.

Chang, Y. C., George, S. J., and Hsu, S. (2005). Oral allergy syndrome and contact urticaria to apples. Journal of the American Academy of Dermatology 53(4): 736–737.

Ciardiello, M. A., Palazzo, P., Bernardi, M. L., Carratore, V., Giangrieco, I., Longo, V., Melis, M., Tamburrini, M., Zennaro, D., Mari, A., and Colombo, P. (2010). Biochemical, immunological and clinical characterization of a cross-reactive nonspecific lipid transfer protein 1 from mulberry. Allergy 65(5): 597–605.

Crespo, J. F., Retzek, M., Foetisch, K., Sierra-Maestro, E., Cid-Sanchez, A. B., Pascual, C. Y., Conti, A., Feliu, A., Rodriguez, J., Vieths, S., and Scheurer, S. (2006). Germin-like protein Cit s 1 and profilin Cit s 2 are major allergens in orange (Citrus sinensis) fruits. Molecular Nutrition & Food Research 50(3): 282–290.

Cudowska, B., Kaczmarski, M., and Restani, P. (2005). Immunoblotting in the diagnosis of cross-reactivity in children allergic to birch. Rocz Akad Med Bialymst 50: 268–273.

D'Amato, G., Spieksma, F. T., Liccardi, G., Jager, S., Russo, M., Kontou-Fili, K., Nikkels, H., Wuthrich, B., and Bonini, S. (1998). Pollen-related allergy in Europe. Allergy 53(6): 567–578.

De Knop, K. J., Verweij, M. M., Grimmelikhuijsen, M., Philipse, E., Hagendorens, M. M., Bridts, C. H., De Clerck, L. S., Stevens, W. J., and Ebo, D. G. (2011). Age-related sensitization profiles for hazelnut (Corylus avellana) in a birch-endemic region. Pediatric Allergy and Immunology: Official Publication of the European Society of Pediatric Allergy and Immunology 22(1 Pt 2): e139–149.

Diaz-Perales, A., Lombardero, M., Sanchez-Monge, R., Garcia-Selles, F. J., Pernas, M., Fernandez-Rivas, M., Barber, D., and Salcedo, G. (2000). Lipid-transfer proteins as potential plant panallergens: cross-reactivity among proteins of Artemisia pollen, Castanea nut and Rosaceae fruits, with different IgE-binding capacities. Clinical and Experimental Allergy: Journal of the British Society for Allergy and Clinical Immunology 30(10): 1403–1410.

Ebner, C., Birkner, T., Valenta, R., Rumpold, H., Breitenbach, M., Scheiner, O., and Kraft, D. (1991). Common epitopes of birch pollen and apples—studies by western and northern blot. The Journal of Allergy and Clinical Immunology 88(4): 588–594.

Egger, M., Mutschlechner, S., Wopfner, N., Gadermaier, G., Briza, P., and Ferreira, F. (2006). Pollen-food syndromes associated with weed pollinosis: an update from the molecular point of view. Allergy 61(4): 461–476.

Egger, M., Hauser, M., Mari, A., Ferreira, F., and Gadermaier, G. (2010). The role of lipid transfer proteins in allergic diseases. Current Allergy and Asthma Reports 10(5): 326–335.

Fah, J., Wuthrich, B., and Vieths, S. (1995). Anaphylactic reaction to lychee fruit: evidence for sensitization to profilin. Clinical and Experimental Allergy: Journal of the British Society for Allergy and Clinical Immunology 25(10): 1018–1023.

Fernandes, H., Michalska, K., Sikorski, M., and Jaskolski, M. (2013). Structural and functional aspects of PR-10 proteins. The FEBS Journal 280(5): 1169–1199.

Flinterman, A. E., Akkerdaas, J. H., den Hartog Jager, C. F., Rigby, N. M., Fernandez-Rivas, M., Hoekstra, M. O., Bruijnzeel-Koomen, C. A., Knulst, A. C., van Ree, R., and Pasmans, S. G. (2008). Lipid transfer protein-linked hazelnut allergy in children from a non-Mediterranean birch-endemic area. The Journal of Allergy and Clinical Immunology 121(2): 423–428 e422.

Foetisch, K., Son, D. Y., Altmann, F., Aulepp, H., Conti, A., Haustein, D., and Vieths, S. (2001). Tomato (Lycopersicon esculentum) allergens in pollen-allergic patients. European Food Research and Technology 213(4-5): 259–266.

Gadermaier, G., Harrer, A., Girbl, T., Palazzo, P., Himly, M., Vogel, L., Briza, P., Mari, A., and Ferreira, F. (2009). Isoform identification and characterization of Art v 3, the lipid-transfer protein of mugwort pollen. Molecular Immunology 46(10): 1919–1924.

Gadermaier, G., Hauser, M., Egger, M., Ferrara, R., Briza, P., Santos, K. S., Zennaro, D., Girbl, T., Zuidmeer-Jongejan, L., Mari, A., and Ferreira, F. (2011). Sensitization prevalence, antibody cross-reactivity and immunogenic peptide profile of Api g 2, the non-specific lipid transfer protein 1 of celery. PLoS One 6(8): e24150.

Gaier, S., Marsh, J., Oberhuber, C., Rigby, N. M., Lovegrove, A., Alessandri, S., Briza, P., Radauer, C., Zuidmeer, L., van Ree, R., Hemmer, W., Sancho, A. I., Mills, C., Hoffmann-Sommergruber, K., and Shewry, P. R. (2008). Purification and structural stability of the peach allergens Pru p 1 and Pru p 3. Molecular Nutrition and Food Research 52 Suppl 2: S220–229.

Gamboa, P. M., Caceres, O., Antepara, I., Sanchez-Monge, R., Ahrazem, O., Salcedo, G., Barber, D., Lombardero, M., and Sanz, M. L. (2007). Two different profiles of peach allergy in the north of Spain. Allergy 62(4): 408–414.

Garcia-Blanca, A., Aranda, A., Blanca-Lopez, N., Perez, D., Gomez, F., Mayorga, C., Torres, M. J., Diaz-Perales, A., Perkins, J. R., Villalba, M., Blanca, M., and Canto, G. (2015). Influence of age on IgE response in peanut-allergic children and adolescents from the Mediterranean area. Pediatric Allergy and Immunology: Official Publication of the European Society of Pediatric Allergy and Immunology 26(6): 497–502.

Garcia-Selles, F. J., Diaz-Perales, A., Sanchez-Monge, R., Alcantara, M., Lombardero, M., Barber, D., Salcedo, G., and Fernandez-Rivas, M. (2002). Patterns of reactivity to lipid transfer proteins of plant foods and Artemisia pollen: an *in vivo* study. International Archives of Allergy and Immunology 128(2): 115–122.

Geroldinger-Simic, M., Zelniker, T., Aberer, W., Ebner, C., Egger, C., Greiderer, A., Prem, N., Lidholm, J., Ballmer-Weber, B. K., Vieths, S., and Bohle, B. (2011). Birch pollen-related food allergy: clinical aspects and the role of allergen-specific IgE and IgG4 antibodies. The Journal of Allergy and Clinical Immunology 127(3): 616–622 e611.

Gomez, F., Aranda, A., Campo, P., Diaz-Perales, A., Blanca-Lopez, N., Perkins, J., Garrido, M., Blanca, M., Mayorga, C., and Torres, M. J. (2014). High prevalence of lipid transfer protein sensitization in apple allergic patients with systemic symptoms. PLoS One 9(9): e107304.

Hartz, C., San Miguel-Moncin Mdel, M., Cistero-Bahima, A., Fotisch, K., Metzner, K. J., Fortunato, D., Lidholm, J., Vieths, S., and Scheurer, S. (2007). Molecular characterisation of Lac s 1, the major allergen from lettuce (*Lactuca sativa*). Molecular Immunology 44(11): 2820–2830.

Hauser, M., Roulias, A., Ferreira, F., and Egger, M. (2010). Panallergens and their impact on the allergic patient. Allergy, Asthma, and Clinical Immunology: Official Journal of the Canadian Society of Allergy and Clinical Immunology 6(1): 1.

Hauser, M., Asam, C., Himly, M., Palazzo, P., Voltolini, S., Montanari, C., Briza, P., Bernardi, M. L., Mari, A., Ferreira, F., and Wallner, M. (2011). Bet v 1-like pollen allergens of multiple Fagales species can sensitize atopic individuals. Clinical and Experimental Allergy: Journal of the British Society for Allergy and Clinical Immunology 41(12): 1804–1814.

Hauser, M., Egger, M., Wallner, M., Wopfner, N., Schmidt, G., and Ferreira, F. (2008). Molecular properties of plant food allergens: a current classification into protein families. The Open Immunology Journal 1: 1–12.

Hoffmann-Sommergruber, K., O'Riordain, G., Ahorn, H., Ebner, C., Laimer Da Camara Machado, M., Puhringer, H., Scheiner, O., and Breiteneder, H. (1999). Molecular characterization of Dau c 1, the Bet v 1 homologous protein from carrot and its cross-reactivity with Bet v 1 and Api g 1. Clinical and Experimental Allergy: Journal of the British Society for Allergy and Clinical Immunology 29(6): 840–847.

Hurlburt, B. K., Offermann, L. R., McBride, J. K., Majorek, K. A., Maleki, S. J., and Chruszcz, M. (2013). Structure and function of the peanut panallergen Ara h 8. The Journal of Biological Chemistry 288(52): 36890–36901.

Julka, S., Kuppannan, K., Karnoup, A., Dielman, D., Schafer, B., and Young, S. A. (2012). Quantification of Gly m 4 protein, a major soybean allergen, by two-dimensional liquid chromatography with ultraviolet and mass spectrometry detection. Analytical Chemistry 84(22): 10019–10030.

Karamloo, F., Scheurer, S., Wangorsch, A., May, S., Haustein, D., and Vieths, S. (2001). Pyr c 1, the major allergen from pear (Pyrus communis), is a new member of the Bet v 1 allergen family. Journal of Chromatography B, Biomedical Sciences and Applications 756(1-2): 281–293.

Karlsson, A. L., Alm, R., Ekstrand, B., Fjelkner-Modig, S., Schiott, A., Bengtsson, U., Bjork, L., Hjerno, K., Roepstorff, P., and Emanuelsson, C. S. (2004). Bet v 1 homologues in strawberry identified as IgE-binding proteins and presumptive allergens. Allergy 59(12): 1277–1284.

Kelso, J. M. (1995). Oral allergy syndrome? The Journal of Allergy and Clinical Immunology 96(2): 275.

Kelso, J. M., Jones, R. T., and Yunginger, J. W. (1998). Anaphylaxis after initial ingestion of rambutan, a tropical fruit. The Journal of Allergy and Clinical Immunology 102(1): 145–146.

Kelso, J. M. (2000). Pollen-food allergy syndrome. Clinical and Experimental Allergy: Journal of the British Society for Allergy and Clinical Immunology 30(7): 905–907.

Kleine-Tebbe, J., Vogel, L., Crowell, D. N., Haustein, U. F., and Vieths, S. (2002). Severe oral allergy syndrome and anaphylactic reactions caused by a Bet v 1-related PR-10 protein in soybean, SAM22. The Journal of Allergy and Clinical Immunology 110(5): 797–804.

Kofler, S., Asam, C., Eckhard, U., Wallner, M., Ferreira, F., and Brandstetter, H. (2012). Crystallographically mapped ligand binding differs in high and low IgE binding isoforms of birch pollen allergen bet v 1. Journal of Molecular Biology 422(1): 109–123.

Kondo, Y., and Urisu, A. (2009). Oral allergy syndrome. Allergology International 58(4): 485–491.

Kos, T., Hoffmann-Sommergruber, K., Ferreira, F., Hirschwehr, R., Ahorn, H., Horak, F., Jager, S., Sperr, W., Kraft, D., and Scheiner, O. (1993). Purification, characterization and N-terminal amino acid sequence of a new major allergen from European chestnut pollen—Cas s 1. Biochemical and Biophysical Research Communications 196(3): 1086–1092.

Krishnan, K., and Moens, P. D. J. (2009). Structure and functions of profilins. Biophysical Reviews 1(2): 71–81.

Lauer, I., Miguel-Moncin, M. S., Abel, T., Foetisch, K., Hartz, C., Fortunato, D., Cistero-Bahima, A., Vieths, S., and Scheurer, S. (2007). Identification of a plane pollen lipid transfer protein (Pla a 3) and its immunological relation to the peach lipid-transfer protein, Pru p 3. Clinical and Experimental Allergy: Journal of the British Society for Allergy and Clinical Immunology 37(2): 261–269.

Le, T. M., Bublin, M., Breiteneder, H., Fernandez-Rivas, M., Asero, R., Ballmer-Weber, B., Barreales, L., Bures, P., Belohlavkova, S., de Blay, F., Clausen, M., Dubakiene, R., Gislason, D., van Hoffen, E., Jedrzejczak-Czechowicz, M., Kowalski, M. L., Kralimarkova, T., Lidholm, J., DeWitt, A. M., Mills, C. E., Papadopoulos, N. G., Popov, T., Purohit, A., van Ree, R., Seneviratne, S., Sinaniotis, A., Summers, C., Vazquez-Cortes, S., Vieths, S., Vogel, L., Hoffmann-Sommergruber, K., and Knulst, A. C. (2013a). Kiwifruit allergy across Europe: clinical manifestation and IgE recognition patterns to kiwifruit allergens. The Journal of Allergy and Clinical Immunology 131(1): 164–171.

Le, T. M., van Hoffen, E., Lebens, A. F., Bruijnzeel-Koomen, C. A., and Knulst, A. C. (2013b). Anaphylactic versus mild reactions to hazelnut and apple in a birch-endemic area: different sensitization profiles? International Archives of Allergy and Immunology 160(1): 56–62.

Lessof, M. H. (1996). Pollen-food allergy syndrome. The Journal of Allergy and Clinical Immunology 98(1): 239–240.

Liccardi, G., and D'Amato, G. (1994). Oral allergy syndrome in a subject with a highly relevant monosensitization to egg. The Journal of Allergy and Clinical Immunology 94(5): 931–932.

Liu, F., Zhang, X., Lu, C., Zeng, X., Li, Y., Fu, D., and Wu, G. (2015). Non-specific lipid transfer proteins in plants: presenting new advances and an integrated functional analysis. Journal of Experimental Botany 66(19): 5663–5681.

Lombardero, M., Garcia-Selles, F. J., Polo, F., Jimeno, L., Chamorro, M. J., Garcia-Casado, G., Sanchez-Monge, R., Diaz-Perales, A., Salcedo, G., and Barber, D. (2004). Prevalence of sensitization to Artemisia allergens Art v 1, Art v 3 and Art v 60 kDa. Cross-reactivity among Art v 3 and other relevant lipid-transfer protein allergens. Clinical and Experimental Allergy: Journal of the British Society for Allergy and Clinical Immunology 34(9): 1415–1421.

Lopez-Torrejon, G., Ibanez, M. D., Ahrazem, O., Sanchez-Monge, R., Sastre, J., Lombardero, M., Barber, D., and Salcedo, G. (2005). Isolation, cloning and allergenic reactivity of natural profilin Cit s 2, a major orange allergen. Allergy 60(11): 1424–1429.

Lucas, J. S. A., Grimshaw, K. E. C., Collins, K., Warner, J. O., and Hourihane, J. O. (2004). Kiwi fruit is a significant allergen and is associated with differing patterns of reactivity in children and adults. Clinical and Experimental Allergy 34(7): 1115–1121.

Luttkopf, D., Ballmer-Weber, B. K., Wuthrich, B., and Vieths, S. (2000). Celery allergens in patients with positive double-blind placebo-controlled food challenge. The Journal of Allergy and Clinical Immunology 106(2): 390–399.

Mauro, M., Russello, M., Incorvaia, C., Gazzola, G., Frati, F., Moingeon, P., and Passalacqua, G. (2011). Birch-apple syndrome treated with birch pollen immunotherapy. International Archives of Allergy and Immunology 156(4): 416–422.

Mittag, D., Akkerdaas, J., Ballmer-Weber, B. K., Vogel, L., Wenising, M., Becker, W. M., Koppelman, S. J., Knulst, A. C., Helbling, A., Hefle, S. L., van Ree, R., and Vieths, S. (2004). Ara h 8, a Bet v 1-homologous allergen from peanut, is a major allergen in patients with combined birch pollen and peanut allergy. The Journal of Allergy and Clinical Immunology 114(6): 1410–1417.

Mittag, D., Vieths, S., Vogel, L., Wagner-Loew, D., Starke, A., Hunziker, P., Becker, W. M., and Ballmer-Weber, B. K. (2005). Birch pollen-related food allergy to legumes: identification and characterization of the Bet v 1 homologue in mungbean (Vigna radiata), Vig r 1. Clinical and Experimental Allergy: Journal of the British Society for Allergy and Clinical Immunology 35(8): 1049–1055.

Neudecker, P., Schweimer, K., Nerkamp, J., Scheurer, S., Vieths, S., Sticht, H., and Rosch, P. (2001). Allergic cross-reactivity made visible: solution structure of the major cherry allergen Pru av 1. The Journal of Biological Chemistry 276(25): 22756–22763.

Niederberger, V., Pauli, G., Gronlund, H., Froschl, R., Rumpold, H., Kraft, D., Valenta, R., and Spitzauer, S. (1998). Recombinant birch pollen allergens (rBet v 1 and rBet v 2) contain most of the IgE epitopes present in birch, alder, hornbeam, hazel, and oak pollen: a quantitative IgE inhibition study with sera from different populations. The Journal of Allergy and Clinical Immunology 102(4 Pt 1): 579–591.

Oberhuber, C., Bulley, S. M., Ballmer-Weber, B. K., Bublin, M., Gaier, S., DeWitt, A. M., Briza, P., Hofstetter, G., Lidholm, J., Vieths, S., and Hoffmann-Sommergruber, K. (2008). Characterization of Bet v 1-related allergens from kiwifruit relevant for patients with combined kiwifruit and birch pollen allergy. Molecular Nutrition & Food Research 52 Suppl 2: S230–240.

Ortolani, C., Ispano, M., Pastorello, E., Bigi, A., and Ansaloni, R. (1988). The oral allergy syndrome. Annals of Allergy 61(6 Pt 2): 47–52.

Palacin, A., Cumplido, J., Figueroa, J., Ahrazem, O., Sanchez-Monge, R., Carrillo, T., Salcedo, G., and Blanco, C. (2006). Cabbage lipid transfer protein Bra o 3 is a major allergen responsible for cross-reactivity between plant foods and pollens. The Journal of Allergy and Clinical Immunology 117(6): 1423–1429.

Palacin, A., Bartra, J., Munoz, R., Diaz-Perales, A., Valero, A., and Salcedo, G. (2010). Anaphylaxis to wheat flour-derived foodstuffs and the lipid transfer protein syndrome: a potential role of wheat lipid transfer protein Tri a 14. International Archives of Allergy and Immunology 152(2): 178–183.

Pascal, M., Munoz-Cano, R., Reina, Z., Palacin, A., Vilella, R., Picado, C., Juan, M., Sanchez-Lopez, J., Rueda, M., Salcedo, G., Valero, A., Yague, J., and Bartra, J. (2012). Lipid transfer protein syndrome: clinical pattern, cofactor effect and profile of molecular sensitization to plant-foods and pollens. Clinical and Experimental Allergy: Journal of the British Society for Allergy and Clinical Immunology 42(10): 1529–1539.

Pastorello, E. A., Ortolani, C., Farioli, L., Pravettoni, V., Ispano, M., Borga, A., Bengtsson, A., Incorvaia, C., Berti, C., and Zanussi, C. (1994). Allergenic cross-reactivity among Peach, Apricot, Plum, and Cherry in patients with oral allergy syndrome—an *in-vivo* and *in-vitro* Study. The Journal of Allergy and Clinical Immunology 94(4): 699–707.

Pastorello, E. A., Pravettoni, V., Ispano, M., Farioli, L., Ansaloni, R., Rotondo, F., Incorvaia, C., Asman, I., Bengtsson, A., and Ortolani, C. (1996). Identification of the allergenic components of kiwi fruit and evaluation of their cross-reactivity with timothy and birch pollens. The Journal of Allergy and Clinical Immunology 98(3): 601–610.

Pastorello, E. A., and Robino, A. M. (2004). Clinical role of lipid transfer proteins in food allergy. Molecular Nutrition & Food Research 48(5): 356–362.

Pastorello, E. A., Farioli, L., Pravettoni, V., Scibilia, J., Mascheri, A., Borgonovo, L., Piantanida, M., Primavesi, L., Stafylaraki, C., Pasqualetti, S., Schroeder, J., Nichelatti, M., and Marocchi, A. (2011). Pru p 3-sensitised Italian peach-allergic patients are less likely to develop severe symptoms when also presenting IgE antibodies to Pru p 1 and Pru p 4. International Archives of Allergy and Immunology 156(4): 362–372.

Pauli, G., Bessot, J. C., Braun, P. A., Dietemann-Molard, A., Kopferschmitt-Kubler, M. C., and Thierry, R. (1988). Celery allergy: clinical and biological study of 20 cases. Annals of Allergy 60(3): 243–246.

Price, A., Ramachandran, S., Smith, G. P., Stevenson, M. L., Pomeranz, M. K., and Cohen, D. E. (2015). Oral allergy syndrome (pollen-food allergy syndrome). Dermatitis: Contact, Atopic, Occupational, Drug 26(2): 78–88.

Reindl, J., Anliker, M. D., Karamloo, F., Vieths, S., and Wuthrich, B. (2000). Allergy caused by ingestion of zucchini (Cucurbita pepo): characterization of allergens and cross-reactivity to pollen and other foods. The Journal of Allergy and Clinical Immunology 106(2): 379–385.

Reindl, J., Rihs, H. P., Scheurer, S., Wangorsch, A., Haustein, D., and Vieths, S. (2002). IgE reactivity to profilin in pollen-sensitized subjects with adverse reactions to banana and pineapple. International Archives of Allergy and Immunology 128(2): 105–114.

Reuter, A., Lidholm, J., Andersson, K., Ostling, J., Lundberg, M., Scheurer, S., Enrique, E., Cistero-Bahima, A., San Miguel-Moncin, M., Ballmer-Weber, B. K., and Vieths, S. (2006). A critical assessment of allergen component-based *in vitro* diagnosis in cherry allergy across Europe. Clinical and Experimental Allergy: Journal of the British Society for Allergy and Clinical Immunology 36(6): 815–823.

Rihs, H. P., Chen, Z., Rueff, F., Petersen, A., Rozynek, P., Heimann, H., and Baur, X. (1999). IgE binding of the recombinant allergen soybean profilin (rGly m 3) is mediated by conformational epitopes. The Journal of Allergy and Clinical Immunology 104(6): 1293–1301.

Rodriguez-Perez, R., Fernandez-Rivas, M., Gonzalez-Mancebo, E., Sanchez-Monge, R., Diaz-Perales, A., and Salcedo, G. (2003). Peach profilin: cloning, heterologous expression and cross-reactivity with Bet v 2. Allergy 58(7): 635–640.

Rossi, R. E., Monasterolo, G., Operti, D., and Corsi, M. (1996). Evaluation of recombinant allergens Bet v 1 and Bet v 2 (profilin) by Pharmacia CAP system in patients with pollen-related allergy to birch and apple. Allergy 51(12): 940–945.

Salcedo, G., Sanchez-Monge, R., Barber, D., and Diaz-Perales, A. (2007). Plant non-specific lipid transfer proteins: an interface between plant defence and human allergy. Biochimica et Biophysica Acta 1771(6): 781–791.

Sampson, H. A. (1999). Food allergy. Part 1: immunopathogenesis and clinical disorders. The Journal of Allergy and Clinical Immunology 103(5 Pt 1): 717–728.

San Miguel-Moncin, M., Krail, M., Scheurer, S., Enrique, E., Alonso, R., Conti, A., Cistero-Bahima, A., and Vieths, S. (2003). Lettuce anaphylaxis: identification of a lipid transfer protein as the major allergen. Allergy 58(6): 511–517.

Sanchez-Lopez, J., Tordesillas, L., Pascal, M., Munoz-Cano, R., Garrido, M., Rueda, M., Vilella, R., Valero, A., Diaz-Perales, A., Picado, C., and Bartra, J. (2014). Role of Art v 3 in pollinosis of patients allergic to Pru p 3. The Journal of Allergy and Clinical Immunology 133(4): 1018–1025.

Sanchez-Monge, R., Blanco, C., Lopez-Torrejon, G., Cumplido, J., Recas, M., Figueroa, J., Carrillo, T., and Salcedo, G. (2006). Differential allergen sensitization patterns in chestnut allergy with or without associated latex-fruit syndrome. The Journal of Allergy and Clinical Immunology 118(3): 705–710.

Sankian, M., Varasteh, A., Pazouki, N., and Mahmoudi, M. (2005). Sequence homology: a poor predictive value for profilins cross-reactivity. Clinical and Molecular Allergy: CMA 3: 13.

Santos, A., and Van Ree, R. (2011). Profilins: mimickers of allergy or relevant allergens? International Archives of Allergy and Immunology 155(3): 191–204.

Scala, E., Till, S. J., Asero, R., Abeni, D., Guerra, E. C., Pirrotta, L., Paganelli, R., Pomponi, D., Giani, M., De Pita, O., and Cecchi, L. (2015). Lipid transfer protein sensitization: reactivity profiles and clinical risk assessment in an Italian cohort. Allergy 70(8): 933–943.

Scheurer, S., Metzner, K., Haustein, D., and Vieths, S. (1997). Molecular cloning, expression and characterization of Pru a 1, the major cherry allergen. Molecular Immunology 34(8-9): 619–629.

Scheurer, S., Son, D. Y., Boehm, M., Karamloo, F., Franke, S., Hoffmann, A., Haustein, D., and Vieths, S. (1999). Cross-reactivity and epitope analysis of Pru a 1, the major cherry allergen. Molecular Immunology 36(3): 155–167.

Scheurer, S., Wangorsch, A., Haustein, D., and Vieths, S. (2000). Cloning of the minor allergen Api g 4 profilin from celery (Apium graveolens) and its cross-reactivity with birch pollen profilin Bet v 2. Clinical and Experimental Allergy: Journal of the British Society for Allergy and Clinical Immunology 30(7): 962–971.

Scheurer, S., Wangorsch, A., Nerkamp, J., Skov, P. S., Ballmer-Weber, B., Wuthrich, B., Haustein, D., and Vieths, S. (2001). Cross-reactivity within the profilin panallergen family investigated by comparison of recombinant profilins from pear (Pyr c 4), cherry (Pru av 4) and celery (Api g 4) with birch pollen profilin Bet v 2. Journal of Chromatography B 756(1-2): 315–325.

Scheurer, S., Lauer, I., Foetisch, K., San Miguel Moncin, M., Retzek, M., Hartz, C., Enrique, E., Lidholm, J., Cistero-Bahima, A., and Vieths, S. (2004). Strong allergenicity of Pru av 3, the lipid transfer protein from cherry, is related to high stability against thermal processing and digestion. The Journal of Allergy and Clinical Immunology 114(4): 900–907.

Seutter von Loetzen, C., Hoffmann, T., Hartl, M. J., Schweimer, K., Schwab, W., Rosch, P., and Hartl-Spiegelhauer, O. (2014). Secret of the major birch pollen allergen Bet v 1: identification of the physiological ligand. The Biochemical Journal 457(3): 379–390.

Sinha, M., Singh, R. P., Kushwaha, G. S., Iqbal, N., Singh, A., Kaushik, S., Kaur, P., Sharma, S., and Singh, T. P. (2014). Current overview of allergens of plant pathogenesis related protein families. The Scientific World Journal 2014: 543195.

Sloane, D., and Sheffer, A. (2001). Oral allergy syndrome. Allergy Asthma Proc 22(5): 321–325.

Song, J. J., Zhang, H. Y., Liu, Z. G., and Ran, P. X. (2007). Cloning of the panallergen profilin from lychee fruit and its cross-reactivity with birch pollen profilin Bet v 2. Food Agricultural Immunology 18(2): 129–138.

Sun, T., Li, S., and Ren, H. (2013). Profilin as a regulator of the membrane-actin cytoskeleton interface in plant cells. Frontiers in Plant Science 4: 512.

Tordesillas, L., Pacios, L. F., Palacin, A., Cuesta-Herranz, J., Madero, M., and Diaz-Perales, A. (2010). Characterization of IgE epitopes of Cuc m 2, the major melon allergen, and their role in cross-reactivity with pollen profilins. Clinical and Experimental Allergy: Journal of the British Society for Allergy and Clinical Immunology 40(1): 174–181.

Tuft, L., and Blumstein, G. I. (1942). Studies in food allergy: II. Sensitization to fresh fruits: Clinical and experimental observations. Journal of Allergy 13(6): 574–582.

Uasuf, C. G., Villalta, D., Conte, M. E., Di Sano, C., Barrale, M., Cantisano, V., Pace, E., Gjomarkaj, M., Gangemi, S., and Brusca, I. (2015). Different co-sensitizations could determine different risk assessment in peach allergy? Evaluation of an anaphylactic biomarker in Pru p 3 positive patients. Clinical and Molecular Allergy: CMA 13: 30.

Valenta, R., Duchene, M., Pettenburger, K., Sillaber, C., Valent, P., Bettelheim, P., Breitenbach, M., Rumpold, H., Kraft, D., and Scheiner, O. (1991). Identification of profilin as a novel pollen allergen; IgE autoreactivity in sensitized individuals. Science (New York, N.Y.) 253(5019): 557–560.

Valenta, R., Hochwallner, H., Linhart, B., and Pahr, S. (2015). Food allergies: the basics. Gastroenterology 148(6): 1120–1131 e1124.

Vallier, P., Dechamp, C., Vial, O., and Deviller, P. (1988). A study of allergens in celery with cross-sensitivity to mugwort and birch pollens. Clinical Allergy 18(5): 491–500.

van Ree, R., Fernandez-Rivas, M., Cuevas, M., van Wijngaarden, M., and Aalberse, R. C. (1995). Pollen-related allergy to peach and apple: an important role for profilin. The Journal of Allergy and Clinical Immunology 95(3): 726–734.

Vanek-Krebitz, M., Hoffmann-Sommergruber, K., Laimer da Camara Machado, M., Susani, M., Ebner, C., Kraft, D., Scheiner, O., and Breiteneder, H. (1995). Cloning and sequencing of Mal d 1, the major allergen from apple (Malus domestica), and its immunological relationship to Bet v 1, the major birch pollen allergen. Biochemical and Biophysical Research Communications 214(2): 538–551.

Vieths, S., Scheurer, S., and Ballmer-Weber, B. (2002). Current understanding of cross-reactivity of food allergens and pollen. Annals of the New York Academy of Sciences 964: 47–68.

Wangorsch, A., Jamin, A., Foetisch, K., Malczyk, A., Reuter, A., Vierecke, S., Schulke, S., Bartel, D., Mahler, V., Lidholm, J., Vieths, S., and Scheurer, S. (2015). Identification of Sola l 4 as Bet v 1 homologous pathogenesis related-10 allergen in tomato fruits. Molecular Nutrition & Food Research 59(3): 582–592.

Werfel, T., Asero, R., Ballmer-Weber, B. K., Beyer, K., Enrique, E., Knulst, A. C., Mari, A., Muraro, A., Ollert, M., Poulsen, L. K., Vieths, S., Worm, M., and Hoffmann-Sommergruber, K. (2015). Position paper of the EAACI: food allergy due to immunological cross-reactions with common inhalant allergens. Allergy 70(9): 1079–1090.

Westphal, S., Kempf, W., Foetisch, K., Retzek, M., Vieths, S., and Scheurer, S. (2004). Tomato profilin Lyc e 1: IgE cross-reactivity and allergenic potency. Allergy 59(5): 526–532.

Wopfner, N., Willeroidee, M., Hebenstreit, D., van Ree, R., Aalbers, M., Briza, P., Thalhamer, J., Ebner, C., Richter, K., and Ferreira, F. (2002). Molecular and immunological characterization of profilin from mugwort pollen. Biological Chemistry 383(11): 1779–1789.

Xue, B., and Robinson, R. C. (2013). Guardians of the actin monomer. European Journal of Cell Biology 92(10-11): 316–332.

Yamamoto, T., Asakura, K., Shirasaki, H., and Himi, T. (2015). Oral allergy syndrome following soy milk ingestion in patients with birch pollen allergy. Nihon Jibiinkoka Gakkai Kaiho 118(9): 1124–1132.

Zuidmeer, L., and van Ree, R. (2007). Lipid transfer protein allergy: primary food allergy or pollen/food syndrome in some cases. Current Opinion in Allergy and Clinical Immunology 7(3): 269–273.

CHAPTER 14

Biotechnology

Methods for Assessing Potential Allergenicity of Novel Proteins According to Global Regulations

Christal C. Bowman[1,*] and *Scott McClain*[2]

Introduction

Biotechnology can introduce dietary proteins that are considered novel and for which there is little to no prior consumption. The expectation from a regulatory standpoint is that the novel protein be assessed for potential allergenicity before it can enter the food supply by way of a biotech crop or novel food product. Potential identity of an existing allergen as a novel food protein, cross-reactivity of the novel protein with existing allergens, and the potential for the protein to become a *de novo* sensitizer are addressed. This assessment of potential allergenicity is based on two principles. The first is that there are well understood and accepted precepts for identifying existing allergens, and that the amino acid sequences of those allergens are known. The second is that characterizing biotech proteins are based on standardized approaches to determine the biophysical features of those proteins, so that comparisons with known allergens are possible. Characterizing several features together remains the basis of risk assessment because there is no single feature or holistic animal model that can predict risk for the several distinct structural protein classes of allergens.

[1] Bayer CropScience LLP, a division of Bayer: 2 T.W. Alexander Dr., Research Triangle Park, NC 27709, USA.
[2] Syngenta Crop Protection, LLC: 3054 E. Cornwallis Road, Research Triangle Park, NC 27709, USA.
Email: scott.mcclain@syngenta.com
* Corresponding author: christal.bowman@bayer.com

For the first generation of biotech protein products, food allergy has been assessed through a weight-of-evidence approach. The approach utilizes the data from the characterization studies to build an overall conclusion of risk. In practical terms, this means that no single study would discount the possibility that a protein is safe. For example, pepsin susceptibility results may show that a biotech protein survives a minute or two longer than what has typically been shown for biotech proteins in the past. This result, however, should not indict the protein as having a risk if all the other characterizations show a lack of risk for allergy under the weight-of-evidence approach. If applied properly, allergy risk would be concluded as low or negligible if the following are true (1) the protein has a history of safe exposure, (2) the protein is unlike allergens at the sequence level, and (3) the protein is in no other way similar to allergens and therefore is not likely to have allergenic potential based on pepsin characterization alone. The source organism has traditionally been important in identifying the select set of the population allergic to specific proteins within that organism. However, the source organism is not, of itself, a predictor of clinical risk for a particular protein. Allergenic foods, animals, etc. contain both allergens and non-allergens.

It is important to understand how the concept of characterizing an allergen feature or biophysical characteristic is performed (protocols), when it is performed (hypothesized to yield relevant data), and how the data is interpreted for use in allergy risk assessment. For example, characterizing a feature such as protein susceptibility to pepsin enzyme has its goal to determine the time by which the original, intact test protein is no longer present. The interpretation of this type of data is then compared to what is expected for most known allergens. In this sense, the characterization is a relative comparison. What it is not is a test. The biotech protein that is characterized cannot "pass" or "fail" because there is no universally prescriptive rule for pepsin digestion to which all allergens adhere. In fact, several allergens are very sensitive to exposure to pepsin but retain their ability to sensitize and elicit allergy.

The key to building a suite of characterization studies that are valuable across many different assessments for different proteins is ensuring consistency with standardized protocols. The best attempt at this has been the original Simulated Gastric Fluid (SGF) Pharmacopeia protocols (USP, 1995, 2000) and later, the protocol for novel proteins outlined in Thomas *et al.* (2004) that describes how to characterize pepsin sensitivity for purified proteins. Although there has been interest in recent years in building a true model of gastric digestion, that of Thomas *et al.* (2004) remains a standard for a protocol as a screening tool for novel proteins and their degradation by pepsin under repeatable conditions. Again, this is not a test; its purpose is to measure time under which a protein is exposed to pepsin and to identify when the intact protein is no longer intact. Ultimately, the time-to-digestion is compared to what is expected of most allergens; i.e., allergens typically resist degradation and non-allergens degrade rapidly.

Other steps performed to assess potential allergy risk are similar to SGF in that they are screening activities designed to rapidly identify potential hazards of concern Identifying true hazards necessitates more scrutiny, and hazards alone do not predict risk. This is particularly true of allergy hazard identification. This is because, as with SGF, not all known allergens fall neatly into either a "yes" or "no" category for possessing a particular characteristic. In the case of comparing biotech proteins to allergen sequences, the bioinformatics approach is understood also to be one of interpreting probability. That is, the probability that a known allergen and a biotech protein share enough similar amino acid residues, and that those residues themselves are biochemically similar, is enough to be interpreted as risk of allergic cross-reactivity. In some respects, this comparison has been treated as a test because regulatory guidance has been in place (Codex, 2003, 2009) with relatively definitive thresholds of 35% exact matching residue count over an overlap of 80 or more residues. Those comparisons exceeding these dual criteria would be deemed as having a hazard and thus, fail this part of the safety assessment. In reality, even just this part of an overall risk assessment is more complicated. Allergen bioinformatics is relatively new, but bioinformatics and biosystematics have a much longer history with work in this field dedicated to improving its use specifically for biotech proteins with the goal of a more standardized and reliable approach to interpreting the data. In the final analysis, understanding that bioinformatics is not a predictive tool for allergy hazard (or risk) is critical; it is a step, usually the first step, in determining more definitive studies to identify allergy risk.

In this chapter, we will outline details of protocols that offer standardized approaches to allergy characterization for GM or novel proteins intended for use in food (Fig. 14.1).

Starting with allergen identification, the formation and use of identity criteria will be discussed. We will also address how the data from characterization studies of biotech proteins rely on allergen identity and how this data is built into a thorough risk assessment of allergenic potential.

Allergen Discovery

The identification of proteins as allergens is a critical step in understanding the nature of allergenicity (the probability of eliciting a clinical allergic reaction) and necessary for making comparisons between novel proteins of unknown allergenicity and proteins of known allergenicity. In the most obvious sense, a protein is considered an allergen when there is evidence that people are allergic to it. Therefore, it is clinical evidence that supports the categorization of a protein as an allergen (and including it in a database of allergens as discussed below). This process of identification typically begins by carefully recording a case history of exposure to a source organism (pollen from a specific tree, or a specific food). The protein allergen must then be found to bind serum IgE from that of the same patient(s). Ideally, the patient will have demonstrated

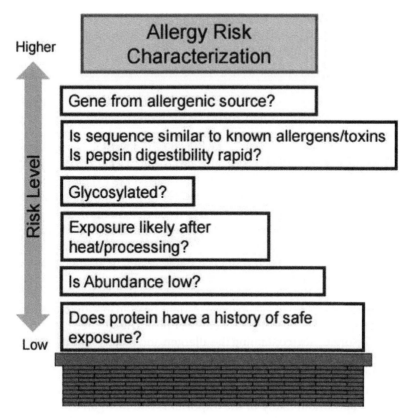

Fig. 14.1: Schematic representation of the characterization studies that support the allergy evaluation of GM proteins. The risk is lowered when GM proteins are demonstrated to show a lack of shared similarity with allergens.

a positive reaction in a double-blind placebo-controlled food challenge to confirm clinically relevant symptomology to the source of the protein. Positive skin-prick tests can also add to the evidence of allergy to the protein source, and although these are less reliable than the food challenge, they are the key for gauging reactivity to aeroallergens.

Direct testing of the patient with purified protein is fairly rare, so component-resolved diagnosis, or identification of the individual offending proteins, is generally conducted through *in vitro* experimentation. This usually involves running the food extract on an electrophoretic gel to separate proteins and visualize protein bands, for example, determining which of those bands is recognized by patient IgE. Proteins can then be sequenced. Of course, IgE is necessary for allergic elicitation, but *in vitro* observations of its binding to a particular protein are not sufficient to predict allergic reactions. Therefore, the clinical relevance of IgE binding ideally should be verified with cell-based testing (basophil activation test). IgE binding can also be non-specific, so proper experimental controls for non-specific binding are critical. For a more detailed explanation of strategies for allergen discovery, see Abdel Rahman *et al.* (2012).

Bioinformatics

As bioinformatic approaches have matured, their use in identifying relevant similarity among allergens and their use for biotech safety assessments has become more important. Bioinformatic assessments are performed throughout the lifespan of a biotech product, from early-phase research and development to post-market surveillance. This is primarily because it is recognized that new allergens are periodically identified and added to existing databases of allergens. One of the most important aspects of both the allergen database concept and bioinformatics is that it lets the assessment of allergy risk for biotech proteins step past the initial 1990s idea of exclusively identifying the allergen source organism. The reason for a focus on organism was the lack of collated and curated allergen sequence databases. One of the symptoms of this was the identification of a known allergen, the Brazil nut 2S albumin, in a prospective biotech soybean product (Nordlee *et al.*, 1996), which reinforced the source organism bias of allergy hazard identification in sourcing genes from allergenic foods. Without sequence identification and associated biosystematics analysis, the organism (containing the allergen and mostly non-allergens) was the only way to identify the hazard.

Today, we have examples of curated allergen databases and a well-characterized description of the structural protein families that contain allergens. In addition, many of the important food allergen organisms have undergone extensive, if not complete genome sequencing. Together, this supports a good understanding of exactly which sequences are allergens, and it also helps to clearly identify which sequences are not allergens. If using soybean as an example, under the original hazard identification paradigm, simply using (i.e., transferring) a soybean's endogenous gene (a non-allergen) as a biotech protein would have been categorized as having a risk because soybean is a known allergenic food. Today, for all practical purposes, both the known allergens and the known non-allergens can be identified in soybean. Therefore, the hazard identification for the risk of moving a known allergen from soybean into another organism (to be used as food) rests on comparing the protein of interest to a reliable allergen database, or, simply characterizing the protein for its annotated name and function. This paradigm puts the focus of hazard identification on the annotated name of the protein, its characterized function and its presence (or lack thereof) in an allergen database. If it is clearly not an allergen (does not belong to a named structural class of allergens) and has a history of expression in other foods (i.e., a history of safe exposure), a protein from soybean would retain the same negligible risk of allergy as the homologous protein from an organism that contains no allergens.

This leads to more fully characterizing the history of safe exposure. In using the soybean example, since most if not all of the soybean allergens have been identified there is reasonable assurance that the rest of the endogenous soybean proteins are safe from an allergy perspective. Along with a lack of presence in an allergen database, this is considered empirical data supporting the case that a protein of interest is not an allergen and is unlikely to become an allergen. An extension of this would be the characterization of the homologous proteins that are from the same structural family and have the same function, but are expressed in other organisms that are safely consumed. In a sense, there would be overwhelming evidence for the lack of allergenic potential for a protein from soybean if it was a ubiquitous protein; a well-described Krebs cycle enzyme for example that is expressed in all commonly consumed plant foods.

Rationale for applying allergen characterization study protocols to novel genes and their proteins

The history of novel protein bioinformatic safety assessment guidance resides in FAO/WHO and Codex documentation from the early 2000s. Much of this guidance was focused on establishing whether a protein was a known allergen or, based on criteria for shared similarity: similar enough in amino acid sequence with existing allergens to be cross-reactive. In addition to these criteria-based guidelines, the organism providing the source of a novel gene/protein was treated as an inherent risk factor. The premise being that an undiscovered protein could be an allergen and that a "novel" protein from that organism could be one of these new allergens. However, in the interim, there has been a thorough curation of known allergens into databases against which a novel protein can be compared. As discussed above, this allows specific identification of the criteria-based similarity between a protein and a known allergen, including the organism. In conjunction with an allergen database, Genbank (NCBI) helps provide the details of a specific gene sequence, including the source organism and the ability to identify homologous sequences in other organisms (i.e., taxonomic distribution). A clear characterization of the gene and the function of the gene's protein along with clear characterization of any similarity with known, specific allergens delineates allergens from non-allergens. Clearly, not all proteins are allergens and therefore, the full genomic documentation of organisms, especially crops, and other plant foods, is an important keystone that provides a basis for removing the source organism itself as a risk factor for an otherwise non-allergen protein. From a safety perspective, this helps to alleviate the contention that any protein from an organism that contains allergens is an allergen by association only.

Protocol outline for comparing a biotech protein to allergens

The purpose of comparing a biotech protein to known allergens is to establish whether that protein is a known allergen or whether there is a risk of cross-reactivity with an allergen. The first key element in setting up a comparative analysis between a protein requiring an assessment and allergens is to have allergens organized and annotated into a database. There are a number of examples of varying standards and purposes. For example, the IUIS has good scientific support from experts in the field of allergy disease and focuses on the nomenclature that helps in identifying groups of proteins that are allergens. At the University of Nebraska, the AllergenOnline database is an example of sequences that have been reviewed for clinical evidence of allergy. Another database for which the sequence search implements advanced search algorithm tools equipped to handle the increasing number of available NCBI entries is under development. Called the Comprehensive Protein Allergen Resource, or COMPARE database, sequences in this database will also be included based on clinical evidence of allergy. Good curation and annotation allow for interpretation of any alignments between the biotech protein and one or more allergens.

The next step is to establish acceptance criteria for the alignments that may occur between a protein under review and any allergens. The most recent novel food and feed safety guidance was updated globally under *Codex Alimentarius* (Codex, 2009). The bioinformatic comparison criteria are that any alignments with exact matching amino acids (identity) would be a concern if the rate was greater than 35%. In addition, this percentage was only of concern if the sequence overlap was 80 or more amino acids. This set of two criteria was an attempt to recognize that smaller, overlapping portions of proteins are unlikely to identify enough similarity arbitrarily at 35% shared amino acids to indicate a risk of cross-reactivity. These criteria are still considered the standard today.

The acceptance criteria are critical in interpreting the algorithmic alignment output. However, the protocol for setting up the comparison is important as well. The algorithms generally considered relevant are FASTA and BLAST. The BLAST package of sequence comparison programs is recognizable through GenBank and NCBI. However, for allergen comparison, the FASTA program has more consistently been used over the last 15 years. Both provide a localized (localized within the full-length proteins) determination of sequence similarity. From this software, the two key criteria are easily reviewable, and both offer more sophisticated assessments of the quality and significance of the alignments. This has been reviewed in terms of best practices (Ladics *et al.*, 2011) and specific modeling of allergen alignments to determine the best use of the FASTA program has also been performed (Mirsky *et al.*, 2013; Silvanovich *et al.*, 2009).

The FASTA program has key criteria that help determine whether alignments between a protein and allergens will produce a significant alignment; i.e., one that exceeds the criteria. There are many parameters, but the most important are the "word size" and the scoring allotment of alignments based on any gaps allowed in a sequence during alignment pairing. The gaps are gauged by the "gap penalty" and the "gap extension" parameters. Together, these are typically set at word size = 2, gap penalty = 10–12, and gap extension = 2.

Other parameters that help with consistency are "Z" and "z". The uppercase Z tells the scoring of alignments to be normalized to a given allergen database size. Given that the number of new allergens added each year is small, the Z parameter can be kept the same, which helps limit variation in the probability score that helps determine the significance of the alignments. One last parameter that provides an upper limit to those alignments that will be judged based on the alignments and their key criteria (e.g., identity, similarity, E-value) is the E-value limiter. The FASTA program has to have a limit beyond which alignments will not be considered and displayed. Traditionally, the default value has been 10. Although unnecessary, this value can be acceptable if it is recognized that both the authors of FASTA and specific work with allergens have determined that output E-values are much lower where relevant homology between two proteins occurs; typically from 0.01–0.000001 (Pearson and Lipman, 1988; Silvanovich *et al.*, 2009).

Celiac Disease

Recently, a review of non-IgE-mediated food protein diseases and the diagnostic approaches to identify the clinical presence in affected patients was performed (Manchester, 2013). Gluten associated pathologies are most frequently associated with celiac disease of the gut. Celiac disease is also the best understood in terms of the cellular mechanisms and the discrete peptides of gluten proteins that act on T-cells (Koning, 2003). Also recently, a list of these peptides has been formed into a searchable database to provide a supplemental database that can be used to assess sequence matches to any other protein (Goodman *et al.*, 2016). The intent of a peptide database is to identify matches between a GM protein and a peptide known to have the capacity to act as a causative celiac disease agent.

Until now, non-IgE-mediated disease risk for a GM protein has been assessed as a function of both identifying the source organism and performing characterization studies (e.g., bioinformatic comparisons, SGF, etc.). As with IgE-mediated allergens, clarifying risk by identifying the source organism does not hold the same weight as it did before the advent of sequence databases. Celiac disease risk, in particular, is tied very closely with a very select set of foods; namely wheat, barley and rye. There is limited evidence that a low-expressing protein, avenin, may also implicate oat; a cereal grain with a more removed taxonomic similarity to wheat, barley and rye. In summary, if a GM protein is not from a celiac source organism then there is no identified hazard associated with celiac disease potential. Given the clear identification of specific celiac-triggering proteins in wheat, barley and rye, a more specific assessment can be pursued to exonerate all of the other proteins expressed in wheat, barley, rye and oat.

Serum Screening; When Appropriate

Exceeding the threshold for shared identity with a known allergen (> 35% over 80 amino acids) triggers specific serum screening studies to determine if there is cross-reactivity with the known allergen. Serum IgE antibody binding protocols require the availability of well-characterized sera from patients with clinically validated allergy to the food and demonstrated IgE binding to the specific allergen (Thomas *et al.*, 2007). Serum screening is also performed when the source of the gene is allergenic, in case additional allergens in that source have not been identified. Sera for this purpose need to come from patients allergic to the food in general but not necessarily any specific protein within that food. According to *Codex* guidelines, a negative result in this assay is not sufficient to conclude that there is no hazard; undefined, additional testing using cells from allergic patients or skin prick testing is recommended (Codex, 2009). Much of the guidance in regulatory documents is based on the study of known allergens but is limited in indicating the utility of sera for putative and unconfirmed allergens. This guidance is also in conjunction with bioinformatics guidance that was written prior to the formation of databases and established informatics methods.

In most cases, it is understood that lack of IgE binding towards a specific protein is confirmation enough that the informatics sequence similarity was not indicative of a hazard for cross-reactivity. The only caveat being if the similarity were occurring in a region of allergen sequence shown to be a specific IgE binding motif whereby cross-reactivity with a novel protein may be hypothesized to occur. Serum screening is still recommended as a way to investigate cross-reactivity that might occur due to the source organism of a GM protein having an indirect taxonomic relationship with a taxonomic group containing allergens. In this instance the recommendation is to test sera from patients allergic to other broadly related sources (e.g., monocots or insects); this is termed targeted serum screening as opposed to specific serum screening, but its utility has been questioned, and it would be difficult to support as a confirmatory test for allergy risk.

Amylase: A Case Study

Presented here is a case study of an alpha-amylase enzyme developed as a GM protein to provide carbohydrate hydrolysis to support maize use in ethanol production. The amylase (AMY797E) was developed as a chimeric, reassembled protein, as sourced from the thermophilic taxonomic domain, *Archae*. The protein was constructed from three of the wild-type isoforms of the alpha-amylase gene from the genera, *Thermococcales*. As with all GM proteins, AM797E, was evaluated for allergy safety using a weight-of-evidence approach (Goodman, 2008; Ladics and Selgrade, 2009). There were no indications of allergy from the hazard characterization studies and exposure considerations, and the maize crop which expresses AMY797E has received regulatory approval in most global regions for either import and/or cultivation.

One legacy of the early attempts to define the informatics sequence assessment guidelines holds that the exact match of eight or more amino acids with an allergen warrants further study; serum screening being the presumptive method considered. The AMY797E protein shares a match with a putative allergen, Per a 3.01, from the American cockroach (*Periplaneta americana*). The Per a 3.01 allergen is recognized as part of the AllergenOnline database (Goodman *et al.*, 2016).

As noted by the regulatory approvals, the eight amino acid match was not considered an allergy hazard for AMY797E and the case study herein provided added evidence for those regulatory regions deeming it necessary. Several considerations were made to distinguish whether this type of sequence similarity indicated a hazard, prior to considering serology as the most definitive assessment of cross-reactivity risk.

First, the characterization of the cockroach allergen was considered with regard to any known IgE binding epitopes that might have suggested the eight amino acid match was indicative of a clinically relevant location within the protein sequence/structure. Shown in Fig. 14.2 is the location of the eight amino acid match relative to the research by the laboratory identifying the Per a 3.01 allergen(s) (Wu *et al.*, 1990; Wu and Lan, 1988; Wu *et al.*, 1995; Wu *et al.*, 1996; Wu *et al.*, 2003).

The conclusion from this assessment was that (a) the eight amino acid match alone was highly unlikely to identify a functionally relevant epitope

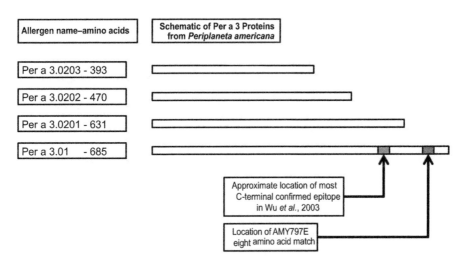

Fig. 14.2: Schematic representation of *Periplaneta americana* Per a 3 allergen isoforms and the location of the eight amino acid identity match between AMY797E and Per a 3.01 relative to the known, most C-terminal Per a 3.01 epitope.

and (b) in the case of Per a 3.01, the likelihood remained low due to the lack of overlap with the described IgE binding epitope.

Second, production of the allergen, in purified form, was evaluated. A full-length protein is typically specified as a recombinant protein to as high a purity as practically possible for use in IgE binding studies. This was the case with Per a 3.01 given that collection of the proper cockroach species, and purification of milligram amounts of the protein from the organisms was impractical.

Third, in attempting to consider the application of a serology screening test design, access to serum from cockroach allergic patients was the primary focus. Identification of a clinician(s) that has access to patients who are willing to make sera available is the primary relationship required to consider serology screening. The clinician has to survey and screen appropriate patients and acquire consent to draw, store and ship sera to the laboratory where screening is performed.

In the first consideration (IgE epitope overlap), there was no hypothesis that the eight amino acid match was a safety concern regarding cross-reactivity. And, since the evolution of the modern GM protein allergy assessment process, the eight amino acid match has been deemed as having little value (Goodman *et al.*, 2008; Silvanovich *et al.*, 2006). However, due to the impact of the legacy guidance language (Codex, 2003, 2009), serology screening was undertaken to conclusively demonstrate the lack of relevance for the amino acid match. Utilizing the second and third considerations to draft a test strategy, the AMY797E, in purified form, was compared with a recombinantly produced Per a 3.01 protein (rPer a 3.01). The presence or absence of shared IgE binding was used to assess the validity of the eight amino acid match as a hazard indication for the AMY797E protein.

Study Design: All sera were from subjects known to be allergic to either American (*P. americana*) and/or German (*Blatella germanica*) cockroach species. Most cockroach-allergic subjects had clinical histories of asthma as well as having either skin prick test reactivity to cockroach or had positive IgE reactivity to cockroach antigen(s) as determined by ImmunoCAP or by cockroach-specific IgE ELISA. Sera from subjects negative for cockroach allergy had negative skin prick test reactivity (SPT) to cockroach and/or negative serum IgE reactivity to cockroach. Sera were selected for use in the western blot screening by selecting only those sera that had positive reactivity to cockroach (ImmunoCAP or cockroach specific ELISA). Finally, cockroach allergic sera were qualified for determining IgE binding to AMY797E based on results of a preliminary western blot that tested IgE binding to both an extract of *P. americana* (whole organism) and to rPer a 3.01 protein. Only those sera with demonstrated IgE binding to extract and rPer a 3.01 were used to evaluate IgE binding to AMY797E.

Western blotting methodology was as follows: Briefly, proteins were separated by molecular weight by SDS-PAGE under reducing conditions.

Purified proteins are described briefly in the footnote.[1] Proteins were transferred to PVDF membranes, and non-specific binding sites were blocked with non-fat dry milk before incubation with appropriate test or control serum samples. Bound antibodies (IgG or IgE) were detected with highly specific secondary antibodies which were labeled with the enzyme, horseradish peroxidase, followed by application of chemiluminescent substrate. Emitted light was captured using a Kodak Gel Logic 440 Image Station. The intensity of light is proportional to the abundance of bound antibody. In order to verify sensitivity and specificity of the tests, preliminary tests were performed to demonstrate the identity of the test proteins and the specificity and sensitivity of the anti-IgE reagent.

Specificity and Sensitivity of Anti-IgE Reagent: Purified human IgE and IgG were serially diluted (1:10) and spotted onto identical PVDF membranes with total spot protein content ranging from 1 µg down to 1 pg. The membranes were blocked with non-fat dry milk, then incubated with either 1:1,000 fold diluted anti-human-IgE (horseradish peroxidase labeled) monoclonal antibody or with 1:2,500 fold diluted anti-human IgG (horseradish peroxidase labeled) monoclonal antibody from Southern Biotechnology (Fig. 14.4 B, only human IgE reactivity is shown).

Results: All human serum samples were assessed for binding to rPer a 3.01 protein using a preliminary western blot screen that included the samples of cockroach extract, molecular weight marker, rPer a 3.01 and Rubisco (data not shown). This was to allow selection of serum samples that would afford a meaningful comparison of potential IgE binding between rPer a 3.01 and AMY797E. Out of 48 sera from cockroach allergic donors, only five samples

---

[1] Test Protein

The test protein, AMY797E:

Purified and supplied by Syngenta Biotechnology, Inc. The purity was 62.4%. The protein identity was verified using rabbit anti-AMY797E sera provided by Syngenta (data not shown). AMY797E prepared from plant-produced AMY797E expressed in maize grain and is the mature AMY797E alpha-amylase protein (Fig. 14.3; 50.2 kDa).

Control Materials:

Whole body American cockroach extract intended for skin prick tests was purchased from Greer Laboratories (Lenoir, NC), GB26A03, lot #128870, 1:20 w/v, 50% glycerol. Rubisco (Ribulose 1,5-diphosphate-carboxylase), Sigma Chemical Co. (St. Louis, MO) Product #R8000, 60.9% pure; large and small subunits (Fig. 14.3).

Reference Allergen:

The reference protein was recombinant protein, rPer a 3.01. The rPer a 3.01 was produced by Indoor Biotechnologies, Inc. (IBI), Charlottesville, VANC from a cDNA obtained from *Periplaneta americana* and was cloned into an expression construct in *Pichia pastoris*. The cDNA sequence was verified by IBI and the translation product included the eight amino acid segment that was identical to an eight amino acid segment of AMY797E. The protein identity (Fig. 14.3) was verified using the 2A2-4a mMAb from Dr. Wu (Wu, C.H., Lee, M.F., Tseng, C.Y., 2003. IgE-binding epitopes of the American cockroach Per a 3 allergen. Allergy 58, 986–992.—immunobinding data not shown).

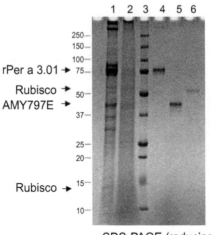

SDS-PAGE (reducing)

Protein Samples

1. Am CR Extract*	(5 µL/Lane)
2. Spent cockroach culture media	(10 µg/Lane)
3. Marker	(2 µL/Lane)
4. rPer a 3.01	(0.5 µg/Lane)
5. AMY797E	(0.5 µg/Lane)
6. RUBISCO	(1.2 µg/Lane)

* Am CR Extract = American Cockroach whole body extract

Fig. 14.3: Coomassie, total protein stained electrophoretic gel displaying locations of the test proteins, rPer a 3.01, AMY797E and control protein, Rubisco.

showed clear and repeatable binding to rPer a 3.01. All five also showed strong IgE binding to a variety of proteins in American cockroach extract (Fig. 14.4 A). The IgE binding to rPer a 3.01 from serum 21 was markedly stronger than the other four and this serum was diluted to 0 1:20 in further tests, compared to 1:10 for the other four sera. These five sera were deemed appropriate as the test sera in evaluating the potential cross-reactivity of rPer a 3.01 and AMY797E. Data were produced at the University of Nebraska.[2]

Rubisco was included as a non-allergen control protein. Faint IgE binding to Rubisco was observed in some blots and indicated that the assay sensitivity was pushed to the extent that non-specific binding was being observed without masking specific binding to the rPer a 3.01. The non-specific binding is likely

[2] Richard E Goodman, PhD FAAAAI, Food Allergy Research and Resource Program, Dept. of Food Science & Technology, 1901 North 21st Street, PO Box 886207. Lincoln, NE 68588-6207, USA. rgoodman2@unl.edu

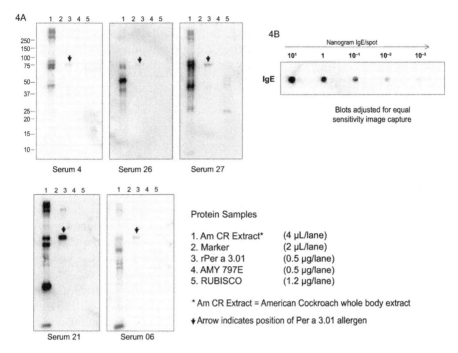

Fig. 14.4: Western blots of rPer a 3.01, AMY797E and control protein, Rubisco, using individual cockroach allergic serum with IgE antibody detection.

due to hydrophobic or charge attraction, rather than epitope-paratope specific recognition that is immunologically relevant for allergy. The interpretation of any sample having IgE binding to Rubisco that is approximately equal to or less than that observed for one of the purified test proteins is that the IgE binding is non-specific for that protein.

Eight non-cockroach allergic (negative) control sera were identified as having minimal non-specific binding and were used to evaluate non-specific binding by the western blot method described herein (data not shown). None of these sera demonstrated reactivity with either Per a 3.01, AMY797E or Rubisco supporting the utility of the specific IgE binding from patient sera to the Per a 3.01 protein.

All five sera showed some level of IgE binding to a band of the same molecular weight as rPer a 3.01 in the cockroach extract (Fig. 14.4A, lane 1). The faint bands that are visible in the Rubisco sample (Fig. 14.4A, lane 5, serum 4 and 27), indicated that appropriate exposure sensitivity was utilized to capture specific IgE binding. None of the five cockroach allergic sera showed any IgE binding to protein at the molecular weight of AMY797E (~ 46 kDa) in lane 4 (Fig. 14.4 A). These results indicate that the eight amino acid sequences shared between rPer a 3.01 and AMY797E does not support IgE-binding and does not indicate a hazard for cross-reactivity for the AMY797E protein. Taken together, this study was also evidence, as was the Ladics *et al.* (2006) work, that short, arbitrary amino acid matches are not an appropriate approach to informatics and that they do not justify serology as a routine technical approach to defining an allergy hazard.

Glycosylation

Many allergens are glycoproteins. The presence of certain types of carbohydrate moieties on the surface of proteins appears to stimulate IgE production when compared with the same proteins lacking glycosylation (Almond *et al.*, 2013). This is likely a result of the stimulation of the mannose receptor on dendritic cells, which functions as a pathogen recognition receptor; it is thought that this enables glycans to stimulate uptake and presentation of antigens on which they are displayed (Al-Ghouleh *et al.*, 2012). The association of glycosylation with allergenicity prompts screening of biotech proteins for the possibility that they will be glycosylated when produced by the plant.

The best-studied mode of glycosylation is the formation of an N-glycosidic linkage to asparagine in the polypeptide chain (Freeze *et al.*, 2012). The necessary (but not sufficient) criterion for protein N-glycosylation is the presence of the sequence N-X~(P)-S/T, where N = asparagine, X~(P) = any amino acid except proline (P), S = serine and T = threonine. Although rare, the sequence motif N-X-C can also be an acceptor site (where N = asparagine, X = any amino acid and C = cysteine). Thus, a search for these consensus sequences is conducted to screen for the potential for glycosylation, but this is not completely predictive. Actual glycosylation is assessed as one of the analyses conducted to establish equivalence between protein expressed *in planta* and protein produced recombinantly to procure the larger quantities required for many of the tests in the safety package (Raybould *et al.*, 2013).

Certain carbohydrate moieties on glycosylated proteins can also serve as targets for IgE binding. Known as Cross-reactive Carbohydrate Determinants, or CCDs, these carbohydrates can be displayed on different proteins and yet recognized by the same IgE antibodies. However, this antibody binding does not seem to have any clinical relevance and is considered to be false positive reactivity (Mari, 2002; van der Veen *et al.*, 1997). The ubiquitous presence of these carbohydrates in most plants and many insects can result in the erroneous identification of certain proteins as important allergens based on recognition by patient sera. However, attributing IgE binding solely to the carbohydrate must be supported through thorough experimentation, and thus it is somewhat difficult to say with certainty that the protein backbone sequence is not relevant. Therefore, allergen databases often contain protein sequences for which there is evidence for carbohydrates being responsible for IgE binding, but it is quite challenging to disprove the allergenicity of the protein sequence itself.

Resistance to degradation by digestive enzymes

In vitro resistance to digestive enzymes, particularly pepsin, is a key part of the safety assessment of proteins used in biotechnology. The rationale for this sort of testing is that a highly digestible protein has limited opportunity to interact with the body after ingestion, whether to exert toxicity or to elicit immune responses. Many, but not all, allergens resist digestion. The imperfect relationship between known allergenicity and observed digestive stability can be attributed to a number of possible factors. The choice of allergens vs. non-allergens is critical for establishing this relationship. Instances where there is disagreement may be due to analysis of aeroallergens, which would not be subject to digestive influence, or proteins that only appear to be allergens on the basis of limited evidence (IgE binding can be a laboratory artifact/ non-specific binding). In addition, of course, there is a fairly large surface between the lips and the stomach where contact with a protein can be made. Importantly, digestibility is only one facet of the weight of evidence approach to allergenicity assessment. However, it is one of the few tools for assessing the potential for *de novo* sensitization. Stability alone cannot be taken as an indicator of allergenicity because stable non-allergens exist, and from an immunologic perspective additional signals are required beyond stability for sensitization to occur (antigen presentation in the absence of costimulation leads to anergy). It is accepted, though, that ingested proteins must survive digestion to at least some extent in order to cause reactions in sensitized individuals. From human and animal *in vivo* studies we know that a peptide must be at least 1.5–3 kDa in size to elicit an immediate-type allergic reaction (Poulsen and Hau, 1987; Van Hoeyveld *et al.*, 1998). The peptide must have at least two IgE binding epitopes available in order to cross-link adjacent IgE molecules and trigger mediator release.

The assays performed for this purpose include incubation of the protein in Simulated Gastric Fluid (SGF) or Simulated Intestinal Fluid (SIF), containing pepsin and pancreatin enzymes, respectively. In some cases these incubations are performed sequentially to mimic transit through the gastrointestinal tract. It is important to note that these assays are not designed to approximate real digestion; they are only a basis for comparison. Results in these assays are largely dependent on the enzyme to substrate ratios and pH; these are known to vary greatly with age, meal size and content, medication use, etc. Additionally, matrix components and prior processing (e.g., heat) are known to alter digestibility differentially for the proteins that have been examined. Such aspects are not generally included, though there is a movement to include matrix components like phosphatidylcholine and use a range of pH conditions and enzyme to substrate ratios. It is not clear whether this effort can solidify the relationship between digestive stability and allergenicity or otherwise enhance the assessment, since the objective of testing purified proteins under highly standard conditions is, again, standardized and reproducible comparison of the protein of interest to known allergens and non-allergens.

In the pepsin resistance assay, the purified protein of interest is incubated for various durations with pepsin in simulated gastric fluid, using a well-established protocol (Astwood *et al.*, 1996; Thomas *et al.*, 2004). Control proteins of known digestive stability are included in this step (e.g., ovalbumin and horseradish peroxidase as slowly and rapidly digested controls, respectively). A broad range of time points (0 to 60 minutes) is utilized initially to capture the general time frame for degradation of the protein. Further experiments are then performed to more finely resolve the time at which the protein degrades (e.g., 0, 0.5, 1, 3, 5, and 7 minutes). The reaction mixtures are visualized using SDS-PAGE and often western blotting. For this step, a "time zero" control containing the protein of interest and the pepsin and a lane with pepsin alone are necessary to differentiate the pepsin bands from the original protein of interest and any digestion fragments arising at later time points. The choice of gel and extent to which mixtures are run on the gel are important considerations because ideally any digestive fragments as small as 1.5 kDa should be visible on the gel. This is difficult in practice, however, and visualizing the full range of sizes with good separation of bands becomes more challenging with a larger protein of interest. Visualization of potential small fragments is also important in the western blot step. Smaller bands are more quickly transferred and can pass through the blotting membrane, and so care should be taken not to transfer for too long or at too high of a voltage. A second membrane can be placed behind the first and stained to ensure no "overtransfer" has occurred. Western blotting confers an advantage in that faint bands that are sometimes not visible in the SDS-PAGE become visible due to the amplifying nature of this assay. One caveat here is that fragments appearing in the SDS-PAGE may not appear in the blot due to loss of epitopes required for recognition by the antibody. In this case, the band in the SDS-PAGE may be sequenced to verify it as a fragment of the protein of interest.

Interpreting the results from the pepsin digestibility assay can be challenging. There is neither a known minimum time frame required for protein exposure for sensitization, nor a known location within the gastrointestinal tract where sensitization occurs. Certainly there seems to be more opportunity for proteins to interact with the immune system within the intestine, where sampling for foreign proteins is highly active, but sampling occurs in other areas of the gastrointestinal tract as well, e.g., the mouth and stomach (Bimczok *et al.*, 2010; Hovav, 2014). Potential improvements to this protocol include those that focus on more discrete time points to determine a more precise measure of pepsin's effect and kinetic-based protocols that have enough time resolution (precision) to determine a half-life of the protein more accurately. In addition, European Food Safety Authority documents have suggestions for more physiologically relevant protocols for SGF, presumably, in hopes the *in vitro* SGF system can more closely model human digestion. It remains uncertain whether this will be more predictive, and any new model will require validation and standardization before it is used in the safety assessment.

Conclusion

Transgenic modification of foods often results in expression of novel proteins, and assessment of potential allergenicity is a key part of the safety assessment of the novel protein. The methods described in this chapter are integral parts of the weight of evidence approach to identifying an allergenic hazard. Each provides information on the characteristics of the novel protein and how they compare with those of known allergens. In assessing a protein's structure and function, as it applies to its use as a GM protein, a history of exposure to that protein is typically part of the characterization. In identifying any food uses for any organisms in which the protein is expressed, dietary exposure in humans and any other mammalians can inform the safety as it pertains to a new use in a different food (crop). This, in effect, is a corollary regarding questions of risk tied to the source organism. If a GM protein is not an allergen or similar to an allergen and, in addition, is a widely distributed (taxonomically) and familiar protein with proven safety, then sourcing a particular homolog of that protein from an allergen-containing food should not warrant concern.

There is no presumption that GM foods are inherently more allergenic than those produced conventionally. To place the expectation of GM protein allergy assessment into context, a far larger number of novel proteins are introduced upon adoption of entirely new foods; typically with little or no history of prior consumption. As recent examples, allergies to introduced foods such as kiwi, lychee, and mealworm have been observed (Dearman *et al.*, 2014; Raap *et al.*, 2007). Interestingly, most allergens identified in these novel foods share similarity (i.e., sequence or structure) with previously identified allergens and often provoke reactions due to cross-reactivity in individuals with existing allergy (D'Avino *et al.*, 2011; FÄR *et al.*, 1995; Ibero *et al.*, 2007; Verhoeckx *et al.*, 2014).

Ultimately, risk assessment of GM proteins and foods rests on a weight of the evidence because the biology of allergy remains limited to a degree that limits the current capacity to perform a quantitative assessment. Thus, the characterization studies of similarity between the GM proteins and allergens are performed and compiled as hazard identifiers and assembled into an assessment that supports the broader risk assessment of GM foods and crops.

Acknowledgements

We gratefully acknowledge the editorial contributions of Drs. Corinne Herouet-Guicheney, Cynthia Stauffer, Doug Wolf, Russ Essner, and Anas Abdel Rahman.

Keywords: Biotechnology, genetic modification, GM foods, allergenicity, bioinformatics, glycosylation, digestibility, cross-reactivity

References

Abdel Rahman, A. M., Helleur, R. J., Jeebhay, M. F., and Lopata, A. L. (2012). Characterization of Seafood Proteins Causing Allergic Diseases. InTech.

Al-Ghouleh, A., Johal, R., Sharquie, I. K., Emara, M., Harrington, H., Shakib, F., and Ghaemmaghami, A. M. (2012). The glycosylation pattern of common allergens: the recognition and uptake of Der p 1 by epithelial and dendritic cells is carbohydrate dependent. PLoS ONE 7: e33929.

Almond, R. J., Flanagan, B. F., Antonopoulos, A., Haslam, S. M., Dell, A., Kimber, I., and Dearman, R. J. (2013). Differential immunogenicity and allergenicity of native and recombinant human lactoferrins: role of glycosylation. European Journal of Immunology 43: 170–181.

Astwood, J. D., Leach, J. N., and Fuchs, R. L. (1996). Stability of food allergens to digestion *in vitro*. Nature Biotechnology 14: 1269–1273.

Bimczok, D., Clements, R. H., Waites, K. B., Novak, L., Eckhoff, D. E., Mannon, P. J., Smith, P. D., and Smythies, L. E. (2010). Human primary gastric dendritic cells induce a Th1 response to *H. pylori*. Mucosal Immunology 3: 260–269.

Codex. (2009). Foods derived from modern biotechnology. pp. 1–85. *In*: C.A. Commission (ed.). Codex Alimentarius (85 ed.) Rome, Italy.

D'Avino, R., Bernardi, M. L., Wallner, M., Palazzo, P., Camardella, L., Tuppo, L., Alessandri, C., Breiteneder, H., Ferreira, F., Ciardiello, M. A., and Mari, A. (2011). Kiwifruit Act d 11 is the first member of the ripening-related protein family identified as an allergen. Allergy 66: 870–877.

Dearman, R. J., Beresford, L., Foster, E. S., McClain, S., and Kimber, I. (2014). Characterization of the allergenic potential of proteins: an assessment of the kiwifruit allergen actinidin. Journal of Applied Toxicology 34: 489–497.

FÄR, J., WÜThrich, B., and Vieths, S. (1995). Anaphylactic reaction to lychee fruit: evidence for sensitization to profilin. Clinical & Experimental Allergy 25: 1018–1023.

Freeze, H., Eklund, E. A., Ng, B., and Patterson, M. C. (2012). Neurology of inherited glycosylation disorders. Lancet Neurology 11: 453–466.

Goodman, R. E. (2008). Performing IgE serum testing due to bioinformatics matches in the allergenicity assessment of GM crops. Food and Chemical Toxicology 46: S24–S34.

Goodman, R. E., Vieths, S., Sampson, H. A., Hill, D., Ebisawa, M., Taylor, S. L., and van Ree, R. (2008). Allergenicity assessment of genetically modified crops—what makes sense? Nature Biotechnology 26: 73–81.

Goodman, R. E., Ebisawa, M., Ferreira, F., Sampson, H. A., van Ree, R., Vieths, S., Baumert, J. L., Bohle, B., Lalithambika, S., Wise, J., and Taylor, S. L. (2016). Allergen online: A peer-reviewed, curated allergen database to assess novel food proteins for potential cross-reactivity. Molecular Nutrition & Food Research 60: 1183–1198.

Hovav, A. H. (2014). Dendritic cells of the oral mucosa. Mucosal Immunology 7: 27–37.

Ibero, M., Castillo, M. J., and Pineda, F. (2007). Allergy to cassava: a new allergenic food with cross-reactivity to latex. Journal of Investigational Allergology & Clinical Immunology 17: 409–412.

Koning, F. (2003). The molecular basis of celiac disease. Journal of Molecular Recognition 16: 333–336.

Ladics, G. S., Bardina, L., Cressman, R. F., Mattsson, J. L., and Sampson, H. A. (2006). Lack of cross-reactivity between the Bacillus thuringiensis derived protein Cry1F in maize grain and dust mite Der p7 protein with human sera positive for Der p7-IgE. Regulatory Toxicology and Pharmacology: RTP 44: 136–143.

Ladics, G. S., and Selgrade, M. K. (2009). Identifying food proteins with allergenic potential: Evolution of approaches to safety assessment and research to provide additional tools. Regulatory Toxicology and Pharmacology 54: S2–S6.

Ladics, G. S., Cressman, R. F., Herouet-Guicheney, C., Herman, R. A., Privalle, L., Song, P., Ward, J. M., and McClain, S. (2011). Bioinformatics and the allergy assessment of agricultural biotechnology products: Industry practices and recommendations. Regulatory Toxicology and Pharmacology 60: 46–53.

Manchester, T. U. o. (2013). Literature review: 'non-IgE mediated adverse reactions to foods'. European Food Safety Authority EN-527: 40.

Mari, A. (2002). IgE to cross-reactive carbohydrate determinants: analysis of the distribution and appraisal of the *in vivo* and *in vitro* reactivity. International Archives of Allergy and Immunology 129: 286–295.

Mirsky, H. P., Cressman Jr, R. F., and Ladics, G. S. (2013). Comparative assessment of multiple criteria for the *in silico* prediction of cross-reactivity of proteins to known allergens. Regulatory Toxicology and Pharmacology 67: 232–239.

Nordlee, J. A., Taylor, S. L., Townsend, J. A., Thomas, L. A., and Bush, R. K. (1996). Identification of a Brazil-nut allergen in transgenic soybeans. The New England Journal of Medicine 334: 688–692.

Pearson, W. R., and Lipman, D. J. (1988). Improved tools for biological sequence comparison. Proceedings of the National Academy of Sciences of the United States of America 85: 2444–2448.

Poulsen, O. M., and Hau, J. (1987). Murine passive cutaneous anaphylaxis test (PCA) for the 'all or none' determination of allergenicity of bovine whey proteins and peptides. Clinical & Experimental Allergy 17: 75–83.

Raap, U., Schaefer, T., Kapp, A., and Wedi, B. (2007). Exotic food allergy: anaphylactic reaction to lychee. Journal of Investigational Allergology & Clinical Immunology 17: 199–201.

Raybould, A., Kilby, P., and Graser, G. (2013). Characterising microbial protein test substances and establishing their equivalence with plant-produced proteins for use in risk assessments of transgenic crops. Transgenic Research 22: 445–460.

Silvanovich, A., Nemeth, M. A., Song, P., Herman, R., Tagliani, L., and Bannon, G. A. (2006). The value of short amino acid sequence matches for prediction of protein allergenicity. Toxicological Sciences 90: 252–258.

Silvanovich, A., Bannon, G., and McClain, S. (2009). The use of E-scores to determine the quality of protein alignments. Regulatory Toxicology and Pharmacology 54: S26–S31.

Thomas, K., Aalbers, M., Bannon, G. A., Bartels, M., Dearman, R. J., Esdaile, D. J., Fu, T. J., Glatt, C. M., Hadfield, N., Hatzos, C., Hefle, S. L., Heylings, J. R., Goodman, R. E., Henry, B., Herouet, C., Holsapple, M., Ladics, G. S., Landry, T. D., MacIntosh, S. C., Rice, E. A., Privalle, L. S., Steiner, H. Y., Teshima, R., van Ree, R., Woolhiser, M., and Zawodny, J. (2004). A multilaboratory evaluation of a common *in vitro* pepsin digestion assay protocol used in assessing the safety of novel proteins. Regulatory Toxicology and Pharmacology 39: 87–98.

Thomas, K., Bannon, G., Herouet-Guicheney, C., Ladics, G., Lee, L., Lee, S. I., Privalle, L., Ballmer-Weber, B., and Vieths, S. (2007). The utility of an international sera bank for use in evaluating the potential human allergenicity of novel proteins. Toxicological Sciences 97: 27–31.

USP, U. P. (1995). The National Formulary, USP XXIII, NF XVIII. US Pharmacopoeia Convention, Inc., Mack Printing Co., Easton, PA, 2053.

USP, U. P. (2000). The National Formulary, USP XXIV, NF XIX. US Pharmacopoeia Convention, Inc., Mack Printing Co., Easton, PA, 2235.

van der Veen, M. J., van Ree, R., Aalberse, R. C., Akkerdaas, J., Koppelman, S. J., Jansen, H. M., and van der Zee, J. S. (1997). Poor biologic activity of cross-reactive IgE directed to carbohydrate determinants of glycoproteins. Journal of Allergy and Clinical Immunology 100: 327–334.

Van Hoeyveld, E. M., Escalona-Monge, M., De Swert, L. F. A., and Stevens, E. A. M. (1998). Allergenic and antigenic activity of peptide fragments in a whey hydrolysate formula. Clinical & Experimental Allergy 28: 1131–1137.

Verhoeckx, K. C. M., van Broekhoven, S., den Hartog-Jager, C. F., Gaspari, M., de Jong, G. A. H., Wichers, H. J., van Hoffen, E., Houben, G. F., and Knulst, A. C. (2014). House dust mite (Der p 10) and crustacean allergic patients may react to food containing Yellow mealworm proteins. Food and Chemical Toxicology 65: 364–373.

Wu, C. H., Lee, M. F., and Liao, S. C. (1995). Isolation and preliminary characterization of cDNA encoding American cockroach allergens. The Journal of Allergy and Clinical Immunology 96: 352–359.

Wu, C. H., Lee, M. F., Liao, S. C., and Luo, S. F. (1996). Sequencing analysis of cDNA clones encoding the American cockroach Cr-PI allergens. Homology with insect hemolymph proteins. The Journal of Biological Chemistry 271: 17937–17943.

Wu, C. H., and Lan, J. L. (1988). Cockroach hypersensitivity: isolation and partial characterization of major allergens. The Journal of Allergy and Clinical Immunology 82: 727–735.

Wu, C. H., Chiang, B. T., Fann, M. C., and Lan, J. L. (1990). Production and characterization of monoclonal antibodies against major allergens of American cockroach. Clinical and Experimental Allergy: Journal of the British Society for Allergy and Clinical Immunology 20: 675–681.

Wu, C. H., Lee, M. F., and Tseng, C. Y. (2003). IgE-binding epitopes of the American cockroach Per a 3 allergen. Allergy 58: 986–992.

CHAPTER 15

Advances in Biosensor Technologies for Food Allergen Monitoring and Diagnosis

Shimaa Eissa,* Raja Chinnappan and
Mohammed Zourob*

Introduction

Food allergy is considered one of the major health issues nowadays (Cianferoni and Spergel1, 2009; Sicherer and Sampson, 2009) that affects millions of people worldwide, especially in industrial countries. Studies have shown that food allergy affects about 4% of the adult population (Sampson *et al.*, 2005) and a higher prevalence amongst children (6–8%) was reported (Roehr *et al.*, 2004). Food allergy is an abnormal immunological response that arises after eating certain kinds of food. This hypersensitivity is mediated by the production of immunoglobulin E (IgE) antibodies in the body of the allergic individual exposed to specific allergen leading to serious health problems. The resulting immunological reactions from the intake of particular allergen depends on the dose and the sensitivity of the consumer (Taylor *et al.*, 2002). No treatment has been discovered for food allergy until now; therefore, sensitive individuals must assure the elimination of the specific allergen from their food. For this reason, the European legislation states that 14 allergenic food ingredient have to be clearly listed on the label of the food product. However, the unintentional contamination of food with allergens that are not listed on the food label can occur during any stage of the food chain. This contamination may happen during food manufacturing due to the use of shared equipment

Department of Chemistry, Alfaisal University, Al Zahrawi Street, Al Maather, Al Takhassusi Road, Riyadh 11533, Saudi Arabia.
Email: rchinnappan@alfaisal.edu
* Corresponding authors: seissa@alfaisal.edu; mzourob@alfaisal.edu

with insufficient cleaning or during transfer or storage processes. In order to avoid cross contact between food ingredients, many industrial institutions have separate production lines for different kinds of products (Taylor *et al.*, 2006). More than 160 food materials can be considered as allergic compounds. Particularly, milk, eggs, wheat, peanuts, tree nuts, soybeans, sesame seed and seafoods (fish, crustaceans and shellfish) are considered the most common allergic food ingredients which cause more than 90% of food allergies worldwide (Hefle *et al.*, 1996). The hazard of the unexpected exposure to hidden allergenic components in processed food has led to a high demand for the development of sensitive tools for allergen detection. Efficient detection methods for the sensitive tracing of allergens in food products and equipment are required for regulatory agencies and food manufacturers for assessing and managing the risk of food contamination with allergens.

Different analytical methods are currently used for allergens detection (Pilolli *et al.*, 2013) such as Enzyme-Linked Immunosorbent Assays (ELISA), enzyme-linked immunoaffinity chromatography, HPLC (High-Performance Liquid Chromatography) and capillary electrophoresis methods with size-exclusion chromatography and laser-induced fluorescence detection. Protein-based methods such as western blot and immunoperoxidase staining are also utilized.

Isolation of allergens from the food is a crucial task. In general, the processed food undergoes many processes for preservation. As a result, changes in the biophysical and immunological properties of the allergic proteins may occur. The common food processes involve thermal (baking, frying, boiling, roasting, etc.) and non-thermal (fermentation, proteolysis, ultrafiltration, etc.) treatments. The thermal food processing influence the allergic potential of the allergen (Jiménez-Saiz *et al.*, 2015; Sathe and Sharma, 2009; Verhoeckx *et al.*, 2015). The allergenicity of the protein is mainly determined by the linear and conformational epitopes. For example, the IgE binding ability of β-lactogloblin significantly decreases after thermal treatment at 90°C (Ehn *et al.*, 2004), whereas the thermal processing enhances the IgE binding affinity of Ara h 1 and Ara h 2 peanut allergens and induce the allergenicity of the peanut (Maleki *et al.*, 2000). On the other hand, diagnosing food allergies is usually done using indirect detection methods of either the allergen-specific IgE antibodies or the mediators released in the blood of the allergic patients. Despite the continuous improvements in the current detection methods, they still do not satisfy current needs because of their high cost and long analysis time. Biosensors are appearing recently as an excellent alternative to the traditional methods that can offer faster detection, lower cost, the capability of automation and high throughput analysis. Particularly, new technologies utilizing novel recognition receptors and transducers to improve the biosensor devices for food allergen detection are being developed. Aptamers are appearing as a new promising biorecognition receptors which can replace antibodies in allergen biosensor platforms (Tran *et al.*, 2013). Moreover, the integration of different nanomaterials into biosensors leads to significant enhancement in the detection signals (Pilolli *et al.*, 2013). Microarray technology has also been implemented in the biosensing platforms which enabled the multiplexed detection of multiple food allergens at the same time (Wang *et al.*, 2011). Here, we discuss several aspects of biosensor developments for allergen monitoring and allergy diagnosis. The recent achievements in the allergen detection will be reviewed. Special attention will be given to the integration of bionanotechnology to the biosensor devices.

Conventional Detection Methods

Allergen analysis

The analysis of food allergen is divided in two major ways: direct methods and the indirect methods. Mass spectrometry and other chromatographic techniques are used for confirmation analysis. The choice of the analytical method depends on the analyte of interest and the required sensitivity. The direct method targets the allergen itself whereas, the indirect method relies on the biomarkers that indicate the presence of a particular allergen in the food. Protein-based analysis methods that involve immunochemical detection techniques such as enzyme-linked immunosorbent assay (ELISA), lateral flow assay (LFD), dipsticks, rocket immune-electrophoresis and dot-immunoblotting are also used (Poms *et al.*, 2004). In other methods, the allergic protein is separated by gel electrophoresis, capillary electrophoresis or HPLC followed by immunoblotting. Indirect methods are mainly DNA-based assays. The target allergen protein is detected by amplification of its encoding gene by Polymerase Chain Reaction (PCR). Accurate and quantitative measurements can be obtained from Real-Time PCR (RT-PCR) methods.

Enzyme-linked immunosorbent assay (ELISA)

ELISA is one of the most common immunological method used for allergen detection in food industries and official food control agencies due to the high sensitivity, specificity and reproducibility (van Hengel, 2007). ELISA tests utilize monoclonal or polyclonal antibodies raised against pure antigens (allergens). Polyclonal antibodies recognize multiple epitopes of the antigen. Therefore, it is preferred in food industries as they can capture the antigen even with minor alteration caused by food processing. Different kinds of commercialized ELISA kits are available in the market (Poms *et al.*, 2004; Schubert-Ullrich *et al.*, 2009). Monaci and Visconti have reviewed the recent development of ELISA kits against different kind of allergens (Monaci and Visconti, 2010). Sandwich ELISA and competitive ELISA approaches are available for the quantification of allergenic proteins from the potentially allergic foods. Sandwich ELISA is the most common method for the detection of allergens in foodstuff (Costa *et al.*, 2015; Peng *et al.*, 2013; Schubert-Ullrich *et al.*, 2009; Werner *et al.*, 2010). However, only limited kits have been validated by the Association Of Analytical Communities (AOAC) internationals. Competitive ELISA is used for the detection of the relatively small amount of allergic proteins in food matrices. Sensitive detection of soybean glycinin has been achieved by the competitive ELISA method with a detection limit of 0.3 ng/ml (Ma *et al.*, 2010). Inductively Coupled Plasma-Mass Spectrometry (ICP-MS) based on the ELISA method has been also been developed. Lanthanide element tagged secondary antibodies is used that can be detected using ICP-MS. Multiple allergen target detection can also achieved by tagging the secondary antibodies with different elements for each target. Careri *et al.* (Careri *et al.*, 2007) have used europium tagged antibody for the detection of peanuts achieving a detection limit of 2 mg/kg. Based on similar detection principle, lateral flow device has also been developed for the rapid detection of food allergens. However, this method is used for qualitative or semi-quantitative measurements. Commercialized rapid allergen tests in various foods have been summarized elsewhere (Schubert-Ullrich *et al.*, 2009).

DNA-based methods

Unlike immunological methods, DNA-based method does not detect the allergic protein directly. However, it detects the genomic DNA which encodes the specific allergen (Prado *et al.*, 2015). Detection of the allergen is achieved by the PCR amplification of its specific DNA. Conventional PCR amplification of allergen-encoding gene by specific primers gives only a qualitative determination of the analytes. Semi-quantitative determination of allergen can be obtained by PCR-ELISA. Although the PCR method is sensitive and quantitative, it fails to detect all the allergens due to degradation of allergen-encoding DNA in the food (Köppel *et al.*, 1998). Simultaneous amplification of many allergen-encoding DNA sequences by PCR is an advantage for the simultaneous detection of multiple analytes using many pairs of primers. Two tetraplex RT-PCR were successfully used for the detection of eight allergens at the same time from hazelnut, peanut, celery, soy, egg, milk, almond and sesame (Köppel *et al.*, 2009). This method is not good for food that contains a high level of protein and low abundance in DNA such as eggs. The main advantage of this method is the stability of the DNA which enables its extraction from food even at denaturing conditions.

Allergen diagnosis

Sensitive and reliable diagnosis methods are important for the proper treatment and protection from the allergen. Two major types of diagnosis are being used: *in vivo* and *in vitro assays*. Both tests have to be performed in parallel in order to achieve high precession. The *in vivo* tests include Skin Prick Test (SPT), oral food challenge and suspicious product elimination diet (Gasilova and Girault, 2015). Although the oral food challenge is considered as a "gold standard", it has a risk of anaphylaxis or other side effects on the patients. SPT is a risk-free and less reliable diagnosis method, in which a small amount of allergen is injected by pricking the patient's skin (Ballmer-Weber, 2014). On the other hand, there are two types of *in vitro* tests, IgE quantification-free based diagnosis and IgE quantification diagnosis. The most popular *in vitro* IgE quantification-free diagnosis is basophil activation test. Flow cytometry is used for the quantification of basophil activation in response to the allergen binding to the IgE antibodies or another effect on the basophil surface (Sanz ML, 2007). Basophil activation test kits are commercially available in the market. In IgE quantification-based tests, the IgE antibodies are used as a universal biomarker for the allergic reactions. Allergy is diagnosed by the quantification of the total amount of IgE antibody or a specific antibody. Other assays for allergy diagnosis have been reviewed elsewhere (Gasilova and Girault, 2015; Hoffmann-Sommergruber *et al.*, 2015; Kulis *et al.*, 2015).

Biosensors in Food Allergens

The biosensor is an emerging technology in the field of the food industry for the detection of allergens from the potentially allergic foods. It appears as excellent alternative to the conventional methods for detection of allergens. Biosensors offer simple and promising ways to overcome the complex processes involved in allergen detection. The biosensor consists of a recognition receptor that is integrated with a transducer which produces a measurable signal upon receptor-analyte binding. Antibody raised against the food allergen, complementary single strand DNA which can be base-paired with the specific sequence of allergen genomic DNA or aptamers (DNA or RNA) selected against the allergen can be used as recognition receptors. The development of point of care, low cost, rapid and real-time biosensors for allergen monitoring and diagnosis is a challenging task. Since the last decade, researchers put considerable efforts to improve the sensitivity of the allergen biosensing platforms (Alves *et al.*, 2015; Pilolli *et al.*, 2013). New materials such as nanoparticles, quantum dots, magnetic materials, carbon nanotubes and graphene (Eissa *et al.*, 2012; Liu *et al.*, 2010; Mairal *et al.*, 2014) that exhibit unique properties have been utilized for designing novel and more sensitive allergen biosensor platforms. Based on the type of transducer, the allergens detection sensors are classified into three major groups: Optical, electrochemical and piezoelectric-based biosensors. Here, we will focus only on the optical and electrochemical biosensors as they are the most applicable for allergen detection and diagnosis.

Optical biosensors

In this type of sensor, the changes in the optical properties are detected by the transducer when the analyte binds to the receptor. Colourimetric, fluorescence and Surface Plasmon Resonance (SPR)-based transducers have been developed for the detection of food allergens (Pilolli *et al.*, 2013).

Absorption spectroscopy is widely used for quantities and qualitative detection of allergen just by monitoring the changes in the optical density of the food samples. These changes can often observed by the naked eyes without the use of any type of equipment (Wang *et al.*, 2011) (Fig. 15.1). Fluorescence-based biosensors are also used frequently due to the high sensitivity, specificity and ease of labelling of the fluorophores. Fluorescence Resonance Energy Transfer (FRET)-based biosensors are used to monitor the change in the conformation of the receptor after allergen binding. Recently, the Rat Basophilic Leukemia cell (RBL-2H3) fluorescence sensor has been developed for the detection of the major fish allergen parvalbumin (Jiang *et al.*, 2014). The main disadvantage of

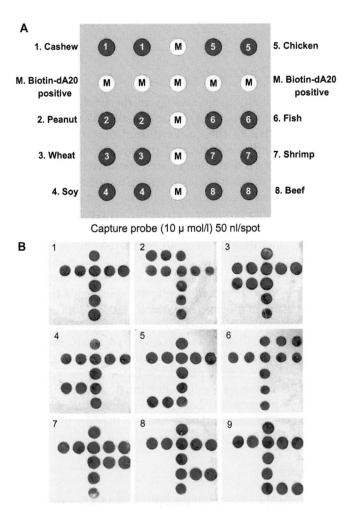

Fig. 15.1: Food allergen detection on a chip with capture probes spotted by a computer-controlled dispenser Reproduced with permission from (Wang *et al.*, 2011). Copyright (2011). American Chemical Society.

Table 15.1: New bionanotechnological innovations in Biosensors for food allergens and allergy diagnosis.

Type of biosensor	Method of detection	Allergen Analyte	Bionanotechnological innovations	Limit of detection	Real sample	Ref.
Immunosensor	Differential pulse voltammetry	β-lactoglobulin	Graphene screen printed electrodes	0.85 pg/ml	cake, sweet biscuit and cheese snacks	(Eissa et al., 2012)
Immunosensor	Differential pulse voltammetry	Ovalbumin	Graphene screen printed electrodes	0.83 pg/ml	Spiked cake sample extract	(Eissa et al., 2013)
Immunosensor	Electrochemical impedance spectroscopy	Ovalbumin	CVD grown monolayer graphene	1 pg/ml	-	(Eissa et al., 2015)
DNA genosensor	Differential pulse voltammetry	Ara h 1	Graphene screen printed electrodes	0.041 fM	peanut milk beverage	
Enzymatic DNA genosensor	chronoamperometry	Ara h 1	chitosan-multiwalled carbon nanotube nanocomposite and spongy gold film	1.3×10^{-17} M	Peanut extract	(Sun et al., 2015b)
Immunosensor	Quartz crystal microbalance	Shrimp	Gold nanoparticles	0.333 µg/ml	Spiked water samples	(Xiulan et al., 2010)
Immunosensor	Quartz crystal microbalance	Gliadin	Gold nanoparticles	1 ppm in foodmatrix	Wheat, barley, oat, rice and digestive biscuit	(Chu et al., 2012)
Immunosensor	Differential pulse voltammetry	casein	Gold nanoparticles/carbon nanotube	50 ng/ml	Cheese	(Cao et al., 2011)
Peptide-based sensor	Surface plasmon resonance	Specific IgE to Ara h 2	microarray	10 pg/ml	Dil. Serum	(Joshi et al., 2014)
Genosensor	Differential pulse voltammetry	Two hazelnut major allergens, Cor a 1.04 and Cor a 1.03	microarray	0.3 and 0.1 nmol L^{-1} for Cor a 1.03 and Cor a 1.04, respectively	Commercial food stuff	(Bettazzi et al., 2008)

Table 15.1 contd. ...

...Table 15.1 contd.

Immunosensor	Imaging surface plasmon resonance	Peanut, Hazelnut, casein, lupine, egg, almond, brazil nut, cashew and pistachio allergens	microarray	0.2–5.0 mg/Kg	Cookies and dark choclate	(Rebe Raz et al., 2010b)
Immunosensor	Fluorescence	Ovalbumin	microarray	1.3 ng/mL	Non-egg pasta extract	(Shriver-Lake et al., 2004)
immunosensor	Surface plasmon resonance	five whey proteins, α-lactalbumin, β-lactoglobulin, bovine serum albumin, lactoferrin and immunoglobulin G	microarray	Varies from 0.05 to 0.52 mg/ml	Raw and processed milk products	(Billakanti et al., 2010)
Immunosensor	resonance enhanced absorption	egg white allergens, ovalbumin and ovomucoid	microarray	1 ng/ml	Whole egg, pasta and cheese tomato and dessert	(Maier et al., 2008)
PCR ampilification/enzymatic sensor	colourimetric	soybean, wheat, peanut, cashew, shrimp, fish, beef and chicken	microarray	0.5 pg of cashew DNA	five different retail samples	(Wang et al., 2011)
Direct sensor	Cyclic voltammetry	Serotonin for allergen diagnosis	Nafion-coated array microelectrode	1 µg/ml	blood	(Okochi et al., 1999)
Immunosensor	Fluorescence	IgG to β-lactoglobulin, IgEs to Ara h 1 and Phl p 1	microarray	—	human serum	(Monroe et al., 2011)
Immunosensor	Localized plasmon array	cat dander (Fel d1), dust mite (Der p1), peanut allergen (Ara h1) and dog dander (Can f1) antibodies	Gold nanoparticle array platform	2 nM	Whole blood	(Olkhov et al., 2012b)
Immunosensor	Fluorescence	allergen-specific Immunoglobin E antibodies and immune cell activation profiling	The arrays were generated using lipid dip-pen nanolithography	—	—	(Sekula-Neuner et al., 2012)

this method is the sensitivity of the fluorescence dyes to the temperature, pH and low the stability over a long time.

Surface plasmon resonance (SPR)

The change in the Refractive Index (RI) at the sensor surface is used for detection when an analyte binds to a receptor. The receptor is immobilized on a thin metal sensor surface, and the RI of the surface is measured using polarized light. A solution of the analyte is added to the immobilized receptor surface; it binds to the receptor, and the change in the RI which reflects SPR angle changes is detected. The sensor signal can be then correlated with the analyte concentration. SPR biosensors are the most popular for detection of allergens in foodstuff. A rapid, real-time SPR based immunosensor for the detection of i (IgG) in bovine and caprine milk has been developed by Crosson *et al.* (Crosson *et al.*, 2010). Rebe Raz *et al.* (Rebe Raz *et al.*, 2010a) have achieved a rapid and quantitative detection of multiple food allergen by imaging surface plasmon resonance (i-SPR) technology integrated with antibody microarray.

Electrochemical biosensors

Electrochemical biosensors are divided into potentiometric, amperometric voltammetry and impedance spectroscopy-based sensors. These sensors offer several advantages over other types of sensors as they are easy to use, low in cost and can be easily miniaturized. Electrochemical-based immunogens has been developed against the peanut allergen, Ara h 1 (Huang *et al.*, 2008). In this method, the antibody against Ara h 1 was immobilized on the gold electrode surface, and changes in the charge transfer resistance and the differential capacitance after addition of analyte have been used for the detection. The sensitivity of the sensor was as low as 0.3 nM. Another electrochemical biosensor has been developed by Singh *et al.* for the detection of the same analyte using nonporous polycarbonate membrane (Singh *et al.*, 2010). This method showed a lower detection limit of 0.04 μg/ml, which is 50% more sensitive than the previously reported value (0.09 μg/ml) (Pollet *et al.*, 2011).

Integration of Nanotechnology in Food Allergen Detection and Allergy Diagnosis

The bionanotechnology revolution resulted in excellent improvements in the biosensor devices for food allergen detection. Novel recognition receptors and transducers to improve the biosensors performance are being developed. Next we will discuss the application of aptamers as new biorecognition receptors (Tran *et al.*, 2013) as well as different nanomaterials in the biosensors for food allergen detection and allergy diagnosis (Pilolli *et al.*, 2013). The multiplexed detection of several food allergens using array biosensor technology will also be presented (Wang *et al.*, 2011).

Aptamer-based biosensors

Despite that antibodies are considered the "gold standard" recognition receptors, their low stability and complicated *in vivo* production limit their widespread applications. Moreover, antibodies usually cross-react with analytes of similar structures. This motivates research for alternative receptors with higher stability and comparable affinity. Aptames are promising receptors that can be used as an alternative to antibodies in biosensors. Aptamers can exhibit extremely high affinities down to pM K_D's (Pagratis *et al.*, 1997) and specificity (Geiger *et al.*, 1996). The selection of aptamers can be achieved through a library screening technique known as "SELEX" (Systematic Enrichment of Ligands by Exponential amplification) or "*in vitro* evolution" from a large library of DNA oligonucleotide molecules of up to 10^{15} different random sequences. With proper separation procedures, target-bound sequences are isolated and subsequently amplified by PCR. The amplified pool enriched with the target-binding sequences is again mixed with the target and the bound sequences are isolated and amplified. This process is repeated for a number of rounds with increasingly stringent binding conditions. The overall SELEX procedure finally results in a step-wise enrichment of target-binding sequences and ultimately yields high-affinity aptamers (Ellington and Szostak, 1990; Geiger *et al.*, 1996). Several aptamers have been selected against different environmental contaminants and food proteins (Cox and Ellington, 2001; McKeague, 2011). However, only a few reports have been published about the use of aptamers in food allergens detection. Egg lysozyme aptamers have been selected and successfully applied for allergen detection using electrochemical biosensors with a detection limit of 36 nM (Huang *et al.*, 2009; Rodríguez and Rivas, 2009). Similarly, DNA aptamers against Lup an 1 allergen have been selected using SELEX by Nadal *et al.* (Nadal *et al.*, 2012) with an affinity of nM range. The same research group has developed a more sensitive aptamer-based biosensor for the detection of beta-conglutin using FRET (Svobodova *et al.*, 2014). Yao *et al.* (Yao *et al.*, 2009) have reported the development of aptamer-based quartz crystal microbalance biosensor array for the detection of IgE in allergic patients serum.

Magnetic nanoparticles-based biosensor

As the allergen content in foodstuffs is usually very low, pre-concentration (Smith *et al.*, 2011) of allergen proteins is a crucial part in their detection. Magnetic nanoparticles are becoming popular for preconcentrating analytes and enables further automated separations from the bulk extracts. Commercially available functionalized magnetic particles with the large surface area can be easily modified with the capture element to improve the sensitivity of the sensor device. Lateral flow immunoassay (LFIA) was developed against the major fish allergen, parvalbumin (Pa) using superparamagnetic nanoparticles (SPMNP). The anti-parvalbumin antibody was immobilized on the particles surface and used for competitive LFIA. Comparable results were obtained with the western blotting method for 29 food samples (Zheng *et al.*, 2012). Spreoni *et al.* (Speroni *et al.*, 2010) have developed new ELISA method using functionalized magnetic particles with antibodies and PAMAM-dendrimers for the detection of Ara h 3/4 peanut allergen. The captured allergens were easily separated from the bulk solution by using a permanent magnet. The use of magnetic particles has enhanced the stability and the sensitivity of the assay compared to the conventional ELISA. Magnetic nanoparticles also play an important role in allergen diagnosis. SPR imaging microarray was developed for the sensitive diagnosis of peanut allergen-IgE antibody by using magnetic particles coated secondary anti-IgE antibody to capture the IgE from serum (Joshi *et al.*, 2014).

Gold nanoparticles

Gold nanoparticles (Au Nps) has been widely used to enhance the analytical performance of the biosensors because of their unique properties. The use of AuNp as transducer facilitates the electron transfer between the immobilized proteins and electrode surfaces in electrochemical sensors. They are also compatible with biomolecules which retain their biological activity upon immobilization.

Electrochemical biosensor for the peanut allergen Ar h 2 has been developed using a film of Ar h 2 peptide sequence immobilized on gold nanoparticle. The sensitivity of the allergen detection improved 100 fold compared to other methods (Liu *et al.*, 2010). Very recently, Bose *et al.* designed gold nanoparticle based colourimetric immunosensors for diagnosis of allergy. The analyte is sandwiched between the IgE and secondary anti-IgE antibody labelled with HRP. Gold (III) chloride was added as a colour developing agent. The colour change from red to blue indicates the presence of allergy which can be seen by naked eye. Simultaneous diagnosis of five allergens in very small volume (25 µl) of serum was shown. Gold nanoparticles are also used to improve the sensitivity of the SPR based biosensors. For example, in a novel immune-sandwich assay, IgE complex sandwiched between an immobilized anti-IgE antibody and anti-IgE apatmer-AuNp was detected by SPR with a detection limit of 1 ng/ml (Wang *et al.*, 2009). Similar work has also been reported by Kim *et al.* (Kim *et al.*, 2010) and the detection limit of IgE was shown to be 20 nM.

Graphene and carbon nanotubes

Graphene is a two-dimensional carbon nanomaterial consisting of Sp^2-hybridized carbon atoms in a hexagonal, honeycomb-like lattice crystal structure. Graphene and their related materials have recently shown to be an ideal material for the development of biosensors. The major advantages of graphene materials are their large surface area, simple preparation and relatively low cost. Due to its unique electronic structure, graphene exhibits excellent electrical and thermal conductivity and high mechanical strength (Geim, 2009; Novoselov *et al.*, 2004). Few graphene-based biosensors have been recently developed for the detection of food allergens. For instance, the detection of the most important milk allergen, β-lactoglobulin in different food matrices on a graphene platform has been reported by Eissa *et al.* (Eissa *et al.*, 2012). In this work, a label-free electrochemical biosensor has been developed employing graphene-modified screen printed carbon electrodes as a transducer surface. The functionalization of graphene electrodes was realized by electrochemical reduction of *in situ* prepared nitrophenyl diazonium salt in acidic aqueous solution. The modification of the graphene surface has been achieved using different electrografting protocols and optimized using cyclic voltammetry as well as X-ray photoelectron spectroscopy. The electrografting approach was shown to be an ideal method to attach monolayer of aryl groups on graphene surface in a controlled manner. The modified graphene electrodes with nitrophenyl groups were further reduced using cyclic voltammetry to produce aminophenyl groups. The formed amino groups were then activated using glutaraldehyde and employed for the covalent attachment of the β-lactoglobulin antibodies. The detection of β-lactoglobulin relied on the gradual decrease of the differential pulse voltammetry reduction peak current of $[Fe(CN)_6]^{3-/4-}$ redox couple due to the blocking of the graphene surface upon β-lactoglobulin binding. This immunogen showed a very good sensitivity and successful applicability in different food samples such as cake, sweet biscuit and cheese snacks. Based on a similar methodology, Eissa *et al.* (Eissa *et al.*, 2013) have reported a sensitive label-free voltammetric immunosensor for the common egg allergen ovalbumin using carboxyphenyl functionalized graphene modified screen-printed carbon electrodes. The electrodes were also functionalized using an electrografting protocol by carboxyphenyl diazonium salt. The antibodies for ovalbumin was then immobilized on the graphene surface via amide bond formation after activating the carboxylic groups on the surface using carbodiimide chemistry. The same research group has also reported another immunosenor for ovalbumin based on functionalized Chemical Vapour Deposited (CVD) monolayer-graphene electrodes (Eissa *et al.*, 2015) (Fig. 15.2). A monolayer of carboxyphenyl groups was attached to the graphene surface as shown by atomic force microscopy. The defect density on the graphene surface is increased with increasing the number of cyclic voltammetry scans used for the electrografting step as was confirmed by Raman spectroscopy. An impedance immunosensor has been fabricated using the developed functionalized CVD graphene with a detection limit of 1 pg/ml.

Multilayer graphene–gold nanocomposite has been used by Sun *et al.* (Sun *et al.*, 2015a) for the fabrication of electrochemical genosensor for the peanut

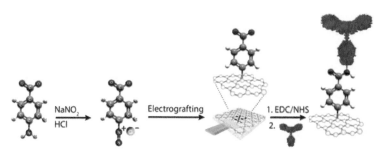

Fig. 15.2: A schematic of the ovalbumin immunosensor fabrication on the CVD monolayer graphene electrode. Reproduced with permission from (Eissa *et al.*, 2015). Copyright (2015) springer.

allergen, Ara h 1 using a stem-loop DNA. Glassy carbon electrodes were used on which alternate monolayers of graphene and gold were electrodeposited. A thiolated stem-loop probe conjugated with biotin from the other terminus was immobilized on the gold deposited layer via self-assembly. A signal-off detection mechanism was utilized based on the conformation change of the immobilized probe DNA upon hybridization with its target sequence. The hybridization leads to opening the stem-loop DNA probe moving its biotin labelled end away from the electrode surface. An increase in the electron transfer resistance and a decrease in the current was then detected. This method enabled the sensitive and selective quantification of Ara h 1 with a detection limit of 0.041 fM. Moreover, selectivity against a single-base mismatch was achieved. The same research group has reported another biosensor for the peanut allergen Ara h 1 using amperometric detection (Sun *et al.*, 2015b). A chitosan-multiwalled carbon nanotube nanocomposite has been used for the electrode fabrication, and a spongy layer of gold was electrodeposited on the surface. The detection was based on an enzymatic amplification using a biotin-labelled stem-loop DNA probe. The biotin is detected by binding with streptavidin–horseradish peroxidase which catalyzes the oxidation of hydroquinone by H_2O_2 to form benzoquinone that can be detected using its electrochemical reduction signal. When the biotin label is in close proximity to the electrode surface, a high current signal is detected from the reduction of the benzoquinone. However, upon target binding the streptavidin–horseradish peroxidase is detached from the carbon nanotube surface leading to a decrease in the current. The method was optimized to achieve a low detection limit of 1.3×10^{-17} mol/L and a very high degree of selectivity. The application of the biosensor for the detection of Ara h 1 in peanuts has also been demonstrated.

High throughput detection

Because of the increasing risk of food contamination with various allergens as a result of using different processed ingredients exported from different countries, the multi-analyte detection is becoming very important. The advances in food technologies have lead to the development of new detection tools with multiplexed and automated capabilities enabling high throughput detection of allergens. Moreover, microarray systems have been used for allergy diagnosis in order to achieve a simultaneous detection of different IgE antibodies against different allergens in the blood of the allergic patient.

Allergenic proteins detection

Several optical methods based on array platforms have been developed for the detection of multiple food allergens employing surface plasmon resonance, fluorescence or colourimetric techniques.

A disposable electrochemical DNA-array platform combined with Polymerase Chain Reaction (PCR) has been developed for the simultaneous detection of the two hazelnut major allergens, Cor a 1.04 and Cor a 1.03 in different commercial food products (Bettazzi *et al.*, 2008). In this work the PCR amplicons obtained from cDNA of the allergen proteins were detected using an electrochemical genosensor based on a screen-printed multielectrode array that contains eight individually addressable gold working electrodes. The electrode surface was first functionalized by mixed self-assembly monolayer of a thiol-modified DNA capture probe and 6-mercapto-1-hexanol. Then the unmodified PCR products were captured at the electrode surface through sandwich hybridization between the DNA capture probe attached to the surface and a biotinylated signalling probes. The signal is then detected using a streptavidin–alkaline phosphatase conjugate via measuring the differential pulse voltammetry oxidation peak of the enzyme-substrate product, α-naphthol.

Surface plasmon resonance is considered one of the major tools for automated, high-throughput analysis of biomolecules. The multiplexing capability of the SPR and the reusability of the biosensor chips leads to a reduction in the assay cost which can compensate for the high cost of the SPR instrument. An imaging surface plasmon resonance microarray platform for the multiplexed immunosensing of 13 major allergens has been developed (Rebe Raz *et al.*, 2010a). The microarray is generated using a continuous flow microfluidic spotter that allowed the sequential functionalization on each spot of the polycarboxylate hydrogel coated SPR Chip. The chip surface was illuminated at different light angles and images were captured for each spot. The application of the SPR microarray platform in different food products such as cookies and dark chocolate has been successfully demonstrated. Shriver-Lake *et al.* (Shriver-Lake *et al.*, 2004) have reported another array biosensor based on fluorescent sandwich immunoassays on the surface of a planar waveguide. The surface was first coated with the capture antibodies followed by running the samples, then fluorescently labelled antibodies to provide the signal. The signal is detected on each spot of the array as an optical image captured by a charged-coupled device camera and then transformed to fluorescence values. The biosensor was successfully applied for the detection of the egg allergen ovalbumin in the buffer and non-egg pasta extract.

Billakanti *et al.* (Billakanti *et al.*, 2010) have also reported the simultaneous quantitative detection of five whey proteins, α-lactalbumin, β-lactoglobulin, bovine serum albumin, lactoferrin and immunoglobulin G using surface plasmon resonance method. The method was used to analyze six samples per assay in various raw and processed milk products. The method was shown to be reproducible with negligible cross-reactivity and the results were comparable with those obtained using liquid chromatography and standard enzyme-linked immunosorbent assays.

Unlike the conventional reflectometry-based surface plasmon resonance, a resonance enhanced absorption optical biosensors may allow the detecting signals to be visible with the naked eye without using complex instrumentation. Few colourimetric array detection methods have been developed for the multiplexed detection of several allergens. Maier *et al.* (Maier *et al.*, 2008) have reported an immunochip biosensor for the detection of the egg white allergens, ovalbumin and ovomucoid in foodstuff. The detection principle was relying on the resonance-enhanced absorption phenomenon using gold nanoparticles in an interferometric setup (Fig. 15.3). Direct and sandwich assay formats were utilized, achieving semi-quantitative detection of egg proteins. The biosensor showed a concentration-dependent colour development that is visible to the naked eye. In the direct assay format, the allergen protein is coated on the sensor surface and the gold nanoparticles labelled antibodies are directly captured on the allergen coated chip. Another silicon-based colourimetric thin-film biosensor chip for the simultaneous detection of eight food allergens including soybean, wheat, peanut, cashew, shrimp, fish, beef and chicken has also been reported (Wang *et al.*, 2011). The detection was based on the PCR amplification of specific allergen DNA followed by indirect enzyme labelled detection assay. The colour was produced on the biosensor surface due to the precipitation of the enzymatic product which modifies the interference pattern of the light.

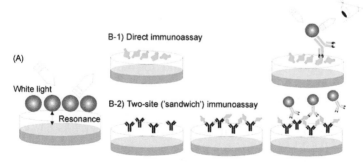

Fig. 15.3: A schematic illustration of the resonance enhanced absorption setup Reproduced with permission from (Maier *et al.*, 2008). Copyright (2008). American Chemical Society.

Allergen diagnosis

Serotonin is a chemical mediator secreted in the blood during the allergic reaction. Therefore, it can be used as a marker for allergen diagnosis. Okochi *et al.* (Okochi *et al.*, 1999) have reported the development of an electrochemical biosensor for serotonin detection using microelectrode array. A drop of blood was enough to carry out the assay. The serotonin was monitored by following it's cyclic voltammetry anodic peak at 350 mV versus a silver/silver chloride electrode on a nation-coated array microelectrode. The results obtained by this electrochemical microarray method were in good agreement with the diagnosis obtained from the amount of IgE antibody.

Immunoglobulin E-mediated mast cell activation plays an important role in the persistence of allergic diseases. Unlike the label-based and end-point assay formats which detect either early signalling or final phase of mast cell activation, Abassi *et al.* (Abassi *et al.*, 2004) have reported the real-time monitoring of the activation events using a microelectronic cell sensor. By integrating the microelectronic cell sensor arrays into the bottom of microtiter plates, the impedance between the cell membrane and sensor surface can be measured.

Various methods have been reported for allergen diagnosis based on the monitoring of allergen-Specific IgE using microarray platforms. These methods require only small volumes of serum. However, because of the variation of probe immobilization on microarrays, the reproducibility of these assays remains a major challenge. Monroe *et al.* (Monroe *et al.*, 2011) have developed a calibrated multiplexed microarray platform based on fluorescence enhancement technique in order to address this problem. This platform has offered several advantages such as the enhancement of the fluorescence emission over a broad range of fluorophores and the capability of performing label-free detection of the probes in each spot while preserving fluorescence enhancement for a particular fluorophore. Moreover, the concentration of the bound protein is directly proportional to the fluorescence signal resulting from the secondary antibody, offering accurate results. This method has been used for the detection of IgG to β-lactoglobulin, IgEs to Ara h 1 and Phl p 1 (timothy grass major allergen) in human serum. The total peanut allergen-specific binding has been detected in the whole serum of patients suffering from peanut allergy using a label-free immunoassay gold nanoparticle array plasmon sensing platform (Olkhov *et al.*, 2012a). The patient's serum was investigated against a four-allergen (cat and dog dander, dust mite and peanut allergen protein Ara h 1). Two secondary IgG- and IgE-specific antibodies were used to identify the IgE and IgG contributions to the total specific binding protein load to Ara h1. The same research group has also reported the detection of allergen-specific antibodies in whole blood and sera using label-free gold nanoparticle localized plasmon array biosensor (Olkhov *et al.*, 2012b). The array sensor surface was first functionalized with four different allergens, cat dander (Fel d1), dust mite (Der p1), peanut allergen (Ara h 1) and dog dander (Can f1). Then an immuno-kinetic assay was utilized to quantify their anti-allergen IgG antibodies based on the change in light scattering. The assay was able to detect the antibodies at a concentration of 25 nM for Fel d1, Der p1 and Ara h 1 allergens. The detection limit was further improved to 2 nM by using a secondary anti-IgG antibodies. The proposed nanoparticle scattering multiplexed arrays platform was shown to be a good point-of-care device for allergen diagnosis in whole blood. Sekula-Neuner et al. (Sekula-Neuner et al., 2012) have developed an allergen arrays for high throughput allergen-specific Immunoglobin E antibodies screening and immune cell activation profiling. The arrays were generated using lipid dip-pen nanolithography in order to enable the direct, nanoscale deposition of functional proteins and the fabrication of biochemical templates for selective adsorption. The nanolithography technique was used for the generation of arrays of the ligand 2,4-dinitrophenyl[1,2-dipalmitoyl-sn-glycero-3-phosphoethanolamine-N-[6-[(2,4 dinitrophenyl) amino]hexanoyl] (DNP)] onto glass surfaces. The authors reported that this set-up would pave the way for multiplexing various lipids with modified terminal groups in order to simultaneously detect multiple allergens. Rusling et al. (Liu et al., 2010) have compared the sensitivity of several electrochemical immunosensors for the detection of antibodies to a peptide sequence from Ara h2 in serum. The biosensors used a synthetic peptide layer of the major IgE-binding epitope from Ara h 2 immobilized on gold nanoparticle-coated pyrolytic graphite electrode. Faradaic and nonfaradaic impedance were compared to amperometric detection. The best response was obtained from the HPR-catalyzed precipitation of the enzyme product onto the electrode sensor that was monitored using nonfaradaic impedance. For more details about the technological innovations for high-throughput methods in allergy diagnosis, we refer the reader to a recent review (Chapman et al., 2015).

Conclusions and Perspectives

Development of highly sensitive, robust, selective, fast and cost-effective biosensors for the detection allergens in foodstuff as well as for food allergy diagnosis is greatly required for consumer protection. In this chapter, we reviewed the recent innovations in biosensor technologies for allergen detection and diagnosis. Selection of new synthetic recognition receptors such as aptamers opens new opportunities for the fabrication of highly stable and selective biosensing platforms. However, only a few aptamers against food allergens have been selected so far. Therefore, the selection of aptamers against various allergen targets should be a major goal in the future.

The majority of the reported biosensors for food allergy were based on optical transduction methods. These methods offered good sensitivity as well as capability of real-time detection of analytes in different complex food matrices. However, the miniaturization of the optical instruments to portable devices remains a major challenge. Electrochemical biosensors are thus more favourable as they can meet market demands for fabrication of compact, portable and low-cost devices. Disposable screen-printed sensors can be employed for the electrochemical measurements as they can be mass produced at low cost. However, the application of electrochemical biosensors in food allergen area has not been reported intensively. More effort should be devoted to the design and fabrication of different electrochemical biosensing platforms for allergen detection. Several reports have shown the integration of nanomaterials in the biosensors for food allergens allowing enhanced sensitivity due to their large surface area and unique properties. Detailed investigation about the use of various nanomaterials exhibiting different properties on biosensors has to be performed in the future. The high throughput detection of multiple-allergen is very promising. Developing such miniaturized biosensor arrays which enables the simultaneous detection of various target analytes will reduce the time and cost of the assays.

Keywords: Aptamer, nanomaterial, graphene, microarrays, multiplexing, allergy diagnosis

References

Abassi, Y. A., Jackson, J. A., Zhu, J., Oconnell, J., Wang, X., and Xu, X. (2004). Label-free, real-time monitoring of IgE-mediated mast cell activation on microelectronic cell sensor arrays. Journal of Immunological Methods 292(1-2): 195–205.

Alves, R. C., Barroso, M. F., González-García, M. B., Oliveira, M. B. P. P., and Delerue-Matos, M. C. (2016). New trends in food allergens detection: towards biosensing strategies. Critical Reviews in Food Science and Nutrition 56(14): 2304–19.

Ballmer-Weber, B. K. (2014). Value of allergy tests for the diagnosis of food allergy. Dig Dis 32(1-2): 84–88.

Bettazzi, F., Lucarelli, F., Palchetti, I., Berti, F., Marrazza, G., and Mascini, M. (2008). Disposable electrochemical DNA-array for PCR amplified detection of hazelnut allergens in foodstuffs. Analytica Chimica Acta 614(1): 93–102.

Billakanti, J. M., Fee, C. J., Lane, F. R., Kash, A. S., and Fredericks, R. (2010). Simultaneous, quantitative detection of five whey proteins in multiple samples by surface plasmon resonance. International Dairy Journal 20(2): 96–105.

Cao, Q., Zhao, H., Yang, Y., He, Y., Ding, N., Wang, J., Wu, Z., Xiang, K., and Wang, G. (2011). Electrochemical immunosensor for casein based on gold nanoparticles and poly(l-Arginine)/multi-walled carbon nanotubes composite film functionalized interface. Biosensors and Bioelectronics 26(8): 3469–3474.

Careri, M., Elviri, L., Mangia, A., and Mucchino, C. (2007). ICP-MS as a novel detection system for quantitative element-tagged immunoassay of hidden peanut allergens in foods. Analytical and Bioanalytical Chemistry 387(5): 1851–1854.

Chapman, M. D., Wuenschmann, S., King, E., and Pomés, A. (2015). Technological innovations for high-throughput approaches to *in vitro* allergy diagnosis. Current Allergy and Asthma Reports 15(7).

Chu, P. -T., Lin, C. -S., Chen, W. -J., Chen, C. -F., and Wen, H. -W. (2012). Detection of gliadin in foods using a quartz crystal microbalance biosensor that incorporates gold nanoparticles. Journal of Agricultural and Food Chemistry 60(26): 6483–6492.

Cianferoni, A., and Spergel, J. M. (2009). Food allergy: review, classification and diagnosis. Allergology International 58: 457–466.

Costa, J., Ansari, P., Mafra, I., Oliveira, M. B. P. P., and Baumgartner, S. (2015). Development of a sandwich ELISA-type system for the detection and quantification of hazelnut in model chocolates. Food Chemistry 173: 257–265.

Cox, J. C., and Ellington, A. D. (2001). Automated selection of anti-protein aptamers. Bioorg Med Chem 9(10): 2525–2531.

Crosson, C., Thomas, D., and Rossi, C. (2010). Quantification of immunoglobulin g in bovine and caprine milk using a surface plasmon resonance-based immunosensor. Journal of Agricultural and Food Chemistry 58(6): 3259–3264.

Ehn, B. -M., Ekstrand, B., Bengtsson, U., and Ahlstedt, S. (2004). Modification of IgE binding during heat processing of the cow's milk allergen β-Lactoglobulin. Journal of Agricultural and Food Chemistry 52(5): 1398–1403.

Eissa, S., Tlili, C., L'Hocine, L., and Zourob, M. (2012). Electrochemical immunosensor for the milk allergen beta-lactoglobulin based on electrografting of organic film on graphene modified screen-printed carbon electrodes. Biosensors and Bioelectronics 38(1): 308–313.

Eissa, S., L'Hocine, L., Siaj, M., and Zourob, M. (2013). A graphene-based label-free voltammetric immunosensor for sensitive detection of the egg allergen ovalbumin. Analyst 138(15): 4378–4384.

Eissa, S., Jimenez, G. C., Mahvash, F., Guermoune, A., Tlili, C., Szkopek, T., Zourob, M., and Siaj, M. (2015). Functionalized CVD monolayer graphene for label-free impedimetric biosensing. Nano Research 8(5): 1698–1709.

Ellington, A. D., and Szostak, J. W. (1990). *In vitro* selection of RNA molecules that bind specific ligands. Nature 346(6287): 818–822.

Gasilova, N., and Girault, H. H. (2015). Bioanalytical methods for food allergy diagnosis, allergen detection and new allergen discovery. Bioanalysis 7(9): 1175–1190.

Geiger, A., Burgstaller, P., von der Eltz, H., Roeder, A., and Famulok, M. (1996). RNA aptamers that bind L-arginine with sub-micromolar dissociation constants and high enantioselectivity. Nucleic Acids Research 24(6): 1029–1036.

Geim, A. K. (2009). Graphene: status and prospects. Science 324(5934): 1530–1534.

Hefle, S. L., Nordlee, J. A., and Taylor, S. L. (1996). Allergenic foods. Critical Reviews in Food Science and Nutrition 36(sup001): 69–89.

Hoffmann-Sommergruber, K., Pfeifer, S., and Bublin, M. (2015). Applications of molecular diagnostic testing in food allergy. Current Allergy and Asthma Reports 15(9): 56.

Huang, H., Jie, G., Cui, R., and Zhu, J. -J. (2009). DNA aptamer-based detection of lysozyme by an electrochemiluminescence assay coupled to quantum dots. Electrochemistry Communications 11(4): 816–818.

Huang, Y., Bell, M. C., and Suni, II. (2008). Impedance biosensor for peanut protein Ara h1. Analytical Chemistry 80(23): 9157–9161.

Jiang, D., Jiang, H., Ji, J., Sun, X., Qian, H., Zhang, G., and Tang, L. (2014). Mast-cell-based fluorescence biosensor for rapid detection of major fish allergen parvalbumin. Journal of Agricultural and Food Chemistry 62(27): 6473–6480.

Jiménez-Saiz, R., Benedé, S., Molina, E., and López-Expósito, I. (2015). Effect of processing technologies on the allergenicity of food products. Critical Reviews in Food Science and Nutrition 55(13): 1902–1917.

Joshi, A. A., Peczuh, M. W., Kumar, C. V., and Rusling, J. F. (2014). Ultrasensitive carbohydrate-peptide SPR imaging microarray for diagnosing IgE mediated peanut allergy. Analyst 139(22): 5728–5733.

Kim, S., Lee, J., Lee, S. J., and Lee, H. J. (2010). Ultra-sensitive detection of IgE using biofunctionalized nanoparticle-enhanced SPR. Talanta 81(4–5): 1755–1759.

Köppel, E., Stadler, M., Lüthy, J., and Hübner, P. (1998). Detection of wheat contamination in oats by polymerase chain reaction (PCR) and enzyme-linked immunosorbent assay (ELISA). Zeitschrift für Lebensmitteluntersuchung und-Forschung A 206(6): 399–403.

Köppel, R., Dvorak, V., Zimmerli, F., Breitenmoser, A., Eugster, A., and Waiblinger, H. -U. (2009). Two tetraplex real-time PCR for the detection and quantification of DNA from eight allergens in food. European Food Research and Technology 230(3): 367–374.

Kulis, M., Wright, B. L., Jones, S. M., and Burks, A. W. (2015). Diagnosis, management, and investigational therapies for food allergies. Gastroenterology 148(6): 1132–1142.

Liu, H., Malhotra, R., Peczuh, M. W., and Rusling, J. F. (2010). Electrochemical immunosensors for antibodies to peanut allergen Ara h2 using gold nanoparticle–peptide films. Analytical Chemistry 82(13): 5865–5871.

Ma, X., Sun, P., He, P., Han, P., Wang, J., Qiao, S., and Li, D. (2010). Development of monoclonal antibodies and a competitive ELISA detection method for glycinin, an allergen in soybean. Food Chemistry 121(2): 546–551.

Maier, I., Morgan, M. R. A., Lindner, W., and Pittner, F. (2008). Optical resonance-enhanced absorption-based near-field immunochip biosensor for allergen detection. Analytical Chemistry 80(8): 2694–2703.

Mairal, T., Nadal, P., Svobodova, M., and O'Sullivan, C. K. (2014). FRET-based dimeric aptamer probe for selective and sensitive Lup an 1 allergen detection. Biosensors and Bioelectronics 54: 207–210.

Maleki, S. J., Chung, S. Y., Champagne, E. T., and Raufman, J. P. (2000). The effects of roasting on the allergenic properties of peanut proteins. The Journal of Allergy and Clinical Immunology 106(4): 763–768.

McKeague, M., Giamberardino, A., and DeRosa, M. (2011). Advances in aptamer-based biosensors for food safety in environmental biosensors. pp. 17–42. In: V. Somerset (ed.). Environmental Biosensors. InTech, Rijeka, Croatia.

Monaci, L., and Visconti, A. (2010). Immunochemical and DNA-based methods in food allergen analysis and quality assurance perspectives. Trends in Food Science & Technology 21(6): 272–283.

Monroe, M. R., Reddington, A. P., Collins, A. D., LaBoda, C., Cretich, M., Chiari, M., Little, F. F., and Ünlü, M. S. (2011). Multiplexed method to calibrate and quantitate fluorescence signal for allergen-specific IgE. Analytical Chemistry 83(24): 9485–9491.

Nadal, P., Pinto, A., Svobodova, M., Canela, N., and O'Sullivan, C. K. (2012). DNA aptamers against the Lup an 1 food allergen. PLoS One 7(4): e35253.

Novoselov, K. S., Geim, A. K., Morozov, S. V., Jiang, D., Zhang, Y., Dubonos, S. V., Grigorieva, I. V., and Firsov, A. A. (2004). Science 306: 666–669.

Okochi, M., Yokouchi, H., Nakamura, N., and Matsunaga, T. (1999). Electrochemical detection of allergen in small-volume whole blood using an array microelectrode: A simple method for detection of allergic reaction. Biotechnology and Bioengineering 65(4): 480–484.

Olkhov, R. V., Kaminski, E. R., and Shaw, A. M. (2012a). Differential immuno-kinetic assays of allergen-specific binding for peanut allergy serum analysis. Analytical and Bioanalytical Chemistry 404(8): 2241–2247.

Olkhov, R. V., Parker, R., and Shaw, A. M. (2012b). Whole blood screening of antibodies using label-free nanoparticle biophotonic array platform. Biosensors and Bioelectronics 36(1): 1–5.

Pagratis, N. C., Bell, C., Chang, Y. F., Jennings, S., Fitzwater, T., Jellinek, D., and Dang, C. (1997). Potent 2'-amino-, and 2'-fluoro-2'-deoxyribonucleotide RNA inhibitors of keratinocyte growth factor. Nature Biotechnology 15(1): 68–73.

Peng, J., Song, S., Xu, L., Ma, W., Liu, L., Kuang, H., and Xu, C. (2013). Development of a monoclonal antibody-based sandwich ELISA for peanut allergen Ara h1 in food. International Journal of Environmental Research and Public Health 10(7): 2897–2905.

Pilolli, R., Monaci, L., and Visconti, A. (2013). Advances in biosensor development based on integrating nanotechnology and applied to food-allergen management. TrAC Trends in Analytical Chemistry 47: 12–26.

Pollet, J., Delport, F., Janssen, K. P., Tran, D. T., Wouters, J., Verbiest, T., and Lammertyn, J. (2011). Fast and accurate peanut allergen detection with nanobead enhanced optical fiber SPR biosensor. Talanta 83(5): 1436–1441.

Poms, R. E., Klein, C. L., and Anklam, E. (2004). Methods for allergen analysis in food: a review. Food Additives and Contaminants 21(1): 1–31.

Prado, M., Ortea, I., Vial, S., Rivas, J., Calo-Mata, P., and Barros-Velázquez, J. (2016). Advanced DNA- and protein-based methods for the detection and investigation of food allergens. Critical Reviews in Food Science and Nutrition 56(15): 2511–2542.

Rebe Raz, S., Liu, H., Norde, W., and Bremer, M. G. (2010a). Food allergens profiling with an imaging surface plasmon resonance-based biosensor. Analytical Chemistry 82(20): 8485–8491.

Rebe Raz, S., Liu, H., Norde, W., and Bremer, M. G. E. G. (2010b). Food allergens profiling with an imaging surface plasmon resonance-based biosensor. Analytical Chemistry 82(20): 8485–8491.

Rodríguez, M. C., and Rivas, G. A. (2009). Label-free electrochemical aptasensor for the detection of lysozyme. Talanta 78(1): 212–216.

Roehr, C. C., Edenharter, G., Reimann, S., Ehlers, I., Worm, M., Zuberbier, T., and Niggemann, B. (2004). Food allergy and non-allergic food hypersensitivity in children and adolescents. Clinical & Experimental Allergy 34(10): 1534–1541.

Sampson, H. A., Muñoz-Furlong, A., Bock, S. A., Schmitt, C., Bass, R., Chowdhury, B. A., Decker, W. W., Furlong, T. J., Galli, S. J., Golden, D. B., Gruchalla, R. S., Harlor Jr, A. D., Hepner, D. L., Howarth, M., Kaplan, A. P., Levy, J. H., Lewis, L. M., Lieberman, P. L., Metcalfe, D. D., Murphy, R., Pollart, S. M., Pumphrey, R. S., Rosenwasser, L. J., Simons, F. E., Wood, J. P., and Camargo Jr, C. A. (2005). Symposium on the definition and management of anaphylaxis: summary report. Journal of Allergy and Clinical Immunology 115(3): 584–591.

Sanz, ML, G. P., and De Weck, A. L. (2007). *In vitro* tests: Basophil activation tests. Drug Hypersensitivity 391–402.

Sathe, S. K., and Sharma, G. M. (2009). Effects of food processing on food allergens. Molecular Nutrition & Food Research 53(8): 970–978.

Schubert-Ullrich, P., Rudolf, J., Ansari, P., Galler, B., Führer, M., Molinelli, A., and Baumgartner, S. (2009). Commercialized rapid immunoanalytical tests for determination of allergenic food proteins: an overview. Analytical and Bioanalytical Chemistry 395(1): 69–81.

Sekula-Neuner, S., Maier, J., Oppong, E., Cato, A. C. B., Hirtz, M., and Fuchs, H. (2012). Allergen arrays for antibody screening and immune cell activation profiling generated by parallel lipid dip-pen nanolithography. Small 8(4): 585–591.

Shriver-Lake, L. C., Taitt, C. R., and Ligler, F. S. (2004). Applications of array biosensor for detection of food allergens. Journal of AOAC International 87(6): 1498–1502.

Sicherer, S. H., and Sampson, H. A. (2009). Food allergy: recent advances in pathophysiology and treatment. Annual Review of Medicine 60(1): 261–277.

Singh, R., Sharma, P. P., Baltus, R. E., and Suni, I. I. (2010). Nanopore immunosensor for peanut protein Ara h1. Sensors and Actuators B: Chemical 145(1): 98–103.

Smith, J. E., Sapsford, K. E., Tan, W., and Ligler, F. S. (2011). Optimization of antibody-conjugated magnetic nanoparticles for target preconcentration and immunoassays. Analytical Biochemistry 410(1): 124–132.

Speroni, F., Elviri, L., Careri, M., and Mangia, A. (2010). Magnetic particles functionalized with PAMAM-dendrimers and antibodies: a new system for an ELISA method able to detect Ara h3/4 peanut allergen in foods. Analytical and Bioanalytical Chemistry 397(7): 3035–3042.

Sun, X., Jia, M., Guan, L., Ji, J., Zhang, Y., Tang, L., and Li, Z. (2015a). Multilayer graphene–gold nanocomposite modified stem-loop DNA biosensor for peanut allergen-Ara h1 detection. Food Chemistry 172: 335–342.

Sun, X., Jia, M., Ji, J., Guan, L., Zhang, Y., Tang, L., and Li, Z. (2015b). Enzymatic amplification detection of peanut allergen Ara h1 using a stem-loop DNA biosensor modified with a chitosan-mutiwalled carbon nanotube nanocomposite and spongy gold film. Talanta 131: 521–527.

Svobodova, M., Mairal, T., Nadal, P., Bermudo, M. C., and O'Sullivan, C. K. (2014). Ultrasensitive aptamer based detection of beta-conglutin food allergen. Food Chemistry 165: 419–423.

Taylor, S. L., Hefle, S. L., Bindslev-Jensen, C., Bock, S. A., Burks, A. W., Jr., Christie, L., Hill, D. J., Host, A., Hourihane, J. O., Lack, G., Metcalfe, D. D., Moneret-Vautrin, D. A., Vadas, P. A., Rance, F., Skrypec, D. J., Trautman, T. A., Yman, I. M., and Zeiger, R. S. (2002). Factors affecting the determination of threshold doses for allergenic foods: how much is too much? The Journal of Allergy and Clinical Immunology 109(1): 24–30.

Taylor, S. L., Hefle, S. L., Farnum, K., Rizk, S. W., Yeung, J., Barnett, M. E., Busta, F., Shank, F. R., Newsome, R., Davis, S., and Bryant, C. M. (2006). Analysis and evaluation of food manufacturing practices used to address allergen concerns. Comprehensive Reviews in Food Science and Food Safety 5(4): 138–157.

Tran, D. T., Knez, K., Janssen, K. P., Pollet, J., Spasic, D., and Lammertyn, J. (2013). Selection of aptamers against Ara h1 protein for FO-SPR biosensing of peanut allergens in food matrices. Biosensors and Bioelectronics 43: 245–251.

van Hengel, A. J. (2007). Food allergen detection methods and the challenge to protect food-allergic consumers. Analytical and Bioanalytical Chemistry 389(1): 111–118.

Verhoeckx, K. C. M., Vissers, Y. M., Baumert, J. L., Faludi, R., Feys, M., Flanagan, S., Herouet-Guicheney, C., Holzhauser, T., Shimojo, R., van der Bolt, N., Wichers, H., and Kimber, I. (2015). Food processing and allergenicity. Food and Chemical Toxicology 80: 223–240.

Wang, J., Munir, A., Li, Z., and Zhou, H. S. (2009). Aptamer–Au NPs conjugates-enhanced SPR sensing for the ultrasensitive sandwich immunoassay. Biosensors and Bioelectronics 25(1): 124–129.

Wang, W., Han, J., Wu, Y., Yuan, F., Chen, Y., and Ge, Y. (2011). Simultaneous detection of eight food allergens using optical thin-film biosensor chips. Journal of Agricultural and Food Chemistry 59(13): 6889–6894.

Werner, M. T., Fæste, C. K., Levsen, A., and Egaas, E. (2010). A quantitative sandwich ELISA for the detection of Anisakis simplex protein in seafood. European Food Research and Technology 232(1): 157–166.

Xiulan, S., Yinzhi, Z., Jingdong, S., Liyan, S., He, Q., and Weijuan, Z. (2010). A quartz crystal microbalance-based immunosensor for shrimp allergen determination in food. European Food Research and Technology 231(4): 563–570.

Yao, C., Qi, Y., Zhao, Y., Xiang, Y., Chen, Q., and Fu, W. (2009). Aptamer-based piezoelectric quartz crystal microbalance biosensor array for the quantification of IgE. Biosensors and Bioelectronics 24(8): 2499–2503.

Zheng, C., Wang, X., Lu, Y., and Liu, Y. (2012). Rapid detection of fish major allergen parvalbumin using super paramagnetic nanoparticle-based lateral flow immunoassay. Food Control 26(2): 446–452.

Index

Printed and bound by CPI Group (UK) Ltd, Croydon, CR0 4YY

01/11/2024

01782624-0006